Asthma: An Issue of Clinics in Chest Medicine

Asthma: An Issue of Clinics in Chest Medicine

Edited by Phillip Johnson

STATES
ACADEMIC PRESS
www.statesacademicpress.com

States Academic Press,
109 South 5th Street,
Brooklyn, NY 11249, USA

Visit us on the World Wide Web at:
www.statesacademicpress.com

ISBN: 978-1-63989-063-7

Cataloging-in-Publication Data

Asthma : an issue of clinics in chest medicine / edited by Phillip Johnson.
p. cm.
Includes bibliographical references and index.
ISBN 978-1-63989-063-7
1. Asthma. 2. Chest--Diseases. 3. Lungs--Diseases. 4. Respiratory intensive care. I. Johnson, Phillip.
RC591 .A78 2022
616.238--dc23

Table of Contents

Preface

In my initial years as a student, I used to run to the library at every possible instance to grab a book and learn something new. Books were my primary source of knowledge and I would not have come such a long way without all that I learnt from them. Thus, when I was approached to edit this book; I became understandably nostalgic. It was an absolute honor to be considered worthy of guiding the current generation as well as those to come. I put all my knowledge and hard work into making this book most beneficial for its readers.

Asthma is an inflammatory disease of the respiratory system that is characterized by easily triggered bronchospasms and reversible airflow obstruction. Bronchospasm is a sudden narrowing of the muscles of the walls of bronchioles. A few of the symptoms of asthma are episodes of coughing, wheezing, shortness of breath and chest tightness. It is caused by a combination of environmental and genetic factors. Environmental factors may include exposure to allergens or air pollution. Some medications such as beta blockers and aspirin can also trigger asthma. Its diagnosis is based on the response to therapy over time, pattern of symptoms and spirometry lung functioning test. Asthma can also be classified as atopic and non-atopic. This book provides significant information of this discipline to help develop a good understanding of asthma. It is compiled in such a manner, that it will provide in-depth knowledge about the clinical aspects of this disease. Researchers and students in this field will be assisted by this book.

I wish to thank my publisher for supporting me at every step. I would also like to thank all the authors who have contributed their researches in this book. I hope this book will be a valuable contribution to the progress of the field.

Editor

1

Asthma in Preschool Children

F. Muñoz-López

Abstract

A proper diagnostic and therapeutic approach in children under 5 years who have symptoms of respiratory distress, of varying intensity, more or less continuously or in acute and repeated episodes must observed. In many cases, the dominant symptom is cough, which has been linked to the existence of asthma ('equivalent asthmatic coughing'). As respiratory symptoms are common to many processes that affect this system, an appropriate differential diagnosis is required before starting treatment, which is often not appropriate.—Concept. Epidemiology—Predisposing factors, risk factors and triggers—Respiratory symptoms addressed from a pathogenic point of view, in order to better understand the possibilities of these symptoms to appear: Pathogenesis of dyspnea, cough, secretion and bronchial breath sounds.—The inflammatory reaction is the pathogenetic basis of asthma, and hence, anti-inflammatories are the most appropriate treatment. But there is no evidence that inflammation is a permanent fact from the start of the disease or that it exists in other respiratory processes. The appropriate methods to assess inflammation in children under 5 years and the evaluation of results in published studies will be presented. The conclusion is that it has been shown that in mild to moderate and sporadic cases, inflammation persists.—Atopy and asthma: onset and evolution—Clinical and allergologic diagnosis—Diagnostic evaluation of the dominant symptoms, relating directly to their pathogenesis.—Exploration of respiratory function, according to age: younger and older than 2 years.—Differential diagnosis based on the dominant symptoms.—Treatment. (a) Etiologic: immunotherapy in <5 years: standards. (b) Pathogenic: anti-inflammatory (corticosteroids). Indications of pre-inflammatory: chromones and anti-leukotriene: montelukast. (c) Treatment regimens: treatment of seizures.

Keywords: preschool children, diagnosis, treatment, immunotherapy, genetic and trigger factors

1. Introduction

Episodes of breathlessness or wheezing are common in preschool children primarily in the first 2 years, being estimated that 50% of infants have episodes of this nature, and their causes are needed to be known. The insufficient development of the immune system opens up to frequent viral infections, but other factors can contribute, such as the home environment, particularly if the mother is a smoker. Given the importance of genetic predisposition, family history of allergic diseases and asthma in particular is always is to be known, taking into account the famous expression 'all that wheezes is not asthma'.

2. Epidemiology

Some anatomical and physiological characteristics of the infant and young child's airways predispose to the development of processes that lead to the narrowing or bronchial obstruction, manifested by common symptoms, such as coughing, dyspnoea and noisy or wheezing breathing.

The *narrower airway calibre* is a basic fact, which contributes to the obstruction due to the inflammation of the mucosa, the smooth muscle constriction or the increased secretion of tracheobronchial mucus glands.

Infant *physiological increase of vagal tone,* which continues during the first years of life, as Montgomery and Tepper [18] demonstrated by methacholine inhalation, is known. Pathologically, bronchial hyperresponsiveness (BHR) is a key element in the pathogenesis of asthma. Having certain anomalies in the protein chain of the beta-receptors of the smooth muscle, such as the substitution of glycine for arginine at position 16 and glutamate for glutamine at position 27, is a characteristic of individuals with atopic predisposition. But in non-predisposed subjects, BHR is usually secondary to the inflammatory reaction that occurs in various circumstances in the bronchial mucosa.

Regarding bronchopulmonary infectious pathology, it is the well-known *immaturity of the immune system,* which in some children continues for several years (infant transient immunodeficiency), facilitating the development of bronchial inflammation processes.

It is not always easy to establish the true diagnosis of asthma in early life, as the evolution of symptoms over the years will confirm the diagnosis by excluding other possible causes of dyspnoea or wheezing, supported by immuno-allergological and respiratory function studies.

In line with these concepts, Martinez et al. [16] distinguish the different phenotypes of the bronchospastic pathology in preschool children, identifying asthma and transient bronchitis (wheezy bronchitis) that encompass various processes suffered by a group of children who, after preschool age, do not show no broncholability, all a consequence of the predisposing factors cited above. However, it is not always easy to determine the phenotype of a particular patient, and in the course of time, as they evolve, the criteria may even have to be modified. Hence, the need to pay attention to the characteristics of the symptoms and their evolution, in addition to a number of circumstances, such as the suffering from other allergic processes by the same child (eczema, allergies to milk proteins), a precocious start of symptoms, or the existence of similar pathologies among siblings, parents or other close relatives, or environmental pollutants, climate, etc. The lack of a family history in approximately 20% of cases adds another obstacle to the diagnosis.

In most children, asthma begins in the first 5 years of life. A study in Spain in 1982 showed that in 76% of asthmatic children, the process had started before 4 years of age. Several studies indicate that between 15 and 35% of preschool children have had an episode of respiratory distress, with or without wheezing or other breathing noises; however, 60–65% of these children would not suffer crises after the third year. The high diagnostic confusion in this group of children with 'transient bronchitis' comes not only from symptomatic similarity but also from the terminology that has been used to label the process. The appearance of these temporary symptoms can be due to various causes, such as viral infections (respiratory syncytial virus (RSV), parainfluenza, influenza), causing bronchiolitis, which may recur, even more in immunodeficient children. Other possible causes can also be household pollutants (tobacco smoke, cleaning chemicals or industrial products) or weather changes (sudden cooling), among other.

3. Predisposing factors, risk factors and triggers

Prevention of diseases is one of the challenges that medicine faces, therefore knowing the risk factors for each of the processes we aim to prevent is essential to carry out effective measures to achieve the proposed objectives. The best known risk factors and triggers that lead to allergic diseases, especially asthma and related bronchopaties, are as follows.

3.1. Atopy: genetic bases

The hereditary component in allergic diseases is well known, being asthma the most important, so that in approximately 70–80% of patients, close family members with the same or other allergy-related pathologies are identified. Allergic (atopic) predisposition is polygenic, that is there are several genes that support polymorphisms, which prompt the abnormal response of the organism to allergens.

In infants and pre-schooler children, the diagnosis of asthma is based on demonstrating the causality of allergic symptoms, and BHR, which is an essential condition for the diagnosis of the disease at any age. Polymorphisms in genes that lead to variants of the β_2-adrenergic receptor in the bronchial smooth muscle are the basis for congenital BHR (primary BHR), which may be also due to the harmful influence of certain exogenous factors such as when smoker women do not drop the habit during pregnancy, thereby harming the normal development of the lung. The existence of congenital BHR is the first precursor of asthma in young children. Moreover, also in these early years, BHR may worsen or appear by the inhalation of pollutants present at home or in the exterior, being this cause of BHR (acquired BHR) the most prominent at later ages.

In children with wheezy bronchitis (transient), such family circumstances are not given, but the causes are different, such as pulmonary immaturity, viral infections or environmental pollution (micro-habitat).

3.2. Foetal immunity and atopy: intrauterine sensitization

The influence of the mother in the transmission of atopic predisposition is greater than the father's, possibly because of the intimate connection between the former and the foetus. Pregnancy maintenance requires an immune environment with predominance of activity of Th2 lymphocytes, which prevents the rejection of the foetus. Thus, the foetus develops in an environment in which cytokines from that lymphocyte subclass, especially interleukin (IL)-4, IL-10 and IL-5, are predominant, increased if the pregnant woman is atopic, suffering or not from any allergic disease. Although IL-13 is a cytokine of the Th2 group, it has been observed that it is produced to a lesser extent in foetuses and neonates at risk of atopic disease, which could be related to the immaturity of the development of the activity of T cells [27]. Along the same lines, low production of IFN-γ by mononuclear cells could be related, thereby reducing the suppression of Th2 activity, defect that is maintained for at least the first 2 years of life [24].

Sensitization to food allergens or pneumoallergens may occur already during pregnancy, as the foetus can produce IgE from the 11th week of gestation, even IgE specific to antigens, as has been shown to occur against parasites (helminths, filaria) in some countries.

What is yet to be clarified is the route by which the allergens that have passed to the mother by inhalation or digestion are brought into contact with the foetus for the immune stimulation that promotes IgE production to occur.

What it is also to be elucidated is the relationship that may exist between the degree of maternal exposure to allergens and the possibility that the foetus becomes sensitized. It does not seem that an environment rich in pneumoallergens cause a greater number of foetuses affected or that the diet of pregnant woman devoid of the most allergenic foods reduce the number of sensitivities.

3.3. Risk factors

Lung development

Regardless of atopic predisposition, various circumstances constitute an added risk for the early onset of asthma, which can also promote the development of wheezing transient bronchitis. Some of these facts can act on the lung during foetal life affecting both the development and maturation of the immune system, but also after birth, especially in the first year of life.

Lung development can be affected by certain circumstances. Prolonged stress of the mother can affect the imbalance of Th1/Th2 activity, due to the excessive production of cortisone that occurs in this emotional condition, since the hormone exerts its immunomodulatory activity in favour of Th2 activity [11]. Similarly, some incidents during pregnancy can affect the development of the lung, such as uterine bleeding, placental insufficiency or other processes that alter the physiology of the uterus favouring premature birth and a consequent low birth weight. Also, prolonged malnutrition of the pregnant mother is detrimental to the overall development of the foetus and particularly of the lung, increasing the risk for prematurity in which many of these pregnancies end.

Smoking during pregnancy and lactation

Among the risk factors that affect lung development in both its structure and mechanisms of immune defence, the greatest interest is focused on the smoking habits of the mother during pregnancy and the first year of life, including also other smokers in the vicinity of the newborn and infant.

There are no doubts about the relationship between smoking and respiratory disease of the small child, with an increase in the prevalence among children of school age. Nevertheless, it is difficult to prove whether the functional changes are already initiated in the foetus or if this occurs later during lactation. Gilliland et al. [9] found decreased respiratory function (FEF_{25-75}) in children whose mothers smoked during pregnancy, but not after birth, suggesting that the injuries already started in the foetus.

Modern methods to assess respiratory function allow the study of BHR already in the first months of life, having shown a slight but real increase in the children of smoking mothers. Regarding immunity, several studies in cord blood appear to show that tobacco produces some changes in the immune response of the foetus, having found higher levels of IgE and a significant production of Th2 cytokines (IL-13, IL-5mRNA, IL-6), after *in vitro* stimulation of lymphocytes with allergens (ovalbumin, mite).

Environmental chemical pollutants

Various common contaminants at home may act as irritants that can cause or increase bronchial reactivity or produce an inflammatory condition of the airways. This may precipitate both sensitization to environmental allergens and be the cause of respiratory symptoms of varying intensity, from irritative cough to wheezing bronchitis. The most common environmental pollutants have a variable influence, in logical dependency on the concentration of chemicals, ventilation, housing characteristics and location (urban, suburban, rural).

It seems less likely that the outside environmental irritants may cause the same problems in young children, perhaps because the degree of exposure is lower than in later ages. However, in big cities or in the vicinity of industrial areas, pollution can be a serious risk, from which only small infants that spend little time outdoors will be protected.

3.4. Trigger factors

Early sensitization

As already mentioned, sensitization to allergens seems possible already during foetal life, although the onset of symptoms of asthma may take some time, depending on the degree of exposure and environmental conditions in addition to the genetic load. But it is after birth when the child is more exposed to common domestic allergens, being mites the most common (*Dermatophagoides pteronyssinus* and *Dermatophagoides farinae*), but sensitization and subsequent development of allergic symptoms in the respiratory tract are associated with atopic predisposition, concentration of allergens and allergenic potency of each of them, and their ability to release the antigens when the particles are deposited on the wet surface of the mucosa, as well as the involvement of adjuvants, as are the aforementioned pollutants or the intercurrent respiratory infections.

Viral infections

Respiratory tract infections caused by viruses are responsible for a high percentage of bronchospasm in young children, for which their characteristic tendency for allergic symptoms in their in upper respiratory tract or even crises of wheezing and/or dyspnoea had already been revealed. But also in non-atopic children, RSV mainly can cause lesions of the bronchial mucosa that facilitate contact with allergens, causing sensitization to them, with a simultaneous increase in broncholability. Also in not-predisposed children, RSV infections and other viruses trigger wheezing crisis or broncho-obstruction, as a pathogenic base for transient or wheezy bronchitis. The cause of these disorders lies in diverse mechanisms, dependent some on the injury of the mucosal epithelium and others on the activation of the cells involved in the immune–allergic response (**Table 1**).

RSV belongs to the *Pneumovirus* genus of the *Paramyxoviridae* family. Through a protein (G), the virus attaches to the surface of target cells, resulting in the fusion of the lipids of the cell membrane by another protein (F), which facilitates the insertion of RNA into the invaded cell. The G protein promotes a Th2 response, whereas the F protein stimulates the production cytokines in Th1 lymphocytes. In connection with the predominance of one or other protein, it has been established the existence of two types of RSV, A and B, whose variety may depend on the different clinical manifestations [13].

The metapneumovirus is responsible for 10–15% of the respiratory infections in children, with the same clinical impact than the VRS, with which shares a certain genotypic and epidemiological similarity. They also belong to the *Paramyxoviridae* family and are genetically similar to the pneumovirus of the avian flu.

The influenza virus A and B, and parainfluenza 1, 2 and 3 are less aggressive but also cause obstructive crisis in atopic and non-atopic children, because they cause desquamation of trachea–larynx–bronchial epithelial cells and bronchial submucosal oedema with infiltration of neutrophils and mononuclear cells, lesions that are reversible within 6 weeks [3].

Moreover, it is possible that in healthy children, RSV infection may be the cause of asthma to be developed later, but is more likely to result in the wheezing bronchitis process that will persist for some time. It is shown that, after severe infection, deterioration of the lung function occurs with increased bronchial reactivity to methacholine or histamine and to physical exercise, as well as the existence of specific IgE antibodies against the virus, which decreases over time, which could be related to the transience of broncho-obstructive crises.

More recently, rhinovirus, with its three subgroups A, B and C, has been identified as the main cause of respiratory infections which will later trigger half of asthma attacks in early childhood. The *in vitro* rhinovirus contact with blood mononuclear cell from adult asthmatics, compared to healthy subjects, demonstrates the production of IL-4 only in patients and less IFNy in these than in controls, with a IFNy(gamma interferon)/IL-4 ratio over three times lower in asthmatics, which shows that rhinoviruses directly induce the activity of Th2 cells, which does not rule out a greater responsibility of rhinoviruses in the pathogenesis of asthma.

Bacterial infections

Unlike viruses, bacteria do not exercise such a harmful function. Some bacterial antigens have an immunomodulatory capacity and repeated infections are what promote the predominance of the activity of Th1 versus Th2 lymphocytes, preventing sensitization to allergens.

Although the protective action against sensitization to pneumoallergens and food in children under 2 years of age seems confirmed, there are studies that nuance the findings, as is the potential coadjuvant effect of endotoxins with sensitization to mites and perhaps other pneumoallergens.

– Epithelial lesions
Increased neuronal sensitivity
Increased penetration of allergens
Decreased ciliary clearance
Neural endopeptidase reduction and increased tachykinins
– Increase in mediators from mast cells
Histamine
Arachidonic acid metabolism: prostaglandins, leukotrienes
– Increase of cellular mechanisms involved in inflammation
Increased production of cytokines
Stimulation of chemotaxis: eosinophils, neutrophils
– Regulation of β_2 receptors
– Production of specific IgE against viruses
Allergic sensitization
Mediators release

Table 1. Mechanisms responsible for bronchobstructive crises caused by viruses.

Moreover, at very low concentrations (10 ng/ml), endotoxins are able to activate alveolar macrophages and promote bronchial inflammation, increasing bronchoreactivity both in asthmatic and healthy people; therefore, it is possible that in the severity of asthma, environmental endotoxin levels may have an outstanding role not only in adults but also from school age, causing especially wheezy bronchitis or non-atopic asthma (6,10).

Conversely, if the asthmatic has a bacterial infection with respiratory location, it is most likely that obstructive symptoms will be intensified by the action of bacterial enterotoxins that act as superantigens, which promote the mechanisms by which the inflammation of the respiratory mucosa is established.

4. Pathogenesis of common symptoms in obstructive bronchopathies

The mechanisms by which the symptoms of asthma occur in preschool children do not differ from those that cause the process at any age. The permeability of the bronchial lumen is maintained by a neuro-chemical mechanism, but airway calibre may be affected either by an imbalance in this mechanism or by the intervention of certain cells and their biochemical mediators involved in the inflammatory reaction, usually triggered in childhood by an allergic reaction or an unfavourable home environment. In the obstruction of the wider bronchi, the dominant mechanism is the constrictor one, of neuro-chemical cause, whereas in the peripheral bronchi (small airways), inflammation is the greatest cause, through cellular mediators that are also constrictors.

BHR and inflammation are the pathogenetic basis of asthma. BHR is usually present already in the newborns of atopic families, although it is true that certain exogenous harmful agents can increase it. Similarly, the regular or intense exposure to these pollutants and also viral infections can cause broncholability in non-predisposed children. This increased broncholability occurs as the result of inflammation that such elements, including allergens, produce in the bronchial mucous membrane. These facts are demonstrated in adults and children from school age, but in preschool children under five, the immediate influence of these exogenous factors is less certain. The injured bronchial epithelium is restored after the aggression that leads to crises of dyspnoea or wheezing, and the permanence of the injury can depend on the intensity of the aggression and the repetition of the same, leading to more or less severe and repeated symptoms. Therefore, there is doubt whether the inflammatory reaction is established from the onset of the first symptoms or whether that permanence occurs after the recurrence of the crisis or after the most serious crises, on which the therapeutic approach may depend. Various conventional methods are used to study bronchial inflammatory reactions, although in younger children, it is not always easy to conduct them. The most common are the following:

Direct methods: (1) Cell study from sputum obtained by bronchoalveolar lavage (BAL), induced sputum, forced cough or aspiration. (2) Bronchial biopsy.

Indirect, non-invasive methods: (1) Exhaled nitric oxide measurement. (2) Exhaled breath condensate: evaluation of several measurements of the inflammation. (3) Blood eosinophilia assessment and eosinophil cationic protein (ECP) in serum levels.

The inflammatory reaction is a key event in the pathogenesis of asthma, as it is evident in adults and children from school age. It seems certain that inflammation is present even in the first episodes of dyspnoea in children who later go on to develop allergic asthma, but there is no unanimity in the recognition of this fact. In the work of Maclennan et al. [14] in preschool children with episodes of severe dyspnoea repeated between 2 and 12 times in the previous year (it is known that from the third episode, asthma can be diagnosed in young children), it is found that a percentage of them had an increased serum IgE levels although it is not significant in relation to a control group.

It is needed to know whether the persistence of inflammation and its intensity corresponds with the frequency and severity of the crisis, that is, if the mucosal lesions are restored after mild episodes that occur at long intervals of time, with implications in the therapeutic approach aimed at preventing recurrences.

5. Initiation and evolution

The precocity of the onset of episodes of respiratory distress may be related to the severity of the process and its evolution over time. Although in some children, the first crisis occurs in the first months of life, the process has a markedly evolutionary nature, not presenting the first crisis of dyspnoea but after a period of time, which varies from child to child.

5.1. Asthma crisis: early onset

For the suspected allergic asthma to be well-founded, it is necessary that the crisis is repeated for at least three times, as it is known that a large number of infants suffer an episode of dyspnoea, possibly of infectious cause, estimating that this happens in between 15 and 32% of children under 5 years, who cannot be labelled as asthmatics until the atopic cause is confirmed, related to the progressive evolution of the process.

The first episodes of dyspnoea are usually caused by viral infections and occur most frequently in the cold months, and it is not uncommon that they are accompanied by light fever. Associated symptoms are similar to asthma: rhinitis, dry cough, shortness of breath, wheezing, dyspnoea, intercostal retractions.

Depending on the intensity and the phase of the crisis, auscultation will show from wheezing to silent areas as well as fine or coarse crackles, indicative of bronchoalveolar involvement.

In any case, it is necessary to make sure there is a bronchiolitis, by RSV, of which prognosis and treatment can differ from that of a simple catarrhal process.

After the first year, it is likely that crises are not triggered by viral infections, but that other environmental factors are responsible, not ruling out weather conditions changes, even in atopic children.

The repetition of three episodes of dyspnoea should alert of the possibility that those are the first manifestations of asthma, which will continue in the following years. It is therefore necessary to assess in each case the various predisposing and boosting elements of atopy and asthma, such as the incidence of allergic disease in parents or close relatives, the coincidence in the child of other allergic processes or the environment in which the patient lives.

5.2. Atopic processes precursors of asthma

In chronological order, but not occurring in all cases, the first manifestation of atopy might be the sensitization to foods, mainly cow's milk when breastfeeding is absent, with symptoms in the first weeks of life. Eczema associated with sensitization to foods, from the third month, and rhinitis, as the first manifestation of respiratory allergy, that usually precedes asthma, both identities related with the persistence and increased intensity of the other two previous allergic processes.

The correlation between early sensitization to foods and later development of asthma is difficult to determine, but in these cases, given the repeated respiratory crisis by possible viral infection, the allergy study must be expanded.

Atopic eczema

Although atopic eczema may be the only manifestation of atopy in many children, there is no question about the relationship between eczema that start of in childhood and asthma, of which the first symptoms sometimes coincide with a cutaneous process, although in most cases, respiratory symptoms appear months or years later, even after skin lesions have disappeared or been attenuated, as it happens in many children before their third year.

To predict the risk of respiratory disease in children with eczema, an early allergologic study is advised. An elevated total serum IgE will be the early sign that will alert of the atopic nature of the process, but skin tests and assessment of serum IgE specific to foods and to the most common aeroallergens at home (mites, animal epithelium), which will alert about the risk of respiratory disease, which will start later.

Besides eczema, it is frequent that allergy to cow milk protein is revealed by digestive (vomiting, diarrhoea) or anaphylactic symptoms, which are also indicative of atopic predisposition and might be a precedent of asthma.

Rhinitis, rhinoconjunctivitis, rhinosinusitis

Not surprisingly, allergic sensitization is initially produced in the respiratory mucosa, as it is directly accessible to airborne allergens present in the air we breathe; and therefore, very often, respiratory pathology of allergic cause starts with symptoms of rhinitis. The frequency and persistence of nasal symptoms in early childhood are well-known fact, and their causes are diverse, from adenoiditis to allergic rhinitis.

Because of the proximity of the conjunctival mucosa, with similar characteristics to the respiratory one, it is not uncommon the concurrence with conjunctivitis (rhinoconjunctivitis). From the second or third year, it is neither uncommon the simultaneous conditioning of maxillary sinusitis, which may be limited to the inflammatory reaction of the mucosa, but that is often complicated by superinfection. Greater doubts arise in the relationship of rhinitis with otitis media present in some children, although it seems that nasal provocation with pollen can cause a dysfunction at the inner ear level.

6. Clinical and allergologic diagnosis

The diagnosis of asthma in the first years of life is based on a thorough questioning (anamnesis) and in the allergologic study. Given the difficulties and controversies surrounding the concept of the disease at a such early age, the issue is to obtain data that, with the smallest possible doubt, may allow on one hand to establish the syndromic diagnosis, that is, the existence of intermittent episodes of bronchial obstruction and, on the other, allergic causality, in most cases, or the responsibility of other exogenous factors able to increase bronchial reactivity, which usually occurs at later ages. When the allergologic study is negative, the questioning may provided valid information to guide diagnosis to some other of the process in which coughing or signs of bronchial obstruction often dominate the case history, having to complete the study in accordance with the suspected diagnosis.

Physical examination is essential, since even if the child is asymptomatic while being examined, important data, such as a chest deformity, the presence of paradoxical breathing with depressed abdomen on inspiration, or the pathologic auscultation when the child breathes deeply, among other information, can be obtained. Moreover, functional exploration will also provide data that can be decisive for the definitive diagnosis.

6.1. Anamnesis

A good interrogation often provides critical data to guide the diagnosis. It should include information about family precedents and medical history, diseases of probable allergic cause cited above, symptomatology, chronology of symptoms, medication use and its effectiveness.

6.2. Other medical history

Primary immunodeficiencies also occur in repeated bronchopaties, by viral or bacterial infections, with symptoms that may remind those of asthma; hence, the need for information on whether there have been relatives with any of these diseases (Wiskott–Aldrich, Hypo or agammaglobulinaemia, Di George, etc.), processes in which predisposition is transmitted by recessive inheritance.

6.3. Symptomatology: chronology

It is not enough to know that the child has episodes of cough or dyspnoea, but it must be also known if the cough is dry or soft, if breathing difficulty improves or worsens after a coughing spell, if there is expectoration, or if it is predominant at night, among other features. It is also necessary to know the intensity of respiratory distress, if it is accompanied with nasal flaring, or if it disrupts sleep. The existence of fever is also a point of great interest because an infectious trigger can be assumed.

The chronology of the succession of symptoms in each episode is another fact of interest, as it is whether dyspnoea appeared abruptly or was preceded by nasal or pharyngeal symptoms, as well as at what time it began, for example, if it was at night or after eating some food. The biggest interest is in the chronology of the process, taking very much into account the age at which symptoms started and whether they were intense from the beginning (mucoviscidosis could be suspected of).

6.4. Medication: use and effectiveness

Usually, when a child presents some of the symptoms that characterize bronchial obstruction, some medication is usually given, and their effectiveness must be critically evaluated, in order to better guide the diagnosis. It is not always possible to reduce or eliminate breathing difficulty with a bronchodilator, when mucous secretion is predominant, or preventing relapse with an inhaled corticoid, when there is no inflammation because the airway obstruction is of another nature.

6.5. Allergologic study

Skin tests

They may already be positive even in the second month of life, to cow's milk protein (casein, β-lactoglobulin). At 4 months, it is possible to show sensitization to other foods, especially egg proteins, increasing the percentage in the coming months, as new foods are introduced. Sensitization to pneumoallergens comes later. It is estimated that approximately 40% of atopic children under 3 years are sensitized to dust mites, reaching 70% in those over 4 years. Figures for animal epithelia range from 3 to 5% in the younger, being 6–8% at around 4–5 years of age. Sensitization to pollens also depends on the place of residence, in relation to the time and intensity of exposure.

The *prick test* is the least traumatic and totally reliable and reproducible technique that has replaced intradermoreaction. It is virtually painless, very well accepted by young children and easily performed with the same technique at any age.

Usually, the study is limited to dust mites, the most common being *Dermatophagoides pteronyssinus* and *Dermatophagoides farinae*, but others can be added, such as *B. tropicalis, Acaro siro* or others that are common in the geographical area of residence: animal epithelia, cat and dog (the most frequent, even if they are not present at home) or other animals with which they may have contact. Fungi can be found anywhere at home. The most important, that allow conducting immunotherapy, are *Alternaria tenuis* and *alternata*, and *Cladoporium* ssp. At homes with high humidity, other fungi must be tested, such as *Aspergillus, Penicillium, Fusarium, Mucor*, etc. Earlier than at 3–4 years of age, sensitization to pollens is unlikely, although there is no objection to include in the list of allergens a mixture of pollen from wild grasses (*Poa pratensis, Festuca, Dactylis glomerata, Lolium perenne, Phleum pratense*) that are most often sensitizing. Other pollens depend on the geographic area in which they reside.

Total serum and specific IgE

From birth, the serum non-specific IgE level increases to reach figures close to those of the adult into adolescence (**Table 2**). IgE has some physiological functions, such as defence against helminth parasites, although it is supposed to participate in other defence mechanisms. In the atopic individual, the regulator mechanism of IgE production is genetically altered by the prevalence of the activity of Th2 lymphocytes already mentioned. Therefore, it is common in these patients to find an elevated serum IgE level, not having yet been specifically produced against any allergen. Hence, the finding of an elevated total serum IgE may be linked to symptoms suggestive of allergic disease, and in consequence, this finding has considerable guidance significance. However, in any case, it must be taken into account that the possibility of elevated total serum IgE, especially if the figure is very high, might be related to other processes such as parasites or certain immunodeficiencies (**Table 3**).

The assessment of total and specific to allergens IgE is based on radioimmunoassay, fluorometric or enzyme techniques. As a first step, in a suspected allergic disease, a method that includes a mixture of allergens that are suspected to be frequent in childhood (food and airborne allergens: Phadiatop® infant, Immuno-CAP, 3gAllergy) can be used, the positivity of which may indicate specific sensitization to any of the antigens included. Subsequently, the allergen that led to the positive test must be identified in order to establish the preventive and specific treatment as appropriate.

Comparing the diagnostic value of skin tests and the specific IgE, it can be said that both are equivalent; however, it is always advisable to check the diagnosis with both tests. To complement the immunoallergologic study, it is required to assess other serum immunoglobulins, IgG, IgM and IgA, as it is not uncommon that the deficit of some of them may favour respiratory infections. It is not unusual that this happens when there is selective deficiency of IgA, a common immunodeficiency (1/700 in the general population and 1/200 people with allergies) that sometimes goes unnoticed by a low clinical expression in most cases.

Eosinophilia: cationic protein

In peripheral blood, increased eosinophils above 500 cells/mm^3 may indicate allergic reaction in any organ system (lung, skin, digestive tract) where the process is in an acute phase or immediate to clinical reaction. The presence of eosinophils in the bronchial exudate or tissue obtained by biopsy reveals the characteristic inflammation of an allergic reaction. When not in these cases, eosinophilia may be normal, and very high levels are usually due to many processes, parasitosis most of the time.

More valuable is the elevation of serum level of the enzymes from eosinophils, mainly ECP, easy to determine. It is necessary to be cautious when assessing the increased serum ECP as a marker of a certain bronchial inflammation, given the variability of the figures that can be found. According to Koller et al. [12], it could be a good marker even after the first episode of dyspnoea, finding a higher ECP in infants which a year later were diagnosed with asthma than in those who did not developed the disease, estimating that figures higher than 20 μg/l could have a strong prognostic value. However, Pohunek et al. [23] found no differences in ECP levels in children under 3, between both diagnoses when children were asymptomatic, as opposite to when they were suffering a crisis. From his work, it can be deducted the interest to assess the enzyme during a bronchobstructive crisis, in yet not diagnosed children, especially during the first episode, for the possibility of establishing prophylactic measures to prevent or delay the establishment of asthma.

Age	**Geometric mean kU/l**	**+1 SD**	**+2 SD**
Umbilical cord	0.3	–	–
6 weeks	0.7	2.1	6.1
3 months	0.8	1.8	3.8
6 months	2.7	6.6	16.3
9 months	2.4	4.2	7.3
12 months	7	21	58
2 years	11	26	61
3 years	11	21	40
4 years	20	37	70
7 years	26	75	221

Table 2. Normal serum IgE levels (Kjellman and Johanson, 1976).

Parasitic infections
Ascaris lumbricoides
Toxocara canis
Entamoeba haemolitica
Echinococcus
Trichinella spiralis
Filaria
Others
Immunodeficiency disorders
Wiskott-Aldrich S.
Di George S.
Hiper IgE S.
Selective IgA deficiency

Table 3. Non-allergic process more frequents in small children that occur with high IgE.

Since allergic rhinitis often precedes the onset of bronchial symptoms, eosinophil count and ECP in nasal mucus can be a good indicator of allergic predisposition and the possible progression of the disease to the lower airways. Presence of allergy will be suspected if the percentage of eosinophils of the total cells of the smear exceeds 10%. In the same sample, ECP and even total and specific IgE can be assessed, in which variation after immunotherapy can be a good indicator of the effectiveness of the treatment [15].

7. Respiratory function exploration

7.1. Children under 2 years of age

In the diagnosis of asthma or of wheezy bronchitis, exploration in the infant has a relative utility. However, the greatest value of early exploration is focussed on distinguishing the processes that occur with breathing difficulties of various kinds, some of bronchopulmonary origin (cystic fibrosis, bronchopulmonary dysplasia, primary ciliary dyskinesia, bronchitis obliterans, malformations) or extrapulmonary (vascular rings, ductus persistence, other heart disease), which can raise the differential diagnosis with severe asthma or resistant to habitual treatment. Exploration in infants should be restricted due to the risk involved in the need to sedate the child, requiring hospital environment, which should be restricted to the following indications, in order to diagnose other possible diseases with apparent symptoms of asthma, although symptoms can have a different origin:

1. Presence of tachypnea, hypoxia, cough or dyspnoea of unexplained causes that cannot be studied with other techniques.
2. Serious and chronic obstructive diseases that do not yield to the usual treatment of corticoids and bronchodilators, both inhaled.
3. Non-characteristic respiratory symptoms, with the likelihood of an extrabronchial origin, in order to assess the origin and severity of the symptoms (e.g. vascular rings).
4. Research, necessary in all diagnostic or therapeutic procedures, but risk must always be assessed and therefore have the corresponding parental consent and approval by ethics committees.

Methodology

The most common method is the rapid thoracoabdominal compression at ordinary volume. As the child breathes normally and at the end of an inspiration, an insufflation of the jacket is provoked to induce maximal forced expiration, thus obtaining the parameter of the maximum flow at functional residual capacity (VmaxFRC). Both the figure obtained and the appreciation of the layout of the flow-volume curve will provide information on the permeability of the airways and the degree of obstruction, if any.

Less suitable is the one based on thoracoabdominal compression provided by a pneumatic jacket, a kind of inflatable vest connected to an air compressor through a non-distensible thick tube. The exhaled airflow is measured with a pneumotachograph of appropriate size that adapts to the mouth through a mask. The biggest drawback is the need to sedate the child with chloral hydrate orally, which is not without risks.

As forced expiration is provoked during a normal respiratory movement, that is ordinary volume, this technique does not provide the value of the forced vital capacity (FVC) obtained with a spirometry, and therefore, no FEV_1 or the FEV_1/FVC ratio and FEV_1% can be obtained. To acquire these values, we must perform the technique known as rapid thoracoabdominal compression with previous insufflation, which is artificially forcing a deep breath, for which, by a compressor connected to an oral–nasal mask, air is blown into child up to the maximum vital capacity and requiring a pressure of 2–3 kPa (20–30 cm H_2O). Afterwards, a rapid inflation of the jacket is performed to provoke the forced expiration. This way, valuable data comparable to those provided by spirometry, can be obtained.

7.2. Children over 2 years of age

Although the following techniques are used in older children who do not cooperate during the exploration, some of them are also used in infants with devices adapted to their size (plethysmograph), requiring sedation of the child. With them, precise information on airway resistance (AWR) and compliance can be obtained.

The AWR is defined by the difference of pressure between both ends of the airways, that is the mouth and alveoli when an air flow of 1 l/s occurs. The circumstantial narrowing of the bronchi increases resistance, deducing the intensity of the obstruction by the degree of the increase in the value of the AWR.

Compliance refers to the intensity of the rigidity of the respiratory system, defined by the increase of the volume produced divided by the increase of the pressure unit, so that the less pressure necessary to produce an equal increase in volume, the higher the compliance.

The resistance can be measured through well-known techniques, such as interruption of flow (Rint), forced oscillation and its oscillometric impulse variation and plethysmography, a technique which also allows the compliance to be known.

Flow interruption (Rint)

The interruption of the airflow during normal breathing causes rapid and complete occlusion of the airways, enabling the measurement of the pressure in the oral cavity immediately before the interruption and during the normal respiratory cycle using a pneumotachograph. The measurement of the alveolar pressure is deduced from the pressure value established in the mouth when the momentary interruption of flow occurs. If this is suddenly interrupted, for a split second, an immediate rise in pressure occurs in the mouth. The pressure measured this way is very similar to that found in the alveoli, allowing the measurement of *resistance*, comparing this pressure with that prevailing in the mouth just before shutting off the flow. The Unit used to measure the resistance is Pascal in litres per second. In short, Rint is the most simple and affordable method to learn the AWR in young children, with the only requirement being that they breathe normally through the tube that is fitted into the mouth, preventing nasal breathing by pinching the nose.

Forced oscillation: impulse oscillometry

Forced oscillometry is based on the application of oscillatory pressure changes and therefore airflow, measuring the resistance from the relationship between the two. Easy to perform, it only requires that the child breathe calmly through a tube—not longer than 1 m—attached to the mouth and a volume of 100 ml, having inserted a pneumotachograph in between. The patient's air flow is superimposed with a oscillanting flow of 2 ml at a frequency of 10 Hz coming from a sinusoidal generator, thereby leading to pressure variations which are not perceived by the child and are proportional to the 'total' patient breathing resistance.

Best results are obtained with a newer variation of this process, the *impulse oscillometry* (IOS). A controlled deviation of the membrane of a loudspeaker, which is adapted to a nozzle, leads to the excitation of the airflow generating pressure impulses, from which ratio, the value of the central airways resistance and the lung elasticity is obtained; and therefore, the values result from the relationship between the exerted pressure and the airflow [4].

Plethysmography

A plethysmograph measures the changes in volume of the thorax. Its principle is the law of Boyle and Mariotte, whereby the volume occupied by a mass of gas, at constant temperature, is inversely proportional to the pressure. By plethysmography, intrathoracic gas volume (TGV) through the volumetric variations of the thorax is measured simultaneously with the AWR, and from these values, conductance can be calculated.

Bronchodynamic tests

The above techniques report on the current state of the permeability of the lower airways but do not provide information on the level of BHR, the increase of which is significant in the diagnosis of asthma. Hence, the need to carry out tests to make it evident, that is bronchoconstrictor (methacholine, histamine) and bronchodilator (β-mimetic) tests. The three technical variations mentioned can be used for this purpose

8. Differential diagnosis based on the dominant symptoms

Many processes that start at preschool age manifest similar symptoms to those of bronchitis or asthma. The too early start of these symptoms, sometimes shortly after birth or in the first months of life, is a matter of warning about the possibility of a process less frequent than those, but even if the process has a late start, the other possible causes of cough or dyspnoea should never be forgotten, avoiding the comfortable position of starting a routine treatment, which may not always be beneficial and could even delay the establishment of appropriate therapeutic measures.

The assessment of cough as a symptom, that in the case of asthma is often maintained between the crises of dyspnoea or wheezing, has some characteristics that can guide to others diagnosis not uncommon at preschool age, with symptoms that may be common to those of asthma, and therefore is mandatory to take them into account in order to conduct a correct differential diagnosis (**Table 4**).

Dominant symptom: cough	Pseudoasthmatic bronchial symptoms	LESS common processes
Maxillary sinusitis	Immunodeficiencies	Congenital anomalies
Adenoids	Bronchiolitis	—Laringo and tracheomalacias
Rhinopharyngitis	Bronchitis obliterans	—Vascular rings
Whooping cough (pertussis)	Wheezy bronchitis	Alpha-1-antitrypsin deficiency
Primary ciliary dyskinesia	Tracheobronchial foreign body	Hypersensitivity pneumonitis
Eosinophilic bronchitis	Mucoviscidosis (cystic pancreatic fibrosis)	Pulmonary hemosiderosis
	Gastroesophageal reflux	Alveolar proteinosis
	Tumour or mediastinal adenopathy	Eosinophilic lung

Table 4. Most significant processes in the differential diagnosis.

9. Practical summary for diagnostic approach

1. Medical history
    a. Family history: allergic pathology, respiratory or genetic pathology.
    b. Own background: allergic comorbidity (eczema, allergies to milk proteins, etc.), recurrent infections
    c. Symptomatology: for each one of the symptoms, it is necessary to specify the characteristics, age of onset, duration, severity, recurrence, association between them.
    d. Environment: smoking, irritating substances, pets, rural area
2. Clinical examination
    a. In a symptomatic stage or during an interval
    b. General inspection: development, nutrition, colour of skin and mucous membranes, acrocyanosis. If there is coughing: characteristics. Nasal or mouth breathing.
    c. Thoracic inspection: circulation, retractions, respiratory rate, dyspnoea. Auscultation: wheezing, rhonchus, crackles, localized or generalized, changing or not present when coughing. Localized hypophonia. Percussion: localized dullness.
    d. Nasopharyngeal: nasal flaring, anterior or posterior rhinorrhea, appearance of mucus. Size and appearance of the tonsils: visible adenoids?
3. Initial Investigations in all cases

a. Complete blood count. ESR

b. Immunoglobulin G, M, A and E

c. Paranasal sinuses X-ray. Adenoid RX if hypertrophy is suspected

4. If all the above rules out the existence of a pathology different of asthma or wheezy bronchitis, continue the study to confirm it.

5. If the above tests fail to lead to that conclusion, if the symptoms are important or if after an initial diagnosis of asthma or bronchitis no improvement is achieved with standard therapy (inhaled bronchodilators and corticoids) the following tests should be made:

   a. Sweat test. Also required in the initial study, if symptoms are of an early onset, severe, with general deterioration or a family history of cystic fibrosis

   b. Esophageal pH monitoring

   c. Thoracis X-ray, front and profile: assessing abnormal masses, adenopathy, condensation, etc. Mediastinal swaying following the suspicion of a foreign body aspiration, especially in children under 3 years

   d. Other imaging techniques based on radiological findings or presumed diagnosis: computed tomography, magnetic resonance, gammagraphy.

   e. Serum antibodies against RSV, influenza, parainfluenza and other

6. If the above tests do not lead to a diagnosis in accordance with the clinical suspicion or in case of uncertainty, it is recommended that, successively:

   a. Lung function study

   b. Serum precipitin against actinomycetes

   c. BAL: hemosiderophages (also in gastric contents), PAS+ protein, eosinophil

   d. Alpha-1-antitrypsin serume

   e. Bronchoscopy

   f. Lung biopsy

10. Treatment

Although asthma treatment at any age is based on the same principles, the characteristics of the disease and the pathophysiology in pre-scholar children require adjusting each of the measures available to the peculiarities of the age.

Overall, these measures aim primarily to combat the cause of the disease, that is *etiological* treatment based, in one part on environmental measures (reduction of household allergens and reducing environmental pollutants) and on the other in desensitization by immunotherapy. The *pathogenic* treatment is based on fighting the bronchial inflammation, trying to prevent or eliminate it, being chromones, anti-leukotrienes and corticoids the appropriate medications, and finally, the *symptomatic* treatment with short-acting bronchodilators, mainly β2-agonists.

10.1. Etiological: specific immunotherapy

Immunotherapy is the only therapeutic procedure, for its widely proven effectiveness, which decreases the sensitivity (desensitization or hyposensitization) to the responsible allergens, in which its mechanisms of action are essential to prevent further sensitization, as is well known (in short, the Th1/Th2 balance).

WHO supports the term 'allergy vaccine' and considers this as the only treatment that can alter the natural course of allergic diseases and also prevent the development of asthma in patients with allergic rhinitis.

Although the age to initiate immunotherapy has been questioned, multiple studies and the own experience show the need for an early start, from the third year of age, provided that the requirements set out in **Table 5** are met.

Recent and extensive literature reviews conclude that it is a serious need to consider the start of immunotherapy in children under 5 years of age that fulfil the required conditions ([7, 8])

— Correct clinical diagnosis
— In case of asthma:
— mild to moderate intensity
— respiratory function within normal limits: parameters not <70% of those foreseen
— Accurate allergologic diagnosis, skin tests and serum specific IgE are sufficient
Exceptionally provocation with allergen will be used
— Right choice of allergen/s to be included
— Extract quality: purity, standardization, coadjutants
— Correct therapeutic regimen monitoring: dose, intervals
— Periodical clinical controls
— Minimum period of 3 years, and at least 1 year without onset of symptoms
— Prescription and control by a allergy and paediatrics expert
—Early onset

Table 5. Premises for immunotherapy for optimal results in paediatrics.

Some of the few problems that can cause subcutaneous immunotherapy could be avoided if administered by sublingual channels, which is virtually risk-free. A problem in young children is the difficulty of successfully administering the pharmaceutical preparation, keeping it under their tongue for the right time, which is likely to be simplified with the most recent preparation in tablets or in atomiser (spray) (WAO).

10.2. Pathogenic: antiinflammatories

Chromones

Under this description, cromolyn sodium and nedocromil are included. Both act by blocking the chloride channels of the membrane in the cells involved in the allergic reaction, especially mast cells and eosinophils, but also epithelial and nerve cells. On the activation of chloride channels depends the crossing of Ca ions into the cell, required for the activation thereof to occur. When these cells are stimulated (allergens, non-specific agents), there is a release of mediators (mast cells) and the commencement of the elements involved in the allergic reaction. When idle, chloride channels are closed and this is what is achieved with chromones, the blocking of the channels, thereby preventing activation of the cells that would lead to the allergic reaction. For this reason, we must consider that chromones act more like preventive agents of inflammation than anti-inflammatories.

Although currently they are less used as inflammation preventives, cromolyn could be indicated in preschool age, before asthma reaches a significant degree of severity, that is in mild intermittent or persistent asthma and in moderate asthma, in which case an inhaled corticoid or salbutamol could be added.

Anti-leukotrienes

These are medications that block the action of cysteinyl leukotrienes that might prevent the onset of one of the most important mechanisms involved in the production of the inflammatory reaction of the bronchial mucosa. They specifically avoid the activity of those on specific receptors localized in bronchial smooth muscle and in bronchoalveolar blood vessels. This is intended to prevent the development of inflammation in the initial period of obstructive bronchial disorders and also contribute to avoid the swelling to persist or increase, once present when asthma has been clinically established.

Knowledge of the receptors of the leukotrienes is a key for the intended purpose. Pharmacological studies have determined that cysteinyl leukotrienes activate at least two types of receptors, named CysLT1 and CysLT2, being the first found in the bronchial muscle and the second in the pulmonary venous system. Depending on the consequences of the activation of these receptors by the corresponding leukotriene, the antagonists used therapeutically will produce diverse positive effects, even more prominent in children than in adults. On one hand, they achieved a discrete bronchodilation resulting as a consequence of counteracting the prolonged constrictor effect of leukotrienes.

In short, anti-leukotrienes behave more like inflammation preventives than as anti-inflammatories, an activity that is better performed by inhaled corticoids, and therefore, both treatments can be used simultaneously.

Of the preparations available (pranlukast, zafirlukast and montelukast), only the latter is indicated in children under 5 years of age, available in chewable tablets and granules. Since the permanence of the inflammatory reaction in all probability depends on the recurrence of episodes of dyspnoea and their intensity, montelukast may prevent the progression of the process in milder cases without resorting to inhaled corticoids. The advantage of oral administration and the single daily dose make this drug of easy acceptance and secure compliance. In asthma of moderate or severe intensity, it will be necessary to combine the treatment with inhaled corticoids.

Several studies confirm the efficacy of the treatment with montelukast in children between 2 and 5 years of age even reducing the number of episodes caused by viral infections (5). Respiratory function improves from the early days of treatment, even in children under 2 years of age as a result of the reduction of the inflammation.

Corticoids

Physiologically, corticoids activate the cytoplasmic receptors that most cells have; the same which corticoids administered therapeutically act upon, with a power that depends on the affinity of each product with these receptors, entering into competition with the natural hormone. They are known to inhibit various cytokines, especially ILs (IL-1, IL-2, IL-3, IL-4, IL5, IL-6 and IL-13), tumour necrosis factor alpha (TNF-α) and the colony stimulating factor in granulocytes and macrophages (GM-CSF), while increasing the IFN-γ and IL-12, that is they reduce the action of Th2 leukocytes, and consequently, the number of basophils, eosinophils and mast cells in bronchial epithelium is reduced. The risk of any side effects resides on the fact that only between 10 and 40% of the drug administered by inhalation reach the bronchi, depending on the inhalation system. The rest of the substance remains in the mouth and is swallowed, getting into the general circulation via the gastrointestinal tract. They are mostly metabolized in the liver, being removed, but another part remains in the bloodstream, reaching the lung, where they produce the same effect as corticoids administered by other means. At the same time, part of the fraction that reached the lung by inhalation passes into the bloodstream, following the same path as the ingested portion. Some of these drawbacks are avoided with ciclesonide, with little oral bioavailability (only 10% of the active molecule is generated in the oropharynx), so that the pharmacotherapy is mainly dependent on deposit and pulmonary absorption.

The most prominent undesirable effects are the hypothalamic–pituitary–adrenal (HPA) axis suppression and growth retardation that, although it seems to be compensated in years not affecting final adult height, it must be considered in order not to fall into the usual trend of increasing doses when the desired effects are not achieved. Prolonged treatments or higher doses may result from severe hypoglycemia to cushingoid features. In children, it is rare that osteoporosis occurs. Depression of immunity caused by corticoids may increase the risk of infections. Other less important effects are of cutaneous nature, such as oral thrush or skin atrophy, less common in children.

A weighting between dose/guideline/efficacy/duration of therapy/adverse effects should be established. Effective maximum doses of inhaled corticoids in children have been established, which is 400 μg/day for beclomethasone dipropionate and budesonide, and 200 μg/day for fluticasone propionate. Despite the better tolerance with ciclesonide, only studies from 4 years of age have been published, with a maximum dose of 160 μg/day. Higher doses of any of them do not improve results and increase the risk of side effects. The daily dose is usually divided into two intakes, but can be simplified without losing efficiency, administering once the total daily dose in the morning, as the physiological hormone production would be reduced if taken at night. In mild-moderate asthma, there is an increased permeability of the airways, and therefore, the drug penetrates with greater ease making the most of the administered dose, hence the recommendation to use lower doses in milder cases.

The oral or intravenous administration of corticoids is reserved for asthma crises of medium or severe intensity, either at home or in hospital. The dose of 1–2 mg/kg/day of prednisone, prednisolone or methylprednisolone should not be prolonged for more than 5 days, but if more time is required, it should be progressively reduced.

Although inhaled corticoids may show a symptomatic improvement, in the long term, the course of the disease does not seem to change; therefore, the duration of the treatment will depend on the results and even a diagnostic review should be considered.

10.3. Symptomatic: bronchodilators

Beta 2-agonists

The indication of short-acting β_2-agonists (salbutamol, terbutaline) is the bronchospasm crisis, whatever its intensity. The most appropriate route of administration is inhalation, achieving improvement in a few minutes, in the case of acute asthma attacks. Continued inhalation is indicated for the inpatient treatment of severe crisis. Other routes of administration are subcutaneous and, above all, continuous intravenous to which we must turn in severe crisis. The oral route may be useful in mild cases or after achieving a significant improvement with the inhaler.

In preschool children, the most common is the metered-dose inhaler (MDI) with a spacer or with a nebulizer when it is necessary to continuously administer the drug. Otherwise, the efficacy appears to be similar with both inhalation systems. Powdered formula, for which there are different systems (turbuhaler, diskhaler, accuhaler), is less useful at this age, because a greater degree of collaboration is required.

Anticholinergics

Ipratropium bromide, is a derivative of atropine, which does not produce the side effects of atropine. Because of its low lipid solubility, it hardly passes biological membranes and produces an effect almost exclusively in the bronchial tree, when administered by inhalation. The recommended dose for all ages is 0.04 mg three or four times daily. The greatest benefits are achieved in asthma attacks triggered by non-specific agents, which may act via vagal.

The bronchodilator action is more deferred with this product, but it remains longer than with the β_2-mimetic, and in some cases might be administered simultaneously, for which there are even preparations with formoterol or salbutamol and ipratropium bromide, although it is preferable to dispense them separately.

11. Therapeutic schemes

11.1. Treatment of crises

The therapeutic approach in episodes of respiratory difficulty should be preceded by a reflection on the different diagnostic possibilities, since various acute processes may manifest common and sometimes confusing symptoms, needing different treatments, care and control. The severity of the case will be visible by observation and by assessing dyspnoea, intercostal, subcostal or supraclavicular retractions, colouring and sensory. The assessment of breath sounds that can be discernible by auscultation is essential for diagnosis as it can indicate the location of the process (trachea, central or peripheral bronchi, alveoli), if bronchospasm, condensation or atelectasis are present, which can be deduced from the presence or prevalence of wheezing, stridor, crackles or coarse crackles, decreased murmur, among other respiratory noises. Other causes of severe respiratory distress that may resemble an asthma attack, should also be considered, especially the frequent aspiration of a foreign body, which requires radiological confirmation, and bronchiolitis, both of a sudden onset and which can also occur in children that already suffer from asthma. Once it is concluded that it is a bronchospasm crisis, its severity will be assessed and of this assessment will depend the therapeutic activities:

1. Mild: β-mimetic inhaled: according to severity: 2 doses × 20 min, maximum 3 doses, or every 4–6–8 h depending on severity; maximum 24–36 h.
2. Moderate: add oral corticosteroids: 1–2 mg/kg/day: 3–4 days
3. In both situations, after the improvement, treatment with β-mimetic continue orally (±1 week) or mucolytic and expectorant, if required.
4. Grave whose intensity, more complex processing conditions outlined in **Table 6**.

<u>*Immediate:*</u>
Oxygen inhalation by flow of a β-mimetic:
Salbutamol: 2.5–5 mg
Terbutaline: 5–10 mg
(Half dose in children under 1 year)
Intravenous hydrocortisone 100 mg
In more severe cases, adding:
Aminophylline e.v.: 5 mg/kg in micro-drip (20 min) followed
continuous infusion of 1 mg/kg/h
(Investigate whether there were received a dose above)
Inhaled ipratropium bromide 0.25 mg (0.125 in infants)

Controls:
Symptomatology
Oximetry: to reach $SaO_2 > 92\%$

<u>*Monitoring*</u>
If no improvement in 15–30 min:
Salbutamol: Continuous inhalation or every 30 min until

to get better. After follow the evolution every 1–4–6 h
Aminophylline: continuous infusion (monitor serum)
Ipratropium bromide: every 6 h
Hydrocortisone repeated every 6 h, or
Methylprednisolone ev: 1–2 mg/kg/day (spread in 4 doses)

If there is no improvement or worse:
Admission to Intensive Care Unit:
Protocol status asthmaticus

Leaving the hospital:
Salbutamol or terbutaline inhaled or oral, to a week
Methylprednisolone oral, decreasing doses, depending on the dose and previously administered treatment days

Medical surveillance: 2–4days

Table 6. Treatment of severe asthma attacks in children under 5 years of age (Abridged outline various guides).

11.2. Maintenance treatment

Pharmacological treatment mainly depends on the frequency and intensity of the symptoms, the severity of which is deduced for each single case (**Table 7**).

When symptoms occur sporadically (occasional episodic) unless there is a crisis, a treatment is not usually needed. When the frequency is higher (frequent episodic), it is recommended to start with montelukast, which will act as an inflammation preventive and if there is a failure to control the symptoms, a low-dose inhaled corticoid will be added.

If symptoms occur more frequently, with intermittent crises (moderate persistent), apart from montelukast, inhaled corticoids without exceeding the maximum recommended dose will be added. If control is not reached, cromolyn sodium nebulizer three times a day will often achieve satisfactory results. Once symptoms are controlled, continue with montelukast and inhaled corticoids.

From the third year of age, when the allergic causality of the process is certain and the responsible allergen has been identified, immunotherapy is the fundamental etiological treatment, provided that the above criteria are met, following WHO recommendations.

Occasional episodic	**Infrequent episodes: 1 every 4–6 weeks or less**
	Asymptomatic intercrisis
Frequent episodic	Over 1 episode in 4–6 weeks
	Intercrisis-isolated symptoms, which do not affect the child's activities or sleep
Moderate persistent	Very frequent exacerbations
	Frequent intercrisis symptoms that interfere with daily activities and sleep
Severe persistent	Daily or nearly daily symptoms, with frequent episodes of respiratory distress
	Disrupted daily activity and sleep

Table 7. Classification of asthma in children under 6 years of age.

Author details

F. Muñoz-López

Address all correspondence to: 5314fml@comb.cat

Former Head of the Department of Pediatric Immunoallergology,Clínic Hospital - Sant Joan de Déu Hospital, Faculty of Medicine University of Barcelona, Spain

References

[1] Antunes J, Borrego LM. Importância da avaliação funcional respiratória em idade precoce. Rev Port Imunoalergologia 2009;17(6):489–505.

[2] Ater D, Bar BE, Fireman N, Fireman E, Shai H, Tasher D, et al. Asthma-predictive-index, bronchial challenge, sputum eosinophils in acutely wheezing preschoolers. Pediatr Pulmonol 2014;49(10):952–959.

[3] Bardin PG, Johnston SL, Pattemore PK. Viruses as precipitants of asthma symptoms. II. Physiology and mechanisms. Clin Exp Allergy 1992;22:809–822.

[4] Bickel S, Pobler J, Lesnick B, Eid N. Impulse oscillometry: interpretation and practical applications. Chest 2014;146:841–847

[5] Bisgaard H, Zielen S, García-García L, Johnston SL, Gilles L, Menten J, et al. Montelukast reduces asthma exacerbations in 2 to 5 year old children with intermittent asthma. Am J Respir Crit Care Med 2005;171:315–322.

[6] Braun-Fahrlander C, Riedler J, Herz U, Eder W, Waser M, Grize L et al. Environmental exposure to endotoxin and its relation to asthma in school-age children. N Engl J Med 2002;347:869–877.

[7] Canonica GW, Bachert C, Hellings P, Ryan D, Valovirta E, Wickman M et al. Allergen immunotherapy (AIT): a prototype of precision medicine. WAO J 2015;8:31

[8] Finegold I. Immunotherapy: when to initiate treatment in children. Allergy Asthma Proc 2007;28:698–705

[9] Gilliland FD, Berhane K, Li YF, Rappaport EB, Peters JM. Effects of early onset asthma and in utero exposure to maternal smoking on childhood lung function. Am J Respir Crit Care Med 2003;167:917–924

[10] Guherin U, Cyrys J, Sedlmeir G, Brunekreef B, Bellander T, Fischer P, et al. Traffic-related air pollution and respiratory health during the 2 years of live. Eur Respir J. 2002; 19:690–698.

[11] Hertzen LC. Maternal stress and T-cell differentiation of the developing immune system: possible implications for the development of asthma and atopy. J Allergy Clin Immunol. 2002;109:923–928.

[12] Koller DY, Wojnarowski C, Herkner KR, Weinländer G, Raderer M, Eichler I et al. High levels of eosinophil cationic protein in wheezing infants predict the development of asthma. J Allergy Clin Immunol 1997;99:752–756.

[13] Lemanske RF, Jr. Viral infections and asthma inception. J Allergy Clin Immunol 2004;114:1023–1026.

[14] Maclennan C, Hutchinson P, Holdsworth S, Bardin PG, Freezer NJ. Airway inflammation in asymptomatic children with episodic wheeze. Pediatr Pulmonol 2006;41:577–583.

[15] Martín-Mateos MA, Monferrer R, Muñoz-López F. Topical nasal immunotherapy. Immunologic response of IgE in nasal secretion after immunotherapy with *Dermatophagoides pteronyssinus*. Allergol Immunopathol 1990;18:223–228.

[16] Martínez FD, Wright AL, Taussig LM, Holberg CJ, Halonen M, Morgan WJ. Asthma and wheezing in the first six year of life. N Engl J Med 1995;332:133–138.

[17] Martota A, Klinner MD, Price MR, Larsen GL, Llu AH. Impulse oscillometry provide an effective measure of lung dysfunction in 4-year-old children at risk for persistent asthma. J Allergy Clin Immunol 2003;112:317–322.

[18] Montgomery GL, Tepper RS, Changes in airway reactivity with age in normal infants and young children. Am Rev Respir Dis 1990;142:1372–1376.

[19] Muñoz-López F. Bronchial hyperresponsiveness and asthma in the pediatric population. Allergol Immunopathol (Madrid) 2014;42:230–234.

[20] Pereira AM, Morais-Almeida M, Santos N, Nunes C. Bousquet J, Fonseca JA . Severity of rhinitis and wheezing in strongly associated in preschoolers: a population-based study. Pediatr Allergy Immunol 2015;26:618–627

[21] Pereira C, Loureiro G, Tavares B, Botelho F. Specific immunotherapy and central immune system. Cap. 19. of Allergic Diseases: 2012; www.intechopen.com.

[22] Pescatore AM, Dogaru CM, Duembgen L, Silverman M, Gailard EA, Spycher BD et al. A simple asthma prediction tool for preschool children with wheeze or cough. J Allergy Clin Immunol 2014;133:111–118.

[23] Pohunek P, Warner W O, Turzícová J, Kudrmann J, Roche WR. Markers of eosinophilic inflammation and tissue re-modelling in children before clinically diagnosed bronchial asthma. Pediatr Allergy Immunol 2005;16:43–51.

[24] Prescoot SL. Allergy: when does it begin and where will it end? Allergy 2003;58:864–7.

[25] Silvestri M, Franchi S, Pistorio A, Petecchia L, Rusconi F. Smoke exposure, wheezing and asthma development: a systematic review and meta-analysis in unselected birth cohorts. Pediatr Pulmonol 2015;50(4):353–62.

[26] Song TW, Kim KW, Kim ES, Park J-W, Sohn MH, Kim K-E. Utility of impulse oscillometry in young children with asthma. Pediatr Allergy Immunol 2008;19:763–8.

[27] Williams TJ, Jones CA, Miles EA, Warner JO, Warner JA. Fetal and neonatal IL-13 production during pregnancy and birth and subsequent development of atopic symptoms. J Allergy Clin Immunol 2000;105:951–9.

[28] WAO Position Paper: Allergen immunotherapy: therapeutic vaccines for allergic diseases. Allergy 1998;53 Suppl. 44:4–42.

[29] Passalacqua G, Compalati E, Canonica GW. Sublingual immunotherapy: clinical indications in the WAO-SLIT position paper. WAO Journal 2010;3(7):216-19.

2

Managing Bronchial Asthma in Underprivileged Communities

Yousser Mohammad and Basim Dubaybo

Abstract

The definition of a primary care facility is the site where the first patient contact occurs. In developing countries, primary healthcare (PHC) facilities are officially healthcare centers, hosting World Health Organization (WHO) programs for tuberculosis and chronic respiratory diseases. In addition, there are many other providers of PHC services, which include emergency departments, general outpatient clinics in public hospitals. Asthma patients may present for treatment in any of these primary care facilities. An international study achieved by the Union showed that 51% of asthma patients in Syria are treated in emergency departments only, many developing countries like Sudan, Algeria, and some African countries had the same use of ER. There are questions about the quality of care provided in these clinics with regard to their adherence to Global Initiatives for Asthma (GINA) guidelines. Evidence suggests that there may be over prescribing of oral corticosteroids and antibiotics and under-prescription of inhaled corticosteroids, so there is a need to improve practice bringing it more into alignment to international guidelines. It may be considered by many that it is not possible to follow guidelines in developing countries and those that have economic and political pressures. However, a pilot program to test the feasibility of a providing systematic follow-up of uncontrolled asthma patients in a general free of charge hospital in Syria showed that it is possible to achieve asthma control following to GINA guidelines even in very deprived community. The same was mentioned by the Union in an international survey for other developing African and Mediterranean countries. WHO launched programs for non-communicable disease including chronic respiratory disease: Practical Approach to lung Health (PAL) and Package of essential no communicable (PEN) disease interventions for primary health care in low-resource settings. The IPCRG also worked on how to improve implementation of guidelines. We will provide the results and following evidence-based recommendations from our field surveys in developing countries, as well comment on international programs. Although much progress has been realized in the diagnosis and management of asthma in developed nations, progress in one variant of asthma, inner city asthma, has been slow. Inner city asthma is that variant of the disease which afflicts residents of urban environments with low socioeconomic conditions, poor housing, and rampant environmental risks. This variant of asthma appears to be more severe, associated with increased psychological burden as well as morbidity and mortality, has a diverse array of predisposing factors, and poses significant challenges in management and treatment. One important aspect of treatment is education which leads to the participation of the patient and the families in the care resulting in a more favorable outcome.

Keywords: asthma, primary care, WHO, chronic respiratory diseases, essential drugs for asthma, inner city, developed nations

Background

This chapter deals with asthma in developing nations and touches on one variant of asthma in the developed world which has significant resemblance to its counterpart in developing nations. The first section is derived from studies in Syria, while the second from the United States.

1. Introduction - Managing bronchial asthma in primary health care

According to the International Study for Asthma and Allergies in Childhood (ISAAC), comparing phase one in 1994 to three in 2000–2003, asthma prevalence expressed by wheezing the last 12 months in 13–14 years old is increasing in developing countries. Asthma prevalence is higher in developed countries, but asthma is more severe in developing countries [1].

The definition of a primary care facility is the site where the first patient contact occurs [2]. If we take Syria as an example of developing county, primary healthcare (PHC) facilities are officially healthcare centers under the control of the Ministry of Health, which among other services provided, host World Health Organization (WHO) programs for tuberculosis and chronic respiratory diseases [3, 4]. In addition, there are many other providers of PHC services which include emergency departments(ED), general outpatient clinics in public hospitals, school health clinics, clinics in workplace settings, and internal and general clinics within the private sector.

Asthma patients may present for treatment in any of these primary care facilities in Syria. A multicenter survey of primary care clinics revealed that 13% of patients aged over 6 years attended with asthma [5]. Another study showed that 51% of asthma patients are treated in ED only, and only 9% are treated in primary care centers [6]. Many developing countries like Sudan, Algeria and some African countries had the same use of ED [6]. The same under-utilization of community primary healthcare services has also been observed in China in 2014 [7].

There are questions about the quality of care provided in these clinics with regard to their adherence to Global Initiatives for Asthma (GINA) guidelines. Evidence suggests that there may be over prescribing of oral corticosteroids and antibiotics and under-prescription of inhaled corticosteroids [5, 6], so there is a need to improve practice bringing it more into alignment to international guidelines.

It may be considered by many that it is not possible to follow guidelines in developing countries and those that have economic and political pressures. However, a pilot program to test the feasibility of a providing systematic follow-up of uncontrolled asthma patients in a general free of charge hospital in Syria showed that it is possible to achieve asthma control following to GINA guidelines even in very poor community [8]. The same was mentioned by the Union in an international survey for other developing African and Mediterranean countries [9], the same in a recent study in Sudan [10].

A Ministry of Health—WHO program for non-communicable diseases in Syria including an intensive courses for asthma and COPD for GPs in health centers has been launched since the beginning of 2015 in a pilot site from Syria. However, unlike developed countries, in Syria, presentations are very personalized, there are no established accredited modules or curriculum for continuing medical education for primary care physicians and nurses. In order to make optimum improvements in care across the country, we need to ensure that high-quality training interventions are made available for healthcare providers who are working in a primary care setting, aiming to increase both their competence and confidence in the essentials of asthma management. This program needs to incorporate accredited educational materials, a process for monitoring and continuous evaluation, and collaborative efforts with an international agency such as the Global Alliance against Chronic Respiratory Diseases (WHO–GARD www.who.int/gard) [8]. A survey conducted by the International COPD Coalition gave the same conclusions about absence of curriculum for education for asthma and COPD [11].

Primary healthcare services are free of charge in Syria, and other developing countries hosting WHO programs, and are staffed by full-time qualified nurses who are supported by part-time physicians, who also provide services in the private sector. In addition, some patients who are able to pay for healthcare may refer themselves directly to private pulmonologists, without being referred from primary care. Since 2006, WHO launched programs for asthma and COPD at primary care level in Syria and other developing countries, and training was undertaken on site [3–5, 8].

In this paper, we share our experience in developing countries and will present first field surveys in developing countries. Second, we will comment on the international programs of WHO and International Primary Care Respiratory Group (IPCRG). And third, we will give our evidence-based recommendations.

2. Discussion

2.1. Field surveys and what we learned

Asthma is under-diagnosed in primary care [5, 6, 8, 12–14]. The Global Alliance against chronic respiratory disease (GARD–WHO: www.who.int/gard) survey on chronic respiratory diseases prevalence and risk factors in Syria revealed that although 27% of the 1599 patients surveyed had evidence of reactive airway disease and reversible obstruction by spirometry, but only 13% had been diagnosed as asthma by the primary care practitioners. Indicating that 50% were under-diagnosed [4]. This finding is not unique to Syria. Under-diagnosis has also been reported in the same GARD survey in Cape Verde [12]. There are several hypotheses for these high rates of under-diagnosis. The condition's variability of symptoms, misdiagnosis such as an infection, some may be mislabeling of patients as COPD when in fact, they may have uncontrolled asthma [5, 15], increasing workload, and demand on services and limited experienced doctors. It is important for practitioners to follow standard diagnostic procedures and good history taking such as recurrent symptoms (wheezing, cough, difficult breathing, and chest tightness) and the presence of triggers. In addition, practitioners should obtain objective tests and look for reversibility of peak expiratory flow rate (PEFR) expressed as increase of 20% and 60 l/min, or 12% increase in forced expiratory volume in one second (FEV1) and 200 ml after short-acting beta agonists (SABA), or a decrease in these measurements after exercise testing. Practitioners could also rely on variability of PEFR or FEV1 between two visits. In situations where spirometry or peak flow meter results are not available, or patients are under 5 years of age, practitioners should rely on clinical history and treatment trials [16]. WHO recommend peak flow meter to be available in the most remote healthcare centers, and referral for spirometry in healthcare centers or hospitals at central level is available [3, 4].

Asthma is under-treated and under-controlled: The GARD–WHO multicentre national survey 2010 for chronic respiratory diseases [5] revealed that only 25% of inhaled corticosteroid (ICS) prescriptions included adequate doses according to the GINA guidelines. In addition, 46% of patients received oral corticosteroids which could be avoided if ICS were prescribed in PHC according to the guidelines. Similarly, 56% of asthma patients received oral antibiotics without a clinical indication. Another important issue is that 56% of asthma patients surveyed have FEV1 < 80% after bronchodilators, which points to poor control [5, 16].

Despite asthma being poorly diagnosed and treated, it is possible to observe improvements in asthma control to the level of published guidelines in underserved areas. In a pilot study conducted on economically deprived patients in an underserved area, we systematically followed up patients with uncontrolled asthma in a general free of charge outpatient clinic in a public hospital 2006–2007 [8]. A trained postgraduate medical student asked every patient questions about the parameters of asthma control, measured PEFR, and ensured prescription of ICS at their first presentation. The student also taught patients proper inhaler technique and educated them about how to avoid risk factors. Weekly follow-up data were collected by the GP. After 3 months, 44 of 66 patients who had not been followed up previously were properly controlled. We conclude that GINA guidelines could be realistic even in underserved areas. In 2006, an international multicenter survey of the Union showed that implementation of asthma guidelines was possible in primary care in developing countries [13]. The same recently in Sudan (2014): In a new model specialized center for asthma, a survey aiming at describing the epidemiological and clinical characteristics of asthma patients concluded that most patients had abnormal spirometry with more than half having an FEV1 that is 60% or less of their predicted normal reading. The majority improved with combined treatment (Formoterol, budesonide) with 60% normalizing their spirometry highlighting the feasibility and applicability of specialized asthma care centers in resource-poor countries [10].

The global initiative for asthma guidelines are based on the level of control [16] such that for each asthmatic presenting to a primary healthcare facility, the general practitioner (GP) should ask standard questions about the clinical control of asthma including:

- Frequency of symptoms
- Need for inhaled bronchodilators
- Frequency of night awakening
- Exercise limitation
- Number of exacerbations.
- values of PEFR or FEV1

To improve care, training should emphasize that: Patients with uncontrolled asthma need to be prescribed low-dose or medium-dose inhaled corticosteroids, educated on inhaler technique, and referred to higher level of care for further assessment if not controlled after follow-up visits [3–5, 16], and referred back to primary care for long-term follow-up and education.

2.1.1. Review of international WHO programs and other programs

WHO–MOH programs: Three programs have been introduced for chronic respiratory diseases (CRD) in Syria since 2006 [3, 4, 11, 16]:

1. Practical Approach to Lung Health (PAL) program, integrating asthma, and COPD care in the National Tuberculosis program, adopting for the first time a referral policy and initiating a respiratory disease dispensary at central level equipped with peak flow, oximetry, and spirometry.
2. The Package for the essential needs for non-communicable diseases (NCD) at primary care level in low resources settings: WHO–PEN program. Integrating all major NCD including CRD at primary care level.
3. GARD program www.who.int/gard Survey on CRD risk factors and prevalence. And the resulting evidence based guidelines, and training. WHO country office is involved.

2.1.2. Other programs

1. The GINA world Asthma day program: Conferences in World Asthma Days are improving asthma care: Make health workers in PHC familiar with asthma symptoms, asthma control, peak flow meter, and corticoid inhalers.
2. Civil societies, in collaborating with the International COPD Coalition www.internationalcopd.org, are helping patients with CRD and allergy is wide-spreading patient education for asthma and COPD, and health education.

3. Educational Program for nurses about asthma and COPD: Two national workshops were run for this purpose in 2004 and 2007 by the Education for health center of Excellence—UK in Syria www.educationforhealth.org, but also in Bangladesh, and many other developing countries, aiming to introduce the role of nurses in national programs.

4. The new intensive course of WHO–MOH mentioned above for non-communicable diseases in Syria and other EMRO countries.

2.1.3. International Primary Care Respiratory Group (IPCRG)

The IPCRG tried to resolve the question on how to deal with asthma and COPD in primary care in developing countries, elaborating a symptomatic approach and algorithms, but they recommend providing primary care in developing countries with PEF and Inhalers [17]. While PAL–WHO went further (Spirometry and referral) [4].

Research priority to improve asthma management in primary care have been investigated by the IPCRG, 2009: Conclusion, primary care research should include awareness about local asthma triggers like biomass fuel, early diagnosis, and management in remote areas where there are no tools for diagnosis, the reliability of medication trial, how to overcome taboos about cultural misbelieves and inhalers, how to make essential drugs available, and how to adapt and evaluate guidelines implementation [18].

PEN–WHO opted for an integrated approach with other NCD; the approach was symptoms and PEAK flow measurements; primary care physician prescribes ICS if asthma; and treat acute attacks with oral corticosteroids and inhaled bronchodilators; referral rules to confirm diagnosis or help for better long-term treatment are stated if failure of control at follow-up visit. Necessary tools are PEF, oximetry, oxygen, and nebulisers or inhalers via spacer [3]

PAL–WHO, integrating CRD with tuberculosis program was very ambitious, referral and spirometry were recommended [4], but unfortunately, there were discontinuity and no evaluation process for the implementation of these programs, in conflict zones.

GARD–WHO was a success with the survey, and following publications and guidelines [5]

2.2. The core messages from the field surveys and international national programs

To empower the role of PHC in controlling asthma and lessen related mortality. Core messages are as follows:

1. The first consultation with the uncontrolled patient is crucial. It is vital that the correct diagnosis is made and good education is delivered. The correct treatment should be initiated at this time which will be an appropriate dose of inhaled corticosteroid and a short-acting reliever inhaler (Bronchodilator). Inhaler technique needs to be taught and the initiation of a self-management plan including what to do in an emergency and whom to contact. A follow-up appointment is important, and the PHC should consider a referral if not controlled during a follow-up visit [19]

2. Prescription of oral corticosteroids on discharge from emergency room, if not hospitalized, is recommended. By contrast, expectorants and antibiotics are often unnecessarily prescribed [5, 13, 19].

3. Methodical follow-up leads to control and is feasible even in poor settings by using standard guideline-based protocols and follow-up records. [8, 13]

4. The core equipment and medicines that health facilities should have include peak flow meter, pulse oximetry, bronchodilator inhalers, spacers (which could be built up in very poor settings/plastic bottle), [20–22], nebulizers and solution of short acting beta agonists (SABA) and if possible anticholinergics, oxygen extractor or oxygen bottle, and systemic corticosteroids.

5. Short-acting beta-agonists (via spacer, which can be built in poor settings using a plastic bottle) is as effective as nebulizer to relieve symptoms, except for very severe attacks [21–23]. The asthma-trained nurses or community healthcare workers key role is to educate patients, particularly in inhaler technique and self-management [23]. This is common practice in many developed countries and the UK and Australia have been leaders in developing nurses to fulfill this role. In the UK, much of the asthma management in primary care is provided by appropriately trained nurses [23].

6. Every uncontrolled asthma patient in spite prescription of ICS and regular follow-up in Primary care should be referred to a specialist or well-trained physician with an interest in asthma and placed in an asthma management plan and then referred back to the PHC for follow-up.

7. A toolbox for general practitioners and nurses should consist of the following:
    - Questions related to symptoms suggestive of asthma diagnosis to face under-diagnosis
    - Asthma control test for initial evaluation and follow up
    - Use of peak flow and table of values
    - Educational photos about inhaler and spacer use (Photos of all available inhalers to educate.)
    - What to do in an emergency
    - Education on how inhaled corticosteroids reverse inflammation
    - A patient self-management plan

8. Every follow-up visit should be the occasion to improve the partnership with patients according to their literacy level of education and cultural believes. A follow-up record to monitor clinical control, PEFR, compliance, and trigger avoidance should be filled at every visit. Education for inhaler technique should be part of every follow-up visit.

9. Including these core elements on the role of primary care in curriculum of medical schools, nursing schools, and pharmacies is recommended.

10. WHO programs of NCD, PEN, and PAL have been introduces in PHC dispensaries in many developing countries including Syria, and training for those programs was done at pilot sites, but the humanitarian crisis in Syria and other conflict zones discontinued progress. Effort should be done to continue [3, 4].

11. Conferences and World Asthma Days as recommended by GINA are improving asthma care: Make health workers in PHC familiar with asthma control, peak flow meter, and corticoid inhalers, but there is a great need for more education, which can also be provided online.

12. Patient organizations are playing a role on patient education and providing free medications [11].

13. According to the GARD Survey results, training sessions for the essential on asthma and COPD are needed for health workers at primary care level. This needs to adapt educational materials.

14. The list of essential medications for asthma, especially inhaled corticosteroids [24], is not available in all countries; in Sudan, a survey pointed this issue [25]. In a general review, researchers reported [26]: Another issue is in some developing countries, the essential medication as listed by WHO is not available. Health services in low-resource countries are poorly adapted to treating chronic diseases. Designed to respond episodically to acute disease, almost all historical investment has focused on infectious diseases. Crucial to the successful management of chronic diseases is an infrastructure designed to support proactive management, providing not only an accurate diagnosis, but also a secure supply of cost-effective drugs at an affordable price. When in very poor health systems, ICS are not available, a variety or a phenotype of severe asthma prevails (defined by WHO as the non-treated severe asthma) [27], while the ATS/ERS definition for severe asthma is asthma refractory to ICS.

15. The WHO issued a guide on prevention and control of non-communicable diseases in: Guidelines for primary healthcare in low-resource settings: 2012, and urged developing countries to follow the directives for chronic respiratory disease as well [28].

3. Inner city asthma - Introduction

Inner city asthma is a variant of asthma that afflicts patients who reside in some of the poorest neighborhoods of some urban localities [29]. These patients frequently have economic and financial difficulties and reside in housing projects that are environmentally poor with increased likelihood of pollution [30]. Several studies have demonstrated that these factors coupled to barriers to appropriate asthma care, as well as reliance on emergency care, poor medication compliance, limited availability of primary and specialty asthma care and poor communication between patient and physicians are responsible for the unique nature of this entity [31–33]. Because of these factors, the character of inner city asthma may be different from that observed in other localities. Different patterns of prevalence, predisposing factor, severity, morbidity, mortality, and management have been observed.

4. Prevalence

Over the past several decades, a gradual increase in the prevalence of asthma has been noted in several industrialized countries [29]. Although some of this increase may be related to changes in health insurance policies resulting in better coverage and increased access to care and improvements in diagnostic testing, other factors may be involved. Some of the increase is attributed, in part, to a gradual increase in prevalence of asthma in individuals of lower socioeconomic status who reside in inner cities [29, 34]. For example, statistical analysis shows that between the years 2001 and 2010, rates of asthma in adolescents in the United States of America have increased at a rate of around 1.4% reaching 9.5% in 2010 [34]. Careful analysis of this phenomenon indicates that this increase was most realized among various minority groups including African-Americans and Hispanics.

African-American children are reported to have a rate of asthma per population that is 1.6 times the level observed in white children [34, 35]. Some Hispanic groups, like children originally from Puerto Ricco, have been reported to have asthma prevalence that is almost 2.4 times that of white children [35, 36]. The prevalence of asthma among children in some Chicago neighborhoods is estimated to be as high as 44%, with the highest rate observed and reported in neighborhoods with a higher proportion of residents of African-American and Hispanic ancestry [37]. In one district of New York City, asthma prevalence was reported 13.2% for Puerto Ricans [38]. Racial background is not the only factor responsible for this disparity. Asthma prevalence varies among various localities with those localities with low income levels manifesting an increase in prevalence irrespective or racial and ethnic mix [29, 33].

5. Severity

Numerous studies have shown that inner city asthma, especially among children, is characterized by increased intensity and poor response to therapy [39]. It is not clear why this population of asthmatics is more difficult to control. Some investigators speculate that a myriad of factors may be involved including environmental, socioeconomic, psychosocial, behavioral, or genetic ones [39, 40]. Other authorities believe that the poor control may be related to inappropriate asthma management practices, limited access to care, poor compliance with therapy, and limited communication between physicians and patients [41, 42]. The practical implications of these observations are that these children have a higher rate of hospital admissions [43] and their condition at the time admission is serious and is frequently described as near fatal [44] which refers to a group of individuals predisposed to acute respiratory failure from their disease state with acidosis and altered mental status.

The increased acuity of inner city asthma has several short-term and long-term implications. The collective cost resulting from loss of work and productivity as well as absenteeism from school and work is hard to measure. The added cost of overutilization of healthcare facilities and emergency department adds to the financial implications of this phenomenon. Overconsumption of pharmaceutical agents and other supportive agents and procedures further increases the overall cost. Finally, the impact on the general health of the individuals, stunted growth, and development of long-term respiratory impairment adds to the overall societal impact.

6. Predisposing factors

The factors contributing to the high prevalence of asthma among inner city residents are varied. Cohen et al. [45] suggest that a key factor in this regard is the poor access to healthcare that patients in urban environments experience. This may be related to a limited number of physicians and healthcare facilities as well as limited availability of safe transportation. Limited access to care has a negative impact on most clinical conditions including the availability of effective prenatal care. Another major predisposing factor which increases the prevalence of asthma in residents of inner cities is exposure to tobacco smoke [45]. Tobacco smoke is known to affect the rate of lung growth, clearance of secretions, and defense mechanisms against particulate matter and infectious agents.

Studies have shown that children living in urban environments have a higher rate of emergency room visits and lower use of inhaled corticosteroids [46]. This may be related to lower rates of diagnosis as shown by the 1999 National Health Interview Study [34]. Specific factors that have been examined include poverty with reduced access to and quality of care [47]. The resultant additional health issues such as prematurity [48, 49] and obesity [29, 50] further confound the problem. In addition, poor housing [51] with exposure to indoor pollutants and environmental tobacco [52] plays a significant role in aggravating the condition. Finally, the psychological impact of the disease in the setting of poor resources worsens the perception among patients, impacts coping, and results in further deterioration in symptomatology [53, 54].

7. Morbidity and mortality

In general, inner city asthma has a higher index of severity, is associated with increased morbidity, and has a higher mortality rate than asthma outside the inner city milieu [29]. Several criteria may be used to evaluate the level of acuity. These include, among others, emergency room visits, hospitalizations, office visits, time lost from work, and absenteeism from school. Research shows that inner city asthma is associated with increased morbidity in each of these criteria. The national database report of 2006 indicated that around 3.5 million visits to physician offices, half a million visits to hospital outpatient departments, an equivalent number of visits to an emergency department, and over 150,000 hospitalizations were related to asthma in this population [55].

Inner city asthma is associated with increased mortality when adjusted for the level of acuity. As far as mortality is concerned, there were 167 deaths from asthma in 2005 among children and adolescents [29, 55]. Interestingly, African-Americans demonstrate a sevenfold increase in mortality, around threefold increase in emergency department visits, threefold increase in hospitalization, but 20% lower nonemergency ambulatory visits than white children. Data on Hispanic children show emergency department visits to be twice that of whites [55].

8. Management

Management of inner city asthma places additional demands on patients and healthcare providers alike. Patients need to be maintained on the usual asthma medications including short-acting and long-acting bronchodilators, inhaled corticosteroids, leukotriene antagonists, and possibly methyl xanthines. In addition, one has to focus on eliminating or minimizing the effect of the predisposing factors listed in the previous paragraphs. Specifically, dealing with poor housing, indoor pollutants, and environmental tobacco makes it necessary for patients and their families to invest in home improvement projects that are costly and demanding. Since this may be beyond the capabilities of several patients, this poses a significant burden on the public health and social safety networks in various cities. These services are already oversubscribed and have limited resources.

Several interventions have focused on the fact that patient and family education are critical to the process of managing and controlling inner city asthma. Patients and their families need to learn the components of quality care so that they can participate in their own care. An important component of this strategy is making sure patients, and their families have the requisite knowledge to reach healthcare providers in a timely and structured manner. Therefore, efforts should focus on educating patients to improve their ability to acquire the knowledge needed to navigate the healthcare system. A family-based intervention performed by a trained counselor has been shown to improve care and decrease morbidity [56]. School-based asthma education is also effective [57]. Emphasis should also be placed on reducing environmental triggers such as the use of pest control [58] services and reduction of exposure to tobacco smoke [59] and weatherizing homes to decrease mold and moisture [60, 61] Good management of inner city asthma requires the same kind of proactive care that has been shown to be effective in other situations. These include guidelines-driven care and assured access to the appropriate controller medication [62] and the addition of a biologic such as omalizumab in selected cases [63].

9. Summary and conclusions

To the pulmonologist, inner city asthma is a complex and challenging entity that requires consolidated management efforts and a comprehensive approach that includes awareness of the unique predisposing factors, the increased acuity, and the need to focus on improved access to care. A multifaceted approach that targets a wide array of risk factors including allergens, indoor pollution, housing quality, and external sources of pollution, such as neighborhood trash collection receptacles must be utilized. Guidelines-based management that is effective in other types of asthma may not be sufficient to provide adequate control. In addition, the structure of the healthcare system must change to allow the needed access and the recognition and management of social factors which impact on asthma management.

Author details

Youssser Mohammad[1,2,3*] and Basim Dubaybo[4]

*Address all correspondence to: ccollaborating@gmail.com

1 Department of Pulmonary and Family Medicine, Syrian Private University, Damascus, Syria

2 Department of Pulmonary, Damascus University, Damascus, Syria

3 Center for Research and Training for CRD, Tishreen University, Latakia, Syria

4 Department of Internal Medicine, Wayne State University School of Medicine, Detroit, Michigan, USA

References

[1] Lai CKW, Beasley R, Crane J, Foliaki S, Shah J, Weiland S, and the ISAAC Phase Three Study Group. Global variation in the prevalence and severity of asthma symptoms: Phase Three of the International Study of Asthma and Allergies in Childhood (ISAAC).Thorax. 2009;64:476–483.

[2] International Classification of Primary Care, Second edition (ICPC-2), available as "print on demand" from OUP website: www.oup.uk

[3] Package of essential noncommunicable (PEN) disease interventions for primary health care in low-resource settings. Geneva, Switzerland: World Health Organization. c2010. Available from: http://whqlibdoc.who.int/ publications/2010/9789241598996_eng.pdf

[4] World Health Organization. Practical approach to lung health. Manual on initiating PAL implementation. Geneva, World Health Organization, 2008. (WHO/HTM/TB/ 2008.410, WHO/NMH/CHP/CPM/08.02).

[5] Mohammad Y, Shaaban R, Yassine F, Allouch J, Daaboul N, Bassam A, Mohammad A, Taha D, Sabba S, Dyban G, Al-Sheih K, Balleh H, Ibrahim M, Al Khaer H, Dayoub M, Halloum R, Fadhil I, Abbas A, KHouri A, Khaltaev N, Bousquet J, Khaddouj M, Suleiman I, Meri M, Bakir M, Naem A, Said H, Al-Dmeirawi F, Myhoub H, Dib G.

Executive summary of the multicenter survey on the prevalence and risk factors of chronic respiratory diseases in patients presenting to primary care centers and emergency rooms in Syria. J Thorac Dis. 2012;4(2):203–205. doi:10.3978/j.issn.2072-1439.2011.11.07.

[6] Burney P, Potts J, Aït-Khaled N, Sepulveda RM, Zidouni N, Benali R, Jerray M, Musa OA, El-Sony A, Behbehani N, El-Sharif N, Mohammad Y, Khouri A, Paralija B, Eiser N, Fitzgerald M, Abu-Laban R.. A multinational study of treatment failures in asthma management. Int J Tuberc Lung Dis. 2008;12(1):13–18.

[7] Yang H, Huang X, Zhou Z, Wang HH, Tong X, Wang Z, Wang J, Lu Z. Determinants of initial utilization of community healthcare services among patients with major non-communicable chronic diseases in South China. Plos One. 2014;9(12):e116051. doi: 10.1371/journal.pone.0116051. eCollection 2014.

[8] http://www.ginasthma.org/Mediterranean

[9] Bousquet J, Dahl R, Khaltaev N. Global alliance against chronic respiratory diseases. Allergy 2007:62:216–223.

[10] Imad H, Yasir G. Pan African Medical Journal Epidemiological and clinical characteristics, spirometric parameters and response to budesonide/formoterol in patients attending an asthma clinic: an experience in a developing country. Pan Afr Respir Med. Pan Afr Med J. 2015; 21: 154.

[11] Mohammad Y, Fink-Wagner A-H, Nonikov D. Assets and needs of respiratory patient organizations: differences between developed and developing countries. J Thorac Dis 2013; 5(6):914–918. doi:10.3978/j.issn.2072-1439.2013.08.72.

[12] Martins P, Rosado-Pinto J, do Céu Teixeira M, Neuparth N, Silva O, Tavares H, Spencer JL, Mascarenhas D, Papoila AL, Khaltaev N, Annesi-Maesano I. Under-report and underdiagnosis of chronic respiratory diseases in an African country. Allergy 2009;64(7):1061–1067.

[13] Ait-Khaled N, Enarson DA, Bencherif N, Boulhbal F, Camara LM, Dagli E, Jankirie TK, Karadag B, Keita B, Ngoran K, Adhiambo J, Ottmanis SE, Pham N, Sow O, Yousser M, Zaidouni N. Implementation of asthma guidelines in health centers of several developing countries. Int J Tuberc Lung Dis. 2006;10(1):104–109.

[14] Shahror N, Bardan H. Prevalence and risk factors of asthma in Damascus school children aged 10–14. Rev Mal Respir. 2006;23:10S109–10S139.

[15] Mohammad Y, Shaaban R, Al-Zahab BA, Khaltaev N, Bousquet J, Dubaybo B. Impact of active and passive smoking as risk factors for asthma and COPD in women presenting to primary care in Syria: first report by the WHO-GARD survey group. Int J Chronic Obstr Pulm Dis. 2013-11-04.

[16] 16-Global Initiative for Asthma. Global Strategy for Asthma management and prevention on www.ginasthma.org accessed.

[17] Levy M, Fletcher M. International primary care respiratory group guidelines. Prim Care Respir J. 2006;15:20–34.

[18] Pinnock H, Thomas M, Tsiligianni I, Lisspers K, Østrem A, Ställberg B, Yusuf O, Ryan D, Buffels J, Cals JW, Chavannes NH, Henrichsen SH, Langhammer A, Latysheva E, Lionis C, Litt J, van der Molen T, Zwar N, Williams S. The International Primary Care Respiratory Group (IPCRG) Research Needs Statement 2010. Prim Care Respir J. 2010;19 Suppl 1:S1–S20.

[19] AAAAI guidelines 2007: Section 3, component 2, education for a partnership on asthma care, pp. 100–106 on www.aaaai.org.

[20] Alhaidera SA, Alshehrib HA, and Al-Eid K. Replacing nebulizers by MDI-spacers for bronchodilator and inhaled corticosteroid administration: Impact on the utilization of hospital resources. International Journal of Pediatrics and Adolescent Medicine. 2014; 1(1):26–30.

[21] Yasmin S, Mollah AH, Basak R, Islam KT, Chowdhury YS. Mymensingh Med J. Efficacy of salbutamol by nebulizer versus metered dose inhaler with home-made non-valved spacer in acute exacerbation of childhood asthma. Mymensingh Med J. 2012;21(1):66–71.

[22] Zar HJ, Levin ME. Challenges in treating pediatric asthma in developing countries. Paediatr Drugs. 2012;14(6):353–359. doi:10.2165/11597420-

[23] Charlton I, et al. Audit of the effect of a nurse run asthma clinic on workload and patient morbidity in a general practice. Br J Gen Pract. 1991;41:227–231.

[24] http://www.who.int/medicines/publications/essentialmedicines/en/index.html: accessed on Juin 2014

[25] El Sony AI, Chiang C-Y, Malik E, Hassanain SA, Hussien H, Khamis AH, Bassilli AF, Enarson DA. Standard case management of asthma in Sudan: a Pilot Project. Public Health Action. PHA 2013;3(3):247–252.

[26] Beran D, Zar HJ, Perrin C, Menezes AM, Burney P. Burden of asthma and chronic obstructive pulmonary disease and access to essential medicines in low-income and middle-income countries. Lancet Respir Med. 2015;3(2):159–170. doi:10.1016/S2213-2600(15)00004-1.

[27] Bousquet J, Baena-Cagnani CE, Mantzouranis E, Bleecker ER, Burney P, et al. Workshop summary. Uniform definition of asthma severity, control, and exacerbations: Document presented for the World Health Organization Consultation on Severe Asthma. J Allergy Clin Immunol 2010;126(5):926–938.

[28] Prevention and Control of Non communicable Diseases: Guidelines for primary health care in low-resource settings. Geneva: WHO, 2012.

[29] Gergen PJ, Togias A. Inner city asthma. Immunol Allergy Clin N Am 2015;35:101–114.

[30] Forno E, Celedón JC. Asthma and Ethnic Minorities: Socioeconomic Status and Beyond. Curr Opin Allergy Clin Immunol. 2009;9(2):154–160. PMCID: PMC3920741

[31] Akinbami L. The state of childhood asthma, United States, 1980–2005. Adv Data. 2006;(381):1–24

[32] Sarver N, Murphy K. Management of asthma: new approaches to establishing control. J Am Acad Nurse Pract 2009;21:54–65.

[33] Celano MP, Linzer JF, Demi A, Bakeman R, Smith CO, Croft S, et al. Treatment adherence among low-income, African American children with persistent asthma. J Asthma 2010;47:317–22. NIHMSID: NIHMS94525

[34] Moorman JE, Akinbami LJ, Bailey CM, et al. National surveillance of asthma: United States, 2001–2010. Vital Health Stat 2012;3:1–67.

[35] Akinbami LJ, Moorman JE, Garbe PL, et al. Status of childhood asthma in the United States, 1980–2007. Pediatrics 2009;123(Suppl 3):S131–45.

[36] Carter-Pokras OD, Gergen PJ. Reported asthma among Puerto Rican, Mexican-American, and Cuban children, 1982 through 1984. Am J Public Health 1993;83:580–582.

[37] Gupta RS, Zhang X, Sharp LK, et al. Geographic variability in childhood asthma prevalence in Chicago. J Allergy Clin Immunol 2008;121:639–645.e1.

[38] Ledogar RJ, Penchaszadeh A, Garden CC, et al. Asthma and Latino cultures: different prevalence reported among groups sharing the same environment. Am J Public Health 2000;90:929–935.

[39] Breysse J, Dixon S, Gregory J, et al. Effect of weatherization combined with community health worker in-home education on asthma control. Am J Public Health 2014;104:e57–e64.

[40] Takaro TK, Krieger J, Song L, et al. The breathe-easy home: the impact of asthma-friendly home construction on clinical outcomes and trigger exposure. Am J Public Health 2011;101:55–62.

[41] Szefler SJ, Mitchell H, Sorkness CA, et al. Management of asthma based on exhaled nitric oxide in addition to guideline-based treatment for inner-city adolescents and young adults: a randomised controlled trial. Lancet 2008;372:1065–1072.

[42] Busse WW, Morgan WJ, Gergen PJ, et al. Randomized trial of omalizumab (anti-IgE) for asthma in inner-city children. N Engl J Med 2011;364:1005–1015.

[43] Scott L, Morphew T, Bollinger ME, Samuelson S, Galant S, Clement L, O'Cull K, Jones F, and Jones CA. Achieving and maintaining asthma control in inner-city children. J Allergy Clin Immunol 2011;128:56–63.

[44] Bryant-Stephens T. Asthma disparities in urban environments. J Allergy Clin Immunol 2009;123:1199–1206.

[45] Cohen RT, Canino GJ, Bird HR, et al. Area of residence, birthplace, and asthma in Puerto Rican children. Chest 2007;131:1331–1338.

[46] Esteban CA, Klein RB, McQuaid EL, et al. Conundrums in childhood asthma severity, control, and health care use: Puerto Rico versus Rhode Island. J Allergy Clin Immunol 2009;124:238–244, 244.e1–e5.

[47] Information on poverty and income statistics: a summary of 2013 current population survey data. ASPE Issue Brief: Department of Health and Human Services, Office of the Assistant Secretary for Planning and Evaluation; 2013. Available at: aspe.hhs.gov/hsp/13/PovertyandIncomeEst/ib_poverty2013.pdf.

[48] Gessner BD, Chimonas MA. Asthma is associated with preterm birth but not with small for gestational age status among a population-based cohort of Medicaid-enrolled children <10 years of age. Thorax 2007;62:231–236.

[49] Svanes C, Omenaas E, Heuch JM, et al. Birth characteristics and asthma symptoms in young adults: results from a population-based cohort study in Norway. Eur Respir J 1998;12:1366–1370.

[50] Jensen ME, Gibson PG, Collins CE, et al. Diet-induced weight loss in obese children with asthma: a randomized controlled trial. Clin Exp Allergy 2013;43:775–784.

[51] Northridge J, Ramirez OF, Stingone JA, et al. The role of housing type and housing quality in urban children with asthma. J Urban Health 2010;87:211–224.

[52] Akinbami LJ, Kit BK, Simon AE. Impact of environmental tobacco smoke on children with asthma, United States, 2003–2010. Acad Pediatr 2013;13:508–516.

[53] Weil CM, Wade SL, Bauman LJ, et al. The relationship between psychosocial factors and asthma morbidity in inner-city children with asthma. Pediatrics 1999;104:1274–1280.

[54] Bartlett SJ, Kolodner K, Butz AM, et al. Maternal depressive symptoms and emergency department use among inner-city children with asthma. Arch Pediatr Adolesc Med 2001;155:347–353.

[55] Moorman, J.E. et al. National surveillance for asthma–United States, 1980–2004. MMWR Surveill Summ. 2007;56:1–54.

[56] Flores G, Bridon C, Torres S, et al. Improving asthma outcomes in minority children: a randomized, controlled trial of parent mentors. Pediatrics 2009;124:1522–1532.

[57] Bruzzese JM, Sheares BJ, Vincent EJ, et al. Effects of a school-based intervention for urban adolescents with asthma. A controlled trial. Am J Respir Crit Care Med 2011;183:998–1006.

[58] Morgan WJ, Crain EF, Gruchalla RS, et al. Results of a home-based environmental intervention among urban children with asthma. N Engl J Med 2004;351:1068–1080.

[59] Morgan WJ, Crain EF, Gruchalla RS, et al. Results of a home-based environmental intervention among urban children with asthma. N Engl J Med 2004;351:1068–1080.

[60] Akinbami LJ, Moorman JE, Garbe PL, Sondik EJ. Status of childhood asthma in the United States, 1980–2007. Pediatrics 2009;123(suppl 3):S131–S145.

[61] Eakin M, Rand C, Bilderback A, Bollinger M, Butz A, Kandasamy V, Riekert K. Asthma in head start children: effects of the breathmobile program and family communication on asthma outcomesJ Allergy Clin Immunol 2012;129:664–670.

[62] Talreja N, Soubani AO, Sherwin RL, et al. Modifiable factors associated with severe asthma exacerbations in urban patients. Ann Allergy Asthma Immunol. 2012;109:128–132.

[63] Restrepo RD, Peters J. Near-fatal asthma: recognition and management. Curr Opin Pulm Med. 2008;14:13–23.

3

Noninvasive Biomarkers of Asthma

Mirjana Turkalj, Damir Erceg and
Iva Dumbović Dubravčić

Abstract

Asthma is a heterogeneous disease of the lower airways including various types of bronchial inflammation presenting with different phenotypes and endotypes. Therapeutic response of asthmatic phenotypes/endotypes can be predicted by the use of biomarkers of inflammation phenotyping, and in recent years, endotyping of asthmatics allows to predict who will best respond to anti-inflammatory treatment and optimize quality of life of asthmatics by reducing the risk of exacerbations. Based on noninvasive biomarkers of inflammations, several of them have been described that are useful in clinical practice. Some of the noninvasive biomarkers have a particularly important role in the diagnosis and treatment of asthmatics. Monitoring of noninvasive biomarkers, such as fraction of exhaled nitric oxide (FENO), cells in sputum, or biomarkers in exhaled breath condensate (EBC), two main inflammatory phenotypes have been described: eosinophilic phenotype and neutrophilic phenotype. In eosinophilic asthma, as the most prevalent inflammatory phenotype, asthmatics have more than 3% eosinophils in the sputum, elevated levels of FENO, and elevated leukotriene's cytokine levels in EBC. The most extensively studied biomarkers in asthma are TH2 or more generally T2-related asthmatic endotype. Their clinical benefit might be used to phenotype/endotype features of the underlying type of inflammation and selection of asthmatics, particularly with severe or difficult-to-treat asthma, which most likely will respond to additional biological therapy. In this chapter, we summarize the noninvasive biomarkers available for the management of asthmatics.

Keywords: asthma, biomarker, inflammation, phenotype, endotype

1. Introduction

Asthma is a heterogeneous disease which includes a spectrum of different subtypes with different inflammation patterns responding differently to different treatments. The most recently updated GINA guidelines address these issues emphasizing the importance of standardized diagnosis and appropriate treatment strategies according to asthma phenotype and/or endotype [1]. Generally, biomarkers or physiological measures that precisely and conclusively define phenotypes and asthma endotypes are missing or are insufficient. Several biomarkers have been described in asthma, but most of them including noninvasive biomarkers are not commonly available or still need external validation [2]. Many of the potential noninvasive biomarkers will be described in this chapter. Normal ranges and validation need to be established for most of them, and stability over time must be examined in longitudinal studies. The new research is needed about the effects of asthma therapy on biomarker measurements, especially for biomarkers which are proposed to guide different treatments, like therapy with biologics [3]. Finally, and most importantly, the new biomarkers, especially noninvasive, need to be easily sampled and interpreted at the point of care in order to provide and improve the diagnosis and treatment of different asthma subtypes, especially those which are more severe and therapy resistant. The challenge is how to identify "high-quality" biomarkers which have high accuracy and robustness that could predict clinical outcomes and therapy response which is of essential in the application of the concept of precision medicine.

2. Fraction of exhaled nitric oxide (FENO)

Fraction of exhaled nitric oxide (FENO) (or fractional exhaled NO) is currently the most widely used biomarker in the exhaled breath, and it is often increased in asthma, even in mild and asymptomatic condition [4]. Fractional exhaled nitric oxide or the modeling of NO dynamics of the lung can give more information than a single FENO value. The synthesis of NO is mediated by constitutive (endothelial NOS or neuronal NOS) and inducible NO synthase (iNOS). Its production is due to oxidation of L-arginine to L-citrulline. iNOS is the only isoform correlated with exhaled nitric oxide, and FENO has been considered as a marker of eosinophilic inflammation involving small airways [5]. FENO was found to be strongly reduced by treatment with inhaled corticosteroids (ICS) [6]. In a general population of asthmatics, it was found that the FENO threshold that best identified a sputum eosinophil count ≥3% in patients receiving high dose of ICS was 27 ppb [7]. In a recent paper, it was shown that, in severe asthma, FENO, had a lower accuracy than blood eosinophils to identify eosinophilic asthma [8], but increased FENO levels have been associated with a good response to ICS [6], oral corticosteroids, anti-IgE [9], and anti-IL-4 and anti-IL-13 [10, 11]. FENO is established as a marker of inflammation in asthma, but more than 20 years of research have shown that it works in certain asthma endotypes (TH2) [12]. Therefore, there is an increasing need for useful biomarkers with predictive and prognostic value for the progression of the disease in asthmatic patients and their link with clinical treatments.

3. Exhaled breath condensate (EBC)

Exhaled breath condensate (EBC) is the product of cooling and condensation of the exhaled aerosol, collected by tidal breathing during 10–30 minutes into a specially designed cooling device [13]. It represents a potentially very useful method for noninvasive diagnosis of asthma and other pulmonary diseases. EBC consists of three major components, first being distilled water that comes from condensed gas phase of the exhalate. The second component are nonvolatile particles or droplets of different sizes that are aerosolized from the airway lining fluid (ALF), and final components are water-soluble volatiles that are exhaled and absorbed into the condensing breath [14]. Considering the origin of EBC, a large number of inflammation, oxidative stress, nitrosative stress biomarkers, or airway acidification indicators such as pH, adenosine, ammonia, free radicals, hydrogen peroxide, isoprostanes, leukotrienes, prostanoids, nitrogen oxides, peptides, and cytokines can be detected in EBC and have been studied last 20 years [15, 16]. These biomarkers can reflect the underlying state of lower airways as well as lung inflammation and can be altered in patients with asthma.

The collection procedure and requirements for the EBC collection devices as well as the storage and processing are still not standardized and validated due to many factors that influence the final outcome [15]. The final product of the collection is influenced by not only patient factors fluid and food intake timing, concurrent medication or drug intake, age, sex, weight, height, and disease but also external factors as room temperature, collection temperature, and device materials [15]. The volatiles and the nonvolatile particles of the EBC are highly diluted so the detection and analytics of the EBC are challenging tasks, furthermore due to the fact that there is no generally accepted dilution marker detected yet [16, 17].

4. Exhaled breath temperature (EBT)

Exhaled breath temperature (EBT) is a noninvasive method for detecting and monitoring pathological processes based on inflammation in bronchial lumen. According to the fact that heat is one of the cardinal signs of inflammation, the measurement of EBT was developed as a marker of airway inflammation and therefore used in the study of inflammatory respiratory diseases. The use of EBT devices is particularly attractive in patients with asthma who largely exhibit significantly higher EBT values compared with healthy subjects; these patients are therefore encouraged to use these exhaled thermometers in clinical practice for the maintenance of asthma control and in therapeutic management. In the currently available literature, there are almost 200 articles on the use of EBT in asthma and other respiratory diseases. Only few of these studies have assessed EBT measurements, and one recent study provides reliable reference values of EBT in healthy subjects. Despite the potential of EBT, it has not yet reached the clinical setting, partly because of a lack of standardization and validation of the method. However, a recent study deals with these obstacles. There are three groups of external temperatures influenced by EBT in different ways [18]. The first group considered the cases with external temperature ≤ 23°C In this case, the average EBT was 28.268 ± 2.872°C The second group considered cases measured with an external temperature of 23–28°C. In this case, EBT was 30.949 ± 2.511°C. The third group showed that if the test is performed with an external temperature > 28°C, the EBT was 32.558 ± 1.805°C. Authors did not report any influence by other variables, such as weight, height, blood oxygen saturation, lung function, area of residence, work, blood pressure, and axillary temperature, on EBT. Their findings are consistent with data from other authors [19]. There are several potential advantages of EBT measurements: very easy for patients and requires only a few minutes; it is completely noninvasive and is therefore also suitable for children and patients with severe disease. The device is well accepted by patients and ethics committee, it is inexpensive, and it does not affect the underlying airway disease [20].

5. Electronic nose (e-Nose)

Exhaled breath contains thousands of volatile organic compounds (VOCs) in gaseous form that reflect the metabolic process occurring in the host, which may be used as markers of inflammation in the lung or systemically [21]. e-Nose is a portable device, which allows noninvasive, quick, and real-time pattern analysis of VOC spectra. Current e-Nose devices generally consist of an array of chemical sensors that specifically identify VOC mixture. Actually, e-Nose is a system of artificial sensor with chemical sensors that consists of an array for a qualitative and/or quantitative detection and description of VOC profiles or breath prints. Due to poor specificity to individual volatiles, chemical sensor arrays are not generally suitable for identifying single volatiles in complex mixtures of breath. Combining technologies, the high sensitivity of chemical sensor arrays with the high specificity of gas chromatography-mass spectrometry (GC-MS), which could mimic the performance of the natural olfactory system in e-Nose, can be used for identifying breath volatiles, as potential new markers of inflammations in different asthmatic sub-phenotypes [22, 23]. However, e-Nose technology has limitations. The optimal technique for breath collection, sampling, and analysis of single-breath volatiles indicating that future methodological studies are required is unknown. Miniaturized devices based on nanotechnology with micro- or nano-arrays are seen as a key in advancing a new e-Nose device.

Measurement of VOC by e-Nose can discriminate between patients with respiratory disease such as asthma and healthy controls. e-Nose breath prints are associated with the level of airway inflammation and might be useful in the assessment of asthma severity as well as can discriminate patients with fixed asthma from COPD patients with an 88% accuracy [24]. Longitudinal monitoring of exhaled metabolites measured by GC-MS and e-Nose can discriminate loss of asthma control [25]. The usefulness of measurement of VOC profiles by e-Nose in assessing asthma inflammatory phenotypes still needs to be confirmed.

6. Biomarkers in induced sputum

Induced sputum is a relatively noninvasive mode of airway sampling that provides an opportunity for analysis of cellular components and infective agents, including bacteria and viruses, together with fluid-phase constituents [26]. There are several standardized manuals that are available and help to educate health professionals how to perform the technique to the highest standard [27]. The application of induced sputum in the assessment of airway pathology has grown rapidly, especially after 2002, when European Respiratory Society (ERS) published the recommendations for standardization of sputum induction and processing [28, 29]. That is a key component to provide valuable information for clinical decision-making. Sputum is collected after inhalations of hypertonic saline. Although relatively safe, induced sputum requires specialized training, equipment, and laboratory processing. Monitoring lung function during the induction procedure reduces the risk of excessive bronchoconstriction. Patient's active cooperation is needed for collection, making this technique unsuitable for some patients, especially for children below the age of 7 years. Induced sputum provides a rich source of soluble and cellular biomarkers. The sputum eosinophil percentage is a key biomarker which identifies patients who have eosinophilic and non-eosinophilic asthma phenotypes and correlates with severe exacerbations and AHR. Besides eosinophils, other sputum biomarkers are currently in research. Sputum neutrophils are often related to severe non-eosinophilic asthma with fixed airway obstruction. Soluble sputum biomarkers associated with asthma severity are IL-4, IL-5, IL-6, IL-12, IL-13, ECP, LT, TNF-α, CSF, TNF-α, and GM-CSF [30]. Biomarkers such as IL-8 and neurokinin A correlate with exacerbation, while procollagen synthesis peptides, tissue inhibitors of metalloproteinase, or THF-β have been associated with remodeling [31].

The widespread application of induced sputum in asthma proposed several disease phenotypes and defined which of these phenotypes respond to the current therapy. In neutrophilic asthma phenotype, the level of sputum mRNA expression of Toll-like receptors 2 and 4 as well as CD14 was high. Thus, this well-tolerated and safe method provides an additional tool to guide the clinical management of asthmatic patients [32]. To date induced sputum represents the only non-invasive measure of airway inflammation that has a clearly proven role in asthma management.

7. Biomarkers in urine of asthmatics

Urine is an easily accessible and noninvasive collectable biofluid containing many information about the current metabolic status of the body. Metabolic changes in the body of an asthmatic patient are reflected in the metabolite concentrations in urine, and the changes during asthma exacerbation can also be tracked well by urine metabolite analysis. Asthma, especially during exacerbation, causes a high level of oxidative stress due to the pulmonary reaction to exacerbation and resulting formation of reactive oxygen compounds that lead to cell damage. In children with asthma, the levels of LTE4 are increased in urine and are not altered under inhaled corticosteroid (ICS) therapy, but the 5-lipoxygenase inhibitors reduce the urinary LTE4 levels. Eosinophil protein X (EPX) is found in the urine of asthma patients, but the levels of the EPX fall within 3 months after anti-inflammatory therapy induction [33].

Prostaglandin D2 (PGD2) is released from mast cells, and it causes bronchoconstriction and vasodilatation in the airway. PGD2 is metabolized to 9α,11β-PGF2 and excreted in urine. It is also increased in patients with asthma, but its production, thus excretion, may be influenced by corticosteroid therapy [33]. Bromotyrosine (BrTyr) is another biomarker that originates from protein oxidation in eosinophils. Urinary levels of BrTyr are significantly higher in patients with asthma and even higher during exacerbation.

It has been suggested in a few studies with a small number of adult patients that during exacerbation the levels of threonine, alanine, carnitine, acetyl carnitine, and trimethylamine N-oxide were slightly increased, which can be caused not only by the above-described oxidative stress but also by food and drug intake. Some metabolite urine concentrations were lower than usual: acetate, citrate, malonate, and others. Alkane and aldehyde levels were found to be increased in urine; also, the levels of carnitine and acetyl carnitine, which are essential in the process of fatty acid transport into mitochondria, were high in urine of patients with asthma [34]. Other potential biomarkers such as club cell protein 16 (CC16), as a biomarker of epithelial dysfunction, have been studied in urine of patients with asthma. One study in Chinese children showed lower levels of CC16 in asthmatic children [35].

8. Noninvasive biomarkers of asthmatic phenotypes

Over the past decade, the most important advance in the field of asthma has been the recognition of asthma as a syndrome or heterogeneous disease with several clinical presentations or phenotypes. Biomarkers help define the specific pathology of different asthma phenotypes and identify potential therapeutic targets. However, a number of biomarkers have been identified that help define asthma phenotypes most likely than reflect responsiveness to specific therapies. Noninvasive biomarkers such as FENO or sputum cells usually reflect the main inflammatory phenotypes of asthma. Eosinophilic phenotype having more than 3% eosinophils in the sputum is likely to reflect ongoing adaptive immunity in response to allergen. Several biomarkers of eosinophilic asthma, except the percentage of eosinophil, are easily available in clinical practice, such as blood eosinophils, serum-specific IgE, exhaled nitric oxide, or serum periostin level. A significant proportion of asthmatic patients, particularly those with severe disease, do not have a TH2-enhanced phenotype (TH-2 low) [9, 36]. Patients with a non-TH2 phenotype can be further split in two inflammatory phenotypes depending on the level of their airway neutrophilic inflammation: paucigranulocytic and neutrophilic [37]. Neutrophilic asthma as more than 76% neutrophils in the sputum is thought to reflect innate immune system activation in response to pollutants or infectious agents, mixed granulocytic asthma when both inflammatory cells are increased, and paucigranulocytic asthma is thought to be not inflammatory and characterized by smooth muscle dysfunction. Among severe asthmatics, a subgroup characterized by noneosinophilic inflammation was described [38]. We currently lack of user-friendly biomarkers of neutrophilic asthma and airway remodeling. This absence of biomarkers for these patterns of inflammation has made it difficult to recognized subjects who might respond to biologics that target this pathway [38].

9. Noninvasive biomarkers of asthmatic endotypes

Asthma is increasingly recognized as a heterogeneous group of diseases (syndrome) caused by multiple inflammatory pathogenic processes or endotypes. Recently, the definition of the term "endotype," describing a specific pathogenic mechanism leading to the clinical presentation of asthma. Two major asthmatic endotypes have been recognized: TH2-high, manifested by increased eosinophils in the sputum and airways, and TH2-low, with increased neutrophils or a paucigranulocytic cells. Using these classifications and specific biomarkers has led to promising new therapeutics, often biologics, especially for TH2-high asthma. Many studies of asthmatic endotypes have assessed granulocyte populations in induced sputum. Increased percentage of sputum neutrophil usually represents an increase in IL-17-driven neutrophil recruitment or a relative reduction in other inflammatory cells such as eosinophils [39]. Thus, neutrophil activation state rather than number may be a more important indicator of their contribution to asthma severity, as an indicator of TH2-low endotype. From the other side, nitric oxide is produced by the action of iNOS encoded by the *NOS2* gene, and eosinophils are mobilized by chemokines such as eotaxin-3 encoded by the *CCL26* gene, highly correlated with the TH2 domination. Therefore, available noninvasive biomarkers such as sputum cell analysis or FENO can indirectly represent certain type 2-driven inflammation of asthmatic endotype [40]. The TH2-low endotype does not have any readily available point-of-care biomarkers, so TH2-low asthma is often diagnosed based on a lack of TH2-high biomarkers [41]. The TH2-low endotype characterized greater resistance to steroids and the development of therapies. Advances have been made with regard to sputum cytokine analysis and might also help to guide future treatment of severe asthma. Several other noninvasive biomarkers have been described in different asthma endotypes, but most of them are not commonly available or still need external validation [33].

10. Noninvasive biomarkers and asthma control

Asthma is a heterogeneous inflammatory disorder with several different phenotypes and a nonspecific clinical presentation. Even more, the usually used pulmonary function tests are insensitive and often normal or do not correspond to the disease evolvement [33]. Given the different etiology of asthma subtypes, the therapy is adjusted and needs to be evaluated throughout the duration of treatment. For that purpose a number of biomarkers have been studied for the last 30 years.

One of the longest in use is the measurement of the fraction of nitric oxide in exhaled breath (FENO). Nitric oxide (NO) is generated by three nitric oxide synthase isoenzymes, one of them being inducible (NOS2) that produces most of the exhaled NO. In patients with asthma, especially eosinophilic airway inflammation, the NOS2 overexpression can be reduced by inhaled corticosteroid therapy. This effect is used for predicting the efficacy and monitoring of the ICS therapy in patients with asthma [33]. However, the FENO measurement results can be influenced by flow rate, nasal contamination, ambient air, age, height, gender, race, spirometry or exercise before testing, diet, and smoke exposure [42]. In general, low FENO levels seem to be useful in predicting the asthma phenotypes that will respond poorly to ICS treatment [42]. When the asthma is responsive to ICS, the FENO levels correspond in a dose-dependent manner with ICS [42]. Nevertheless, the method still needs to be further evaluated in studies with standardized protocols.

Exhaled breath has recently been studied in a different setting; namely, after cooling the exhaled breath, a condensate (EBC) containing volatile and nonvolatile particles is produced and can be analyzed for existence of numerous biomarkers. The acidity of EBC is high in asthmatics, but after inducing anti-inflammatory therapy, it rapidly returns to normal values [33]. The total nitrite/nitrate levels have been found to be increased in pediatric asthma patients compared to healthy controls; still, the results are conflicting regarding the association to asthma severity [42]. Levels of H_2O_2 increase with asthma severity so it plays a role in monitoring disease control and response to steroid treatment as the levels correspond with inducement of steroid therapy [42]. EBC in patients with asthma contains higher concentrations of 8-isoprostane both in children and in adults, when compared to healthy controls [42]. The level of 8-isoprostane is associated with asthma control and severity and, thus, can be used as a monitoring tool.

In combination with nitric oxide, interferon-gamma (IFN-γ), and interleukin-4 (IL-4) measurements in EBC, the level of 8-isoprostane can be used as a good marker for assessing asthma control [42].

However, there are many indices that the EBC contains biomarkers that could be used as a tool to control asthma progression and therapy adjustments; it is still a method primarily used in research setting. The metabolomic and proteomic methods are required in order to have EBC analysis in clinical use, which subsequently generates low-cost effectiveness of the methods at present [43].

Induced sputum is another source of biomarkers that can be used for asthma disease control. As a method it is safe, noninvasive, and thus usable in pediatrics. It contains cell phase (eosinophils and neutrophils) and supernatant with cytokines. Sputum eosinophil count is a key marker of asthma severity and responsiveness to steroid therapy. The number of eosinophils correlates well with asthma severity and is predictive of asthma exacerbation. Elevated levels of eosinophil cationic protein (ECP), IL-4, IL-5, IL-13, TNF-α, IL-6, IL-12, and granulocyte macrophage colony stimulator factor have been found in sputum supernatant of asthma patients [33]. Several studies have challenged the usage of induced sputum analysis for asthma control, but it seems that the results are contradictory so it needs further testing, and for the moment, the method has not been proven accurate enough to be used for asthma monitoring in childhood asthma [43].

Recently, urine has been studied as one of possible sources of biomarkers for asthma disease monitoring. The studies have, so far, found that only leukotriene E4 and bromotyrosine levels are high and associated with disease severity, exacerbations, and aspirin intake [33].

11. Noninvasive biomarkers and asthma therapy

The use of biomarkers in asthma is restrictive because knowledge of the asthma phenotypes is incomplete. The concept of better endotyping asthma can give precision medicine useful data necessary to develop new therapies. Recent trials evaluating biological therapies targeting IgE, IL-5, IL-4/IL-13, and IL-17 have utilized predictive markers to identify patients who might benefit from therapy. Multiple biomarkers including sputum eosinophil count, blood eosinophil count, FENO, and serum periostin have been used to identify patients with a good response to targeted medications (**Table 1**) [44–47]. Till now, relevant biomarkers that can be useful in the management of asthma are mainly related to TH2 response

	Biological sample	Exhaled air	Sputum		Blood						Urine
Target	**Drug**	**FENO**	**eo**	**neu**	**eo**	**IgE[a]**	**Periostin**	**IL-13**	**IL-17**	**DPP-4**	**LT 4E**
T2 biomarkers											
	Glucocorticoid	•	•								
IgE	Omalizumab	•	•		•		•				
IL-5	Mepolizumab	•			•						
IL-5	Reslizumab		•		•						
IL-5	Benralizumab	•			•						
IL4/IL-13	Dupilumab	•			•		•				
IL-13	Lebrikizumab	•					•				
IL-13	Tralokinumab						•	•			
DPA	Fevipiprant		•							•	
LT	LTA										•
Non-T2 biomarkers											
	Azithromycin	•		•[b]	•						
	Clarithromycin			•							
IL-17	Brodalumab			•[c]							
CXCR2	ACD5096			•[c]							

[a]Determines eligibility for omalizumab, but the level is not predictive for response

[b]Trial did not evaluate sputum neutrophil counts

[c]Trial did not demonstrate clinical improvement

Legend: eo, Eosinophils; neu, neutrophils; IL, interleukin; DPP-4, dipeptidyl peptidase-4; LT 4E, leukotriene 4E; CXCR2, CXC chemokine receptor 2 (Adapted according to Medrek et al. [45])

Table 1. Biomarkers predictive of response to different asthma therapies.

[45]. These biomarkers are considered more steroid-responsive [38]. The eosinophil counts has proven to be useful in the clinical arena in helping to predict short-term response to inhaled corticosteroids (ICS) and tailor the dose of ICS in the severe patients [32]. Sputum eosinophil percentage acts as a key marker and correlates with severe exacerbations and AHR. Also, it can be useful in a panel of biomarkers to select patients who may benefit from IL-5 targeted therapies, including reslizumab, mepolizumab, and benralizumab [48]. Blood eosinophils as surrogate markers for sputum eosinophilia are associated with relevant outcomes and are more readily measureable. New evidence supports fraction of exhaled nitric oxide (FENO)-based treatment algorithms for cost-effective maintenance of asthma control/quality of life. Serum and sputum-derived periostin are biomarkers of lung function decline and associated with eosinophilic airway inflammation. Biomarker panels may improve predictive value as shown for the combination of FENO/urinary bromotyrosine in prediction

of steroid responsiveness. Novel biological therapies are proven effective in biomarker-selected populations. Biomarkers including blood eosinophils and FENO are proven to have utility for the effective administration of steroidal and novel biological therapies in asthma, allowing individualized treatment. According to experience of many investigators, the common cause of persistently elevated FENO despite therapy is poor compliance, but this marker is not validated [6]. The complexity and heterogeneity of the asthma request different approaches of phenotyping patients. Used and clustering omics data will provide a better chance of phenotyping asthma based on disease mechanism with composite set of markers obtained for each endotype. Probably, new biomarkers will replace currently available biomarkers and be more specific for both T2 and non-T2 pathways. According to some authors, novel approach is not based on developing new techniques than combining known biomarkers to increase their predictive values. Personalized medicine will allow more precision therapy and also provide novel targets and new treatment for each defined [46]. The future of personalized medicine will depend of availability of accurate and reliable predictive biomarkers.

12. Noninvasive biomarkers of childhood asthma

Asthma represents the most common chronic respiratory disease in children. Whereas preschool children present with multitrigger and viral wheeze, in school children, asthma is usually classified as allergic and non-allergic. For both, the underlying immunological mechanisms are not yet quite understood. Treatment is still prescribed unrelated of underlying mechanisms, and often asthma control in children has not been achieved. Nevertheless, the spectrum of asthma in clinical presentation is broad, and both symptoms and lung function may not always reflect the underlying airway inflammation or endotype [49]. Therefore, in recent years, following the example of adult asthmatics is trying to differentiate specific asthmatic phenotypes as well as endotypes in children. Several studies aiming to identify endotypes are underway, and their relevance for clinical monitoring and subsequent treatment options is still a subject of discussion [50]. For these reasons, the identification of objective biomarkers of childhood asthma phenotype/endotype, which may guide diagnosis, management, and treatment of asthmatic children and might have a role in the development of personalized approach [51]. That is why the availability of noninvasive and validated biomarkers to study and monitor disease is of relevance especially in childhood asthma [52]. Identification of clinically applicable noninvasive biomarkers such as biomarkers in EBC has been of particular interest in personalized diagnosis and treatment of asthma in children [53]. The utility of noninvasive biomarkers in routine clinical practice for monitoring inflammation in children with asthma is undefined, apart from FENO measurements. Sputum eosinophilia, EBC, and urinary leukotrienes are still not applied in routine clinical practice. Despite the development of new biomarkers or new immunological molecules, the complex puzzle of childhood asthma is still far from being completed (**Table 2**) [54].

Biological sample	Biomarker	Therapy response	Diagnostic	Prognostic
Exhaled air	FENO	x	x	
	EBC		x	x
	EBT		x	
	e-Nose		x	
Sputum	eo	x	x	x
	neu		x	
	IL-4		x	x
	IL-5			x
	IL-6			x
	IL-12			x
	IL-13			x
	ECP		x	x
	LT			x
	TNF-α			x
	CSF			x
	GM-CSF			x
	IL-8			x
	Neurokinin			x
	Metalloproteinase			x
	THF-β			x
	Procollagen synthesis peptides			x
Blood	eo	x	x	x
	IgE	x	x	
	Periostin	x	x	
	IL-13	x	x	
	IL-17	x	x	
	DPP-4	x	x	
Urine	LT E4	x	x	x
	EPX	x	x	
	11β-PGF2	x	x	
	BrTyr		x	x
	CC16		x	

Table 2. Biomarkers in asthma.

13. Conclusion

Over the past decades, a great emphasis has been put into developing and researching biomarkers, as well as noninvasive biomarkers in monitoring of inflammation and treatment of asthmatics. The three most promising biomarkers in clinical practice currently are analysis of cells in induced sputum, FENO, and biomarkers in EBC. In the past years, the progress has been made in the discovery, application, and implementation of new, especially noninvasive biomarkers in asthmatic patients. Although now-available noninvasive biomarkers have marked its benefits, their roles are still too limited and nonspecific for identifying at-risk patients, recognitions of specific asthma pattern (phenotype or endotype), and selection of specific and the most helpful treatment, particularly biologics. In the near future, the role of biomarkers in achieving personalized medicine will be critical.

Conflict of interest

The authors confirm that this article content has no conflict of interest.

Abbreviations

ACQ	Asthma control questionnaire
AHR	Airway hyperreactivity
ALF	Airway lining fluid
BrTyr	Bromotyrosine
CC16	Club cell protein 16
CXCR2	CXC chemokine receptor 2
DPP-4	Dipeptidyl peptidase-4
EBC	Exhaled breath condensate
EBT	Exhaled breath temperature
ECP	Eosinophil cationic protein
e-Nose	Electronic nose
eo	Eosinophils
EPX	Eosinophil protein X
ERS	European Respiratory Society

FENO	Fraction of exhaled nitric oxide
FEV1	Forced expiratory volume in 1 second
FVC	Forced vital capacity
GC-MC	Gas chromatography-mass spectrometry
ICS	Inhaled corticosteroids
IgE	Immunoglobulin E
IL	Interleukin
iNOS	Inducible nitric oxide synthase
LT 4E	Leukotriene 4E
neu	Neutrophils
NO	Nitric oxide
PGD2	Prostaglandin D2
VOC	Volatile organic compound

Author details

Mirjana Turkalj[1,2,3]*, Damir Erceg[1,2,3] and Iva Dumbović Dubravčić[4]

*Address all correspondence to: turkalj@bolnica-srebrnjak.hr

1 Srebrnjak Children's Hospital, Zagreb, Croatia

2 Medical School University of Osijek, Osijek, Croatia

3 Catholic University of Croatia, Zagreb, Croatia

4 Institute for Anthropological Research, Zagreb, Croatia

References

[1] Global Initiative for Asthma (GINA). Global Strategy for Asthma Management and Prevention – Updated 2016. 2016. Available at: http://ginasthma.org/gina-reports/ [Accessed: Jan 19, 2018]

[2] Reddel HK, Bateman ED, Becker A, et al. A summary of the new GINA strategy: A roadmap to asthma control. The European Respiratory Journal. 2015;**46**:622-639

[3] Arron JR, Izuhara K. Asthma biomarkers: What constitutes a 'gold standard'? Thorax. 2015;**70**:105-107

[4] Schleich FN, Seidel L, Sele J, Manise M, Quaedvlieg V, Michils A, et al. Exhaled nitric oxide thresholds associated with a sputum eosinophil count ≥3% in a cohort of unselected patients with asthma. Thorax. 2010;**65**:1039-1044

[5] Hansel TT, Kharitonov SA, Donnelly LE, Erin EM, Currie MG, Moore WM, et al. A selective inhibitor of inducible nitric oxide synthase inhibits exhaled breath nitric oxide in healthy volunteers and asthmatics. The FASEB Journal. 2003;**17**:1298-1300

[6] Dweik RA, Boggs PB, Erzurum SC, Irvin CG, Leigh MW, Lundberg JO, et al. An official ATS clinical practice guideline: Interpretation of exhaled nitric oxide levels (FENO) for clinical applications. American Journal of Respiratory and Critical Care Medicine. 2011;**184**:602-615

[7] Cowan DC, Taylor DR, Peterson LE, Cowan JO, Palmay R, Williamson A, et al. Biomarker-based asthma phenotypes of corticosteroid response. The Journal of Allergy and Clinical Immunology. 2014;**135**(4):877-883

[8] Wagener AH, de Nijs SB, Lutter R, Sousa AR, Weersink EJ, Bel EH, et al. External validation of blood eosinophils, FENO and serum periostin as surrogates for sputum eosinophils in asthma. Thorax. 2015;**70**:115-120

[9] Hanania NA, Wenzel S, Rosen K, Hsieh HJ, Mosesova S, Choy DF, et al. Exploring the effects of omalizumab in allergic asthma: An analysis of biomarkers in the EXTRA study. American Journal of Respiratory and Critical Care Medicine. 2013;**187**:804-811

[10] Humbert M, Busse W, Hanania NA, Lowe PJ, Canvin J, Erpenbeck VJ, et al. Omalizumab in asthma: An update on recent developments. The Journal of Allergy and Clinical Immunology. In Practice. 2014;**2**:525-536

[11] Corren J, Lemanske RF, Hanania NA, Korenblat PE, Parsey MV, Arron JR, et al. Lebrikizumab treatment in adults with asthma. The New England Journal of Medicine. 2011;**365**:1088-1098

[12] Peters MC, Nguyen ML, Dunican EM. Biomarkers of Airway Type-2 inflammation and integrating complex phenotypes to endotypes in asthma. Current Allergy and Asthma Reports. 2016;**16**(10):71. DOI: 10.1007/s11882-016-0651-4

[13] Konstantinidi EM, Lappas AS, Tzortzi AS, Behrakis PK. Exhaled breath condensate: Technical and diagnostic aspects. The Scientific World Journal. 2015:Article ID: 435160

[14] Davis MD, Montpetit A, Hunt J. Exhaled breath condensate – An overview. Immunology and Allergy Clinics of North America. 2012;**32**(3):363-375

[15] Rosias P. Methodological aspects of exhaled breath condensate collection and analysis. Journal of Breath Research. 2012;**6**:027102 (13 p)

[16] Vlašić Ž, Dodig S, Čepelak I, Zrinski Topić R, Živčić J, Nogalo B, Turkalj M. Iron and ferritin concentrations in exhaled breath condensate of children with asthma. The Journal of Asthma. 2009;**46**:81-85

[17] Beck O, Olin AC, Mirgorodskaya E. Potential of mass spectrometry in developing clinical laboratory biomarkers of nonvolatiles in exhaled breath. Clinical Chemistry. 2016; **62**:84-91

[18] Carpagnano GE, Foschino-Barbaro MP, Crocetta C, Lacedonia D, Saliani V, Zoppo LD, et al. Validation of the exhaled breath temperature measure: Reference values in healthy subjects. Chest. 2017;**151**(4):855-860

[19] Popov TA, Dunev S, Kralimarkova TZ, Kraeva S, DuBuske LM. Evaluation of a simple, potentially individual device for exhaled breath temperature measurement. Respiratory Medicine. 2007;**101**(10):2044-2050

[20] Melo RE, Popov TA, Sole D. Exhaled breath temperature, a new biomarker in asthma control: A pilot study. Journal Brasileiro de Pneumologia. 2010;**36**(6):693-699

[21] Fens N, Roldaan AC, van der Schee MP, Boksem RJ, Zwinderman AH, Bel EH, et al. External validation of exhaled breath profiling using an electronic nose in the discrimination of asthma with fixed airways obstruction and chronic obstructive pulmonary disease. Clinical and Experimental Allergy. 2011;**41**:1371-1378

[22] Hye JL, Sang HL, Tae HP, Juhun P, Hyun SS, Tai HP, et al. Nanovesicle-based bioelectronic nose platform mimicking human olfactory signal transduction. Biosensors and Bioelectronics. 2012;**35**(1):335-341

[23] Montuschi P, Santonico M, Penazza G, Mondino C, Mantini G, Martinelli E, et al. Diagnostic performance of an electronic nose, fractional exhaled nitric oxide and lung function testing in asthma. Chest. 2010;**137**:790-796

[24] Montuschi P, Mores N, Trové A, Mondino C, Barnes PJ. The electronic nose in respiratory. Respiration. 2013;**85**:72-84

[25] Brinkman P, van de Pol MA, Gerritsen MG, Bos LD, Dekker T, Smids BS, et al. Exhaled breath profiles in the monitoring of loss of control and clinical recovery in asthma. Clinical and Experimental Allergy. 2017;**47**(9):1159-1169

[26] Weiszha Z, Horvath I. Induced sputum analysis: Step by step. Breathe. 2013;**9**:300-306

[27] Djukanovic R, Sterk PJ. In: Djukanovic R, Sterk PJ, editors. An Atlas of Induced Sputum. An Aid for Research and Diagnosis. London: Parthenon Publishing Group; 2004

[28] Efthimiadis A, Spanevello A, Hamid Q, Kelly MM, Linden M, Louis R, et al. Methods of sputum processing for cell counts, immunohistochemistry and in situ hibridisation. The European Respiratory Journal. Supplement. 2002;**37**:19-23

[29] Djukanović R, Sterk PJ, Fahy JV, Hargreave FE. Standardised methodology of sputum induction and processing. The European Respiratory Journal. Supplement. 2002;**37**:1-2

[30] Diamant Z, Boot JD, Mantzouranis E, Flohr R, Sterk PJ, van Wijk G, et al. Biomarkers in asthma and allergic rhinitis. Pulmonary Pharmacology & Therapeutics. 2010;**23**:468-481

[31] Petsky HL, Cates CJ, Lasserson TJ, Li AM, Turner C, Kynaston JA, et al. A systematic review and meta-analysis: Tailoring asthma treatment on eosinophilic markers (exhaled nitric oxide or sputum eosinophils). Thorax. 2012;**67**:199-208

[32] Bakakos P, Schleich F, Alchanatis M, Louis R. Induced sputum in asthma: From bench to bedside. Current Medicinal Chemistry. 2011;**18**(10):1415-1422

[33] Fatemi F, Saroddiny E, Gheibi A, Mohammadi Farsani T, Kardar GA. Biomolecular markers in assessment and treatment of asthma. Respirology. 2014;**19**:514-523

[34] Loureiro CC, Duarte IF, Gomes J, Carrola J, Barros AS, Gil AM, et al. Urinary metabolomic changes as a predictive biomarker of asthma exacerbation. The Journal of Allergy and Clinical Immunology. 2014;**133**(1):261-263

[35] Ma YN, Wang J, Lee YL, Ren WH, Lv XF, He QC, et al. Association of urine CC16 and lung function and asthma in Chinese children. Allergy and Asthma Proceedings. 2015; **36**(4):59-64

[36] Navratil M, Plavec D, Dodig S, Jelčić Ž, Nogalo B, Erceg D, et al. Markers of systemic and lung inflammation in childhood asthma. The Journal of Asthma. 2009;**46**(8):822

[37] Gauthier M, Ray A, Wenzel SE. Evolving concepts of asthma. American Journal of Respiratory and Critical Care Medicine. 2015;**192**:660-668

[38] Berry A, Busse WW. Biomarkers in asthmatic patients: Has their time come to direct treatment? The Journal of Allergy and Clinical Immunology. 2016;**137**(5):1317-1324

[39] Chen F, Wu W, Millman A, Craft JF, Chen E, Patel N, et al. Neutrophils prime a long-lived effector macrophage phenotype that mediates accelerated helminth expulsion. Nature Immunology. 2014;**15**:938-946

[40] Arron JR, Choy DF, Scheerens H, Matthews JG. Noninvasive biomarkers that predict treatment benefit from biologic therapies in asthma. Annals of the American Thoracic Society. 2013;**10**:206-213

[41] Seys SF. Role of sputum biomarkers in the management of asthma. Current Opinion in Pulmonary Medicine. 2017;**23**(1):34-40

[42] Moschino L, Zanconato S, Bozzetto S, Baraldi E, Carraro S. Childhood asthma biomarkers: Present knowledge and future steps. Paediatric Respiratory Reviews. 2015;**16**(4):205-212

[43] Leung TF, Ko FW, Wong GW. Recent advances in asthma biomarker research. Therapeutic Advances in Respiratory Disease. 2013;**7**(5):297-308

[44] Chung KF. Asthma phenotyping: A necessity for improved therapeutic precision and new targeted therapies. Journal of Internal Medicine. 2016;**279**:192-204

[45] Medrek SK, Parekular AD, Hanania NA. Predictive biomarkers for asthma therapy. Current Allergy and Asthma Reports. 2017;**17**:69

[46] Chung KF. Discovery and validation of new biomarkers for personalizing asthma therapy. In: Szefler SJ, Holguin F, Wechsler ME, editors. Personalizing Asthma Management for the Clinician. Elsevier; 2018. pp. 87-96

[47] Bayes HK, Cowan DC. Biomarkers and asthma management: An update. Current Opinion in Allergy and Clinical Immunology. 2016;**16**:210-217

[48] Pite H, Morais-Almeida M, Mensinga T, Diamant Z. In: Pereira C, editor. Non-invasive Biomarkers in Asthma: Promises and Pitfalls, Asthma – From Childhood Asthma to ACOS Phenotypes. InTech; 2016

[49] Landgraf-Rauf K, Anselm B, Schaub B. The puzzle of immune phenotypes of childhood asthma. Molecular and Cellular Pediatrics. 2016;**3**(1):27

[50] Raedler D, Ballenberger N, Klucker E, Bock A, Otto R, Prazeres da Costa O, et al. Identification of novel immune phenotypes for allergic and nonallergic childhood asthma. The Journal of Allergy and Clinical Immunology. 2015;**135**(1):81-91

[51] Galli SJ. Toward precision medicine and health: Opportunities and challenges in allergic diseases. The Journal of Allergy and Clinical Immunology. 2016;**137**(5):1289-1300

[52] Navratil M, Plavec D, Erceg D, Bulat Lokas S, Živković J, Turkalj M. Urates in exhaled breath condensate as a biomarker of control in childhood asthma. The Journal of Asthma. 2015;**52**:437-446

[53] Maloča Vuljanko I, Turkalj M, Nogalo B, Bulat Lokas S, Plavec D. Diagnostic value of a pattern of exhaled breath condensate biomarkers in asthmatic children. Allergologia et Immunopathologia. 2017;**45**(1):2-10

[54] Lambrecht BN, Hammad H. The immunology of asthma. Nature Immunology. 2015;**16**(1): 45-56

4

Epidemiological Aspects of Rhinitis and Asthma: Comorbidity or United Airway Disease

Sanela Domuz Vujnovic and Adrijana Domuz

Abstract

Bearing in mind the results of the epidemiological studies, the logical question arises whether allergic rhinitis represents an earlier clinical manifestation of allergic airway disease or itself is causative for asthma. Comorbidity or one disease, the diagnosis of allergic rhinitis often precedes the development of asthma. Literature reports that 40–90% of asthmatics have symptoms of allergic rhinitis. The epidemiological evidence also suggests that allergic rhinitis and asthma radially presented one united airway disease with two-stage than two separate diseases. Symptoms of one disease often predominate and are unrecognized or hidden of another disease even if they exist. The epidemiology evidence of comorbidity of allergic rhinitis and asthma confirmed the new concept of the united airway diseases. Despite the evidence of the correlation between allergic rhinitis and asthma, there is some resistance in clinical practice in recognizing this link.

Keywords: asthma, allergic rhinitis, united airway disease, epidemiology, prevalence, comorbidity, respiratory symptoms

1. Introduction

We have to agree with Togias [1] that the respiratory system has been one of the victims of fragmented medical knowledge. The respiratory system is most often viewed as two separate systems, upper and lower. These have resulted in lost opportunities to fully understand the function of the respiratory system [1]. Upper and lower respiratory systems have similarities in histology, physiology, and pathophysiology [2]. The nose warms, filters, and humidifies inhaled air. Impaired air warming and humidification by the nose may cause bronchoconstriction. A reduced function of the nose can be caused by congestion forces the patient to

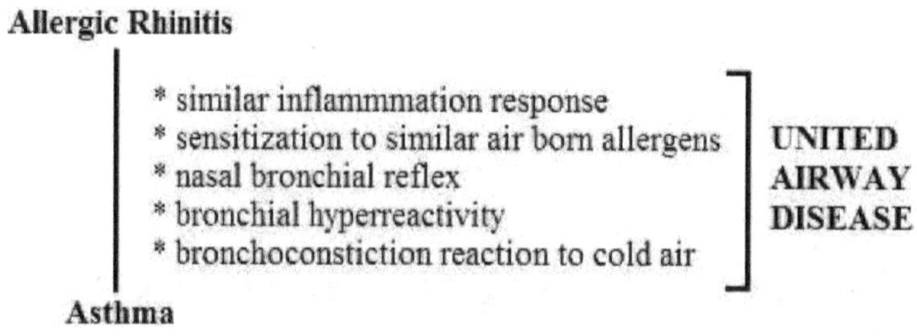

Figure 1. Possible link between asthma and allergic rhinitis.

mouth breathing. Also, there are similarities in inflammation response between allergic rhinitis and asthma [3, 4]. Allergic rhinitis and asthma are frequently associated with sensitization to similar airborne allergens [5]. Some authors suggest the existence of a nasal-bronchial reflex as a cause of bronchial reactivity in a patient with nasal inflammation [6, 7]. That's why recent studies suggest new theory or concept that these two diseases should be viewed as united diseases (**Figure 1**) [8, 9]. The epidemiology evidence of comorbidity of allergic rhinitis and asthma confirmed the new concept of the united airway diseases.

Comorbidity of allergic rhinitis in asthmatics results in frequent emergency visits, asthma exacerbation, asthma-related hospitalizations, and higher asthma-related medical costs [4]. Despite the evidence of the correlation between allergic rhinitis and asthma, there is some resistance in clinical practice in recognizing this link [10]. Also, the guidelines for the treatment of allergic rhinitis and asthma are inconsistently implemented. The consequences of this are a very large number of patients with inadequate diagnosis, no treatment, and poor control of the disease [11, 12].

Most of the epidemiological studies investigate only one allergic disease, asthma or rhinitis. In these studies, another allergic disease was not observed as a comorbidity or a confounding factor. Studies that consider asthma and rhinitis as comorbidity are scarce, but the results of available studies showed that these two diseases are in a high percentage in comorbidity. The percentage of comorbidity showed continuity through different ages of the respondents. A high percentage (70–90%) of rhinitis symptoms in asthmatics was presented in children and the elderly population [13–15].

Despite its high comorbidity, there are surprisingly scarce studies about the treatment of AR in children with asthma or vice versa [14, 15]. Children with allergic rhinitis comorbidity were more likely to have incomplete asthma control in Groot et al. study [15].

2. Epidemiological evidence for the link between allergic rhinitis and asthma

The World Health Organization (WHO) through the Allergic Rhinitis and its Impact on Asthma (ARIA) program tried to understand the possible links between allergic rhinitis and asthma [16]. According to the ARIA study, patients with severe persistent rhinitis more likely have comorbidity with asthma [16]. Epidemiological evidence also suggests coexistence of asthma and allergic rhinitis in the same patients [17]. Symptoms of one disease often predominate and are unrecognized or hidden of another disease even they exist [2]. The epidemiological evidence also suggests that it is radially one disease with two stages than two separate diseases. Underdiagnosis of allergic rhinitis in asthmatics patients is common. Comorbid allergic rhinitis has a clinically relevant effect on asthma, especially on hospitalization and emergency visits [12]. Treating allergic rhinitis in these patients decreased asthma-related medication utilization [17]. Patients with allergic rhinitis also can be underdiagnosed with asthma [12].

2.1. Prevalence of allergic rhinitis and asthma

The prevalence of allergic rhinitis and asthma has increased worldwide over recent decades [13, 18].

Studies appear to indicate that the changes in the prevalence of allergic rhinitis and asthma differ, but they were not designed to show the variation of the link between these two diseases [16]. Epidemiological studies have no standard set of diagnostic criteria for allergic rhinitis or asthma, so it is very difficult to compare the results. Most of the studies used a questionnaire to define a prevalence, or they are self-reported-based study.

2.1.1. Asthma

A number of epidemiologic studies have reported striking differences in asthma prevalence. The largest multicentric study on asthma prevalence in children the International Study of Asthma and Allergies in Children (ISAAC) showed the asthma prevalence increment trend in children in the period from 1994 to 1999 [19]. The lowest asthma prevalence symptoms values in children aged 6–7 years were in the Indian subcontinent, while the highest asthma prevalence symptoms were in Latin America, North America, and Oceania [19, 20]. For the older age group (13–14 years), the lowest prevalence was in the region of Asia and Pacific, Eastern Mediterranean, and the Indian subcontinent, while children from North America had the highest frequency of asthma symptoms [19, 20]. Wheezing prevalence in the last 12 months also had a similar movement trend, with the lowest prevalence in North and Eastern Europe (5%) and the highest in the region of Latin America and Oceania (>20%) [19]. However, a different trend pattern of severe asthma symptom prevalence movement was noticed. Africa, the Indian subcontinent and Eastern Mediterranean had the highest asthma prevalence characterized with a severe form of asthma in children, while children in Latin America had the lowest prevalence of severe asthma symptoms [19]. Twenty-one centers that participated in the multicentric study had the asthma prevalence in children larger than 20%, while seventeen centers had the prevalence lower than 5% [19, 21].

Generally, the prevalence of asthma in children showed the northwest-southeast gradient movement [22]. This kind of trend is especially expressed in eastern continent. The results of ISAAC study show the highest asthma prevalence in English-speaking countries and Latin America and the higher prevalence in West compared to East Europe and the lowest in Asia and Africa regions [19]. The Great Britain has the highest asthma prevalence in children (32%), then Bulgaria, Czech Republic, Ireland, and Norway. The prevalence in Albania and Greek was the lowest (<5%) [19, 21].

Prevalence of asthma among the elderly population was 10.9% in the study by Pite et al. [13]. The prevalence of asthma increased with the number of rhinitis symptoms, from 2.1% in no rhinitis symptoms group to 44.4% in nasal symptoms plus ocular symptoms group [13].

2.1.2. Allergic rhinitis

Allergic rhinitis has increased in prevalence during last decades with the highest prevalence among children and adolescents [7, 23–25].

The prevalence of rhinitis among the 6- to 7-year-old children was 6.4% in Eastern and Northern Europe and 7.3% in Western Europe [26]. Higher prevalence of rhinitis symptom was among older children (13–14 years old) where 10.5% children in Eastern and Northern Europe and 14.5% in Western Europe have rhinitis symptoms. Children from Georgia had the lowest prevalence (2.8%), while children from Polish (18.9%) and Isle of Man (20.2%) had the highest prevalence of rhinitis [26]. It was found that countries with a low prevalence of asthma also had a low prevalence of rhinitis [26]. In addition to the European continent, the highest prevalence of rhinitis was observed in younger children in Latin America (12%) and older children on the African continent (21.7%). The lowest prevalence of rhinitis in the 6- to 7-year-old children was in Africa (3.6%) and the Indian Subcontinent (3.9%) while in older children in the Indian Subcontinent (10%) [26].

The recent studies suggest a higher prevalence of rhinitis among the middle-aged population (20–28%) [23, 25, 27]. Pite et al. study showed that rhinitis was a highly prevalent but under-diagnosed and undertreated disease in the elderly population [13]. About 80% of patients had rhinitis symptoms, but only half of them had a diagnosis and/or treatment [13].

2.2. Comorbidity of allergic rhinitis and asthma

Epidemiological studies show significant comorbidity of these two diseases. Literature reports that 40–90% of asthmatics have symptoms of allergic rhinitis, while patients with allergic rhinitis have significantly less prevalence of asthma symptoms (10–40%) (**Figure 2**) [16, 28].

However, it should be emphasized that the prevalence of allergic rhinitis in asthmatics is significantly higher than in the general population (10–20%). Conversely, there is a significantly higher prevalence of asthma symptoms among patients with allergic rhinitis than the general population (an average of 5–15%). The association between allergic rhinitis and asthma had been examined in several studies. The strength of the association with asthma increased with increased persistence and severity of rhinitis [13]. The prevalence of asthma increased with the number of rhinitis symptoms, from 2.1% in no rhinitis symptoms group to 44.4% in nasal symptoms plus ocular symptoms group [13]. A French study showed that 58% of asthmatics children had symptoms of allergic rhinitis [30]; the Italian study showed even higher percentage (70%) [29]. Prevalence of allergic rhinitis in patients with classic asthma was 50–69% in the study by Tajiri et al. [4]. Among patients with physician-diagnosed asthma, 64% had allergic rhinitis in the study by Eriksson et al. [31]. Symptoms of allergic rhinitis were more common if asthma symptoms were more severe [30, 32]. Children with exercise-induced asthma have a significantly higher prevalence of allergic rhinitis symptoms [32]. The epidemiological evidence consistently demonstrates the coexistence of allergic rhinitis and asthma [17].

The majority of asthmatic patients have seasonal or persistent allergic rhinitis [17, 33]. Also, the presence of allergic rhinitis in asthmatics has been confirmed as a marker of asthma severity [32, 33]. A higher prevalence of allergic rhinitis was observed among children who reported at least four wheezing episodes in the last year or sleep disorders due to acute episodes [32, 34]. Consequently, better asthma control can be achieved if the diagnosis and treatment of allergic rhinitis are adequately done [15]. Comorbidity of allergic rhinitis and other variant forms of asthma (cough variant, exercise-induced) has also been observed in epidemiological studies [4, 32]. Many patients with allergic rhinitis do not have symptoms of classical asthma, but they present with airway hyperresponsiveness and subclinical inflammation of the lower respiratory airway [35]. The results of previous studies showed that almost 50% of patients with bronchial hyperreactivity reported no respiratory symptoms [36]. These patients usually develop asthma but remain underdiagnosed with asthma [12, 28]. Also, allergic rhinitis is not appropriate recognition in patients with asthma [28, 37]. Many patients with allergic rhinitis self-manage the symptoms or do not recognize allergic rhinitis as a condition needing treatment or physicians help [12]. The Portuguese study showed that more than half of patients with rhinitis symptoms had no diagnosis by a physician [13]. This shows that these patients are untreated for allergic rhinitis. It is important to emphasize that patients with mild forms of allergic rhinitis or asthma remain in high percentage without diagnosis and adequate treatment [32]. Esteban et al. found in their study that 53% asthmatics children were underdiagnosed with allergic rhinitis, and asthma was not well controlled in 77% of these children. Only 33% of the children with allergic rhinitis diagnosis were receiving a treatment by ARIA recommendations. Children with poorly controlled allergic rhinitis had poorer asthma control [11].

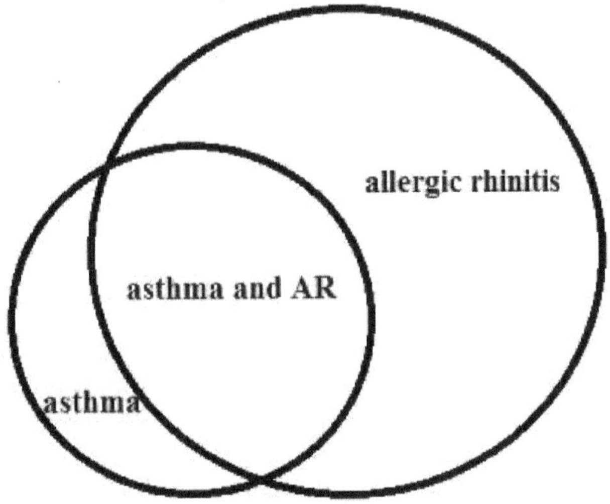

Figure 2. Prevalence and comorbidity of allergic rhinitis and asthma.

Untreated allergic rhinitis in asthmatics contributed to severity symptoms, exacerbation, and uncontrolled asthma [16, 28]. The authors reported that treatment of allergic rhinitis was associated with reduced risk of emergency visits and hospitalization for asthma [3].

3. Allergic rhinitis as risk factor for asthma

Bearing in mind the results of the epidemiological studies, the logical question arises whether allergic rhinitis represents an earlier clinical manifestation of allergic airway disease or itself is causative for asthma [16, 17]. Comorbidity or one disease, the diagnosis of allergic rhinitis often precedes the development of asthma [4, 12]. Studies undoubtedly suggest that allergic rhinitis is a risk factor for asthma [4]. A pathophysiological mechanism which can explain the increased risk of developing asthma in patients with allergic rhinitis is airway hyperresponsiveness. Even 40% of patients with allergic rhinitis showed hyperreactivity to methacholine challenge. Such patients are at greater risk to develop asthma during the next 4–5 years [12]. Also, allergic rhinitis during childhood was associated with increased risk of asthma development in preadolescence and adolescence [28]. The Children's Respiratory Study showed that allergic rhinitis in the first year of life was associated with a risk of developing asthma by 6 years of age [38]. The study by Settipane et al. showed that significantly more (10.5%) of the students diagnosed with allergic rhinitis went on the develop asthma compared with those who did not have allergic rhinitis (3.6%) [39]. The presence of bronchial hyperresponsiveness increased the risk for severe symptoms of allergic rhinitis and asthma and earlier development of asthma in children with allergic rhinitis [12]. It is important to recognize bronchial hyperresponsiveness as a marker of prognostic significance [17]. Epidemiological studies suggest that patients with bronchial hyperresponsiveness without symptoms of classic asthma are more often underdiagnosed with asthma [28].

4. Atopic march

The concept of the atopic march was developed to describe the progression of atopic disorders from atopic dermatitis (AD) in infants to allergic rhinitis and asthma in children [40, 41]. The theory of atopic march implies that young children with atopic dermatitis or food allergy may develop airway allergy such as asthma or allergic rhinitis later in life [40, 42].

The concept of atopic march has been supported by cross-sectional and longitudinal studies [40, 42]. Atopic dermatitis as the first step in the development of atopic march occurs in 45% of children in the first 6 months of life and during the first year of life in 60% of children. In children with atopic dermatitis in the first 2 years of life, an average of 50% of these children develops asthma during subsequent years [42]. The occurrence of only one allergic manifestation, such as recurrent wheeze, eczema, or food allergy, during infancy, was associated with a good prognosis, where over 70% were symptom-free at 8 years of age. Among the children with two or more of any allergic manifestations in infancy, more than half had any allergic disease at 8 years of age [43]. In addition, comorbidity increased from infancy to 8 years of age as a consequence of the increasing prevalence of asthma and allergic rhinitis. Furthermore, the more allergic manifestations a child had in infancy, the greater the risk of allergic disease and comorbidity at 8 years of age [43]. In late adulthood, allergic symptoms generally become less frequent and tend to disappear, but in some, new-onset allergy or asthma may develop in old age [44]. Results of studies showed that the mean age at onset of atopic comorbidities was 1.8 ± 1.0 years for food allergy, 2.2 ± 1.1 years for asthma, 2.3 ± 1.3 years for allergic conjunctivitis, and 2.4 ± 1.3 years for allergic rhinitis [45]. A systematic review of the literature by van der Hulst et al. showed that there is an increased risk of developing asthma by 6 years among children with eczema [46]. The pooled OR for the risk of asthma after eczema, compared with children without eczema, in birth cohort studies was 2.14. In eczema cohort studies, the prevalence of asthma by the age of 6 years was 29.5%. The proportion of children with eczema developing asthma is clearly higher than among those without eczema, and the "rates" for asthma are three- to fourfold higher than in the general population [46]. However, asthma develops in only approximately one in every three children with eczema. Kapoor et al. examined the prevalence of allergic rhinitis and asthma in 2270 children with physician-confirmed AD and found that by 3 years of age, nearly 66% of the subjects reported to have allergic rhinitis, asthma, or both, and the presence of these diseases correlated with poor AD control [47]. These results should be interpreted with caution because of the heterogeneity of the cohorts.

The Tasmanian Longitudinal Health Study investigated the influence of eczema on the development of asthma from childhood to adult life and found that childhood eczema was significantly associated with new-onset asthma in three separate life stages: preadolescence (hazard ratio 1.70; 95% confidence interval 1.05–2.75), adolescence (2.14; 1.33–3.46), and adult life (1.63; 1.28–2.09) [48]. Results from another two cohorts studies, the Melbourne Atopic Cohort Study (MACS) and the LISAplus study, showed that food sensitization in the first 2 years of life increased the risk of subsequent asthma and allergic rhinitis (MACS OR = 8.3 for asthma and aOR = 3.9 for allergic rhinitis; LISAplus OR = 14.4 for asthma and OR = 7.6 for allergic rhinitis) [49].

The risk of developing atopic diseases is complex, and the temporal pattern described in the atopic march may not be a simple progression [40, 43]. Studies found that many individual children do not follow the classical allergic march [49, 50]. For this reason, different patterns of allergic morbidity and the coexistence of the different manifestations, rather than progressive development of one underlying disease, have been suggested [43]. Several studies have suggested that, even though they are associated, the different combinations of allergic manifestations seen over time suggest the coexistence rather than the progressive development of the same underlying disease [43]. Children with early eczema who develop asthma and allergic rhinitis might represent one specific phenotype of eczema, characterized by eczema plus either wheezing or a specific pattern of sensitization [43]. The results of MAS Study showed that children with eczema and without early wheeze were not at increased risk for the development of asthma. These results implied that eczema alone may not be the first most predictive phenotype in the atopic march [51]. Eczema before 2 years of age without the cofactor of wheeze before the age of 3 years and without a specific pattern of atopic sensitization was not associated with an increased risk of wheezing at 7 years of age (adjusted OR 1.11). In addition, the authors suggest that the combination of eczema with early wheeze is a distinct phenotype rather than a representation of a progressive pattern of atopic diseases [51]. However, the risk for development of asthma at 7 years of age among children with early eczema and atopic sensitization to less common antigens but without concomitant wheeze was stronger (adjusted OR, 6.68) than the association between early eczema with early wheezing (adjusted OR, 2.84). This is in consistent with the pattern of the atopic march in which eczema with atopic sensitization presents a higher risk for the development of atopic respiratory disease [52]. The cohort of children with an early-onset AD with a lower rate of sensitization to allergens was associated with a low risk for developing asthma. The cohort of children with multiple sensitizations and with familiar history of asthma had a higher prevalence of asthma than the general population in the study of Amat et al. [53]. Also, studies showed that patients with eczema with specific IgE antibodies to common environmental allergens present by 2 to 4 years of age are at higher risk for progressing in the atopic march to allergic rhinitis and asthma than those with eczema without IgE sensitization [53, 54]. Current evidence suggests that further refining early childhood eczema phenotypes may represent a more robust measure of the first phenotype of the atopic march, with a greater predictive value of identifying those at risk of developing allergic rhinitis and asthma [52].

Likewise, many studies in animal models demonstrate that epidermal barrier dysfunction can be caused by repeated sensitization to allergens to the skin, which leads to phenotypes of AD systemic sensitization and increased risk of allergic rhinitis lung inflammation and airway hyperresponsiveness [43]. A study in a mouse model showed that epicutaneous aeroallergen exposure induces systemic Th2 immunity that predisposes to allergic nasal responses, suggesting that the skin is a potent site for antigen sensitization in the development of experimental allergic rhinitis [43]. Experimental studies showed that epicutaneous sensitization with ovalbumin induced AD and airway hyperresponsiveness to methacholine after challenge with aerosolized ovalbumin [43].

The pathophysiological mechanism of atopic march has been unknown. Skin barrier dysfunctions can explain partly the mechanism of atopic march [50]. Namely, skin barrier defect can promote entry for allergens [50]. Epicutaneous sensitization to aeroallergens has been thought to be responsible, with subsequent migration of sensitized T cell into the nose and airways, for development of allergic upper and lower airway diseases [55]. Sensitization that followed eczema is likely to be a step in the pathophysiological pathway between eczema and asthma [56]. Previous data support the hypothesis that respiratory allergies are secondary to allergic sensitization that occurs after epidermal skin barrier defect [50].

4.1. Conclusion

The atopic march is a useful paradigm to describe the clinically observed progression of atopic diseases in certain children [52]. Whether each step in the march is necessary for progression to the next or further defining of these phenotypes would be more useful in identifying children at risk for developing chronic allergic diseases is still a matter of debate. Allergic manifestations can develop at any point in life. Many children will experience only one or perhaps two atopic manifestations, and the development of these can be interspaced by several years [57]. The progression of allergic disease is not uniform in all atopic children. However, the coexistence of allergic manifestations in the same child has been shown to be more common than expected by chance alone [43]. Also, it is still unclear why some infants with AD outgrow the disease with increasing age, whereas others will march to develop other allergic diseases [41]. Therefore, it is not uncommon that an adult with "new-onset" asthma are unable to remember whether they had allergic diseases in childhood [57]. A better understanding of what places a subset of children with eczema or allergic rhinitis into the risk group for developing asthma is critically important. "Given that most infants with eczema or early wheezing do not develop rhinitis and asthma, further refinement of these early phenotypes or additional risk factors is important for them to be useful" [52]. It is important to define more precise phenotypes of the early stages of the atopic march that may improve its utility in predicting the development of later atopic diseases [52].

Although it has become evident that the mechanisms by which allergen exposure occurs through impaired skin barriers can initiate systemic allergy and predispose individuals to AD, allergic rhinitis, and asthma, the mechanisms of the atopic march are still largely unknown [41]. The findings of studies support the atopic march theory on a population level. But the concept of atopic march is not the strongest factor at the individual level of children with allergic disease [43].

Author details

Sanela Domuz Vujnovic[1*] and Adrijana Domuz[2]

*Address all correspondence to: drdomuz@gmail.com

1 School of Applied Medical Sciences, Prijedor, Republic of Srpska, Bosnia and Herzegovina

2 Primary Health Center, Republic of Srpska, Bosnia and Herzegovina

References

[1] Togias A. Rhinitis and asthma: Evidence for respiratory system integration. The Journal of Allergy and Clinical Immunology. 2003;**111**:1171-1183. DOI: 10.1067/mai.2003.1592

[2] Chawes BLK. Upper and lower airway pathology in young children with allergic- and non-allergic rhinitis. Danish Medical Bulletin. 2011;**58**(5):B4278

[3] Han DH, Rhee C. Comorbidities of allergic rhinitis. In: Pereira C, editor. Allergic Diseases - Highlights in the Clinic, Mechanisms and Treatment. 1st ed. Rijeka: InTech; 2012. pp. 239-254. DOI: 10.5772/1441

[4] Tajiri T, Niimi A, Matsumoto H, Ito I, Oguma T, Otsuka K, et al. Prevalence and clinical relevance of allergic rhinitis in patients with classic asthma and cough variant asthma. Respiration. 2014;**87**(3):211-218. DOI: 10.1159/000355706

[5] Bergeron C, Hamid Q. Relationship between asthma and rhinitis: Epidemiologic, pathophysiologic, and therapeutic aspects. Allergy, Asthma and Clinical Immunology. 2005;**1**(2):81-87. DOI: 10.1186/1710-1492-1-2-81

[6] Braunstahl GJ. The unified immune system: Respiratory tract- nasobronchial interaction mechanisms in allergic airway disease. Journal of Allergy and Clinical Immunology. 2005;**115**(1):142-148. DOI: 10.1016/j.jaci.2004.10.041

[7] Cingi C, Gevaert P, Mosges R, Rondon C, Hox V, Rudenko M, et al. Multi-morbidities of allergic rhinitis in adults: European academy of allergy and clinical immunology task force report. Clinical and Translational Allergy. 2017;**7**:17. DOI: 10.1186/s13601-017-0153-z

[8] Papadopoulou A, Tsoukala D, Tsoumakas K. Rhinitis and asthma in children: Comorbidity or united airway disease? Current Pediatric Reviews. 2014;**10**(4):275-281. DOI: 10.2174/1573396310666141114225203

[9] Bourdin A, Gras D, Vachier I, Chanez P. Upper airway x 1: Allergic rhinitis and asthma: United disease through epithelial cells. Thorax. 2009;**64**(11):999-1004. DOI: 10.1136/thx.2008.112862

[10] Ibiapina Cda C, Sarinho ES, da Cruz Filho AA, Camargos PA. Rhinitis, sinusitis and asthma: Hard to dissociate? Jornal Brasileiro de Pneumologia. 2006;**32**(4):357-366. DOI: 10.1590/S1806-37132006000400015

[11] Esteban CA, Klein RB, Kopel SJ, McQuaid EL, Fritz GK, Seifer R, et al. Underdiagnosed and undertreated allergic rhinitis in Urban School-aged children with asthma. Pediatric Allergy, Immunology, and Pulmonology. 2014;**27**(2):75-81. DOI: 10.1089/ped.2014.0344

[12] Thomas M. Allergic rhinitis: Evidence for impact on asthma. BMC Pulmonary Medicine. 2006;**6**(1):S4. DOI: 10.1186/1471-2466-6-S1-S4

[13] Pite H, Pereira AM, Morais-Almeida M, Nunes C, Bousquet J, Fonseca JA. Prevalence of asthma and its association with rhinitis in the elderly. Respiratory Medicine. 2014;**108**(8):1117-1126. DOI: 10.1016/j.rmed.2014.05.002

[14] Annesi-Maesano I, Sterlin C, Caillaud D, de Blay F, Lavaud F, Charpin D, et al. Factors related to under-diagnosis and under-treatment of childhood asthma in metropolitan France. Multidisciplinary Respiratory Medicine. 2012;**7**(1):24. DOI: 10.1186/2049-6958-7-24

[15] de Groot EP, Nijkamp A, Duiverman EJ, Brand PL. Allergic rhinitis is associated with poor asthma control in children with asthma. Thorax. 2012;**67**(7):582-587. DOI: 10.1136/thoraxjnl-2011-201168

[16] Bousquet J, Khaltaev N, Cruz AA, Denburg J, Fokkens WJ, Togias A, et al. Allergic rhinitis and its impact on asthma (ARIA) 2008 update (in collaboration with World Health Organization, GA(2)LEN and AllerGen). Allergy. 2008;**63**(86):8-160. DOI: 10.1111/j.1398-9995.2007.01620.x

[17] Bousqet J, Hellings PW, Agache I, Bedbrook A, Bachert C, Bergmann KC, et al. ARIA 2016: Care pathways implementing emerging technologies for predictive medicine in rhinitis and asthma across the life cycle. Clinical and Translational Allergy. 2016;**6**:47. DOI: 10.1186/s13601-016-0137-4

[18] D'Amato G, Holgate ST, Pawankar R, Ledford DK, Cecchi L, Al-Ahmad M, et al. Meteorological conditions, climate change, new emerging factors, and asthma and related allergic disorders. A statement of the World Health Organization. World Allergy Organization Journal. 2015;**8**(1):1-52. DOI: 10.1186/s40413-015-0073-0

[19] Lai CK, Beasley R, Crane J, Foliaki S, Shah J, Weiland S. Global variation in the prevalence and severity of asthma symptoms: Phase three of the international study of asthma and allergies in childhood (ISAAC). Thorax. 2009;**64**(6):476-483. DOI: 10.1136/thx.2008.106609

[20] Mallol J, Crane J, von Mutius E, Odhiambo J, Keil U, Stewart A. The ISAAC phase three study group. The international study of asthma and allergies in childhood (ISAAC) phase three: A global synthesis. Allergologia et Immunopathologia. 2013;**41**(2):73-85. DOI: 10.1016/j.aller.2012.03.001

[21] Domuz S. Prevalence of asthma symptoms in children aged 6 to 15 years in the territory of Republic of Sepska [dissertation]. Novi Sad; 2016. 171 p. Available from: nardus.mpn.gov.rs

[22] Pearce N, Douwes J. The global epidemiology of asthma in children. The International Journal of Tuberculosis and Lung Disease. 2006;**10**(2):125-132

[23] Ozdoganoglu T, Songu M. The burden of allergic rhinitis and asthma. Therapeutic Advances in Respiratory Disease. 2012;**6**(1):11-23. DOI: 10.1177/1753465811431975

[24] Zhang Y, Zhang L. Prevalence of allergic rhinitis in China. Allergy, Asthma & Immunology Research. 2014;**6**(2):105-113. DOI: 10.4168/aair.2014.6.2.105

[25] Cibella F, Ferrante G, Cuttitta G, Bucchieri S, Melis MR, Grutta SL, Viegi G. The burden of rhinitis and Rhinoconjunctivitis in adolescents. Allergy, Asthma & Immunology Research. 2015;**7**(1):44-50. DOI: 10.4168/aair.2015.7.1.44

[26] Asher MI, Montefort S, Bjorksten B, Lai CKW, Strachan DP, Weiland SK, et al. Worldwide time trends in the prevalence of symptoms of asthma, allergic rhinoconjunctivitis, and eczema in childhood: ISAAC phases one and three repeat multicountry cross-sectional surveys. Lancet. 2006;**368**:733-743. DOI: 10.1016/S0140-6736(06)69283-0

[27] de Marco R, Cappa V, Accordini S, Rava M, Antonicelli L, Bortolami O, et al. Trends in the prevalence of asthma and allergic rhinitis in Italy between 1991 and 2010. The European Respiratory Journal. 2012;**39**(4):883-892. DOI: 10.1183/09031936.00061611

[28] Egan M, Bunyavanich S. Allergic rhinitis: The "ghost diagnosis" in patients with asthma. Asthma Research and Practice. 2015;**1**:8. DOI: 10.1186/s40733-015-0008-0

[29] Bugiani M, Carosso A, Migliore E, Piccioni P, Corsico A, Olivieri M, et al. Allergic rhinitis and asthma comorbidity in a survey of young adults in Italy. Allergy. 2005;**60**(2):165-170. DOI: 10.1111/j.1398-9995.2005.00659.x

[30] Hamouda S, Karila C, Connault T, Scheinmann P, de Blic J. Allergic rhinitis in children with asthma: A questionnaire-based study. Clinical and Experimental Allergy. 2008;**38**(5):761-766. DOI: 10.1111/j.1365-2222.2008.02953.x

[31] Eriksson J. Prevalence, risk factors and comorbidity of rhinitis, asthma and aspirin-intolerance in West Sweden [thesis]. Gothenburg, Sweden; 2012. Available from: http://hdl.handle.net/2077/32560

[32] Domuz S, Domuz A, Petrovic S. Prevalence and comorbidity of asthma, allergic rhinitis, and eczema among schoolchildren in the republic of Srpska - a cross-sectional study. Srpski Arhiv za Celokupno Lekarstvo. 2017;**145**(1-2):9-13. DOI: 10.2298/SARH151217001D

[33] Camargos PAM, Rodrigues ME, Sole D, Scheinmann P. Asthma and allergic rhinitis as symptoms of the same disease: A paradigm under construction. Jornal de Pediatria. 2002;**78**(2):S123-S128. DOI: 10.1590/S0021-75572002000800003

[34] Sole D, Camelo-Nunes IC, Wandalsen GF, Melo KC, Naspitz CK. Is rhinitis alone or associated with atopic eczema a risk factor for severe asthma in children? Pediatric Allergy and Immunology. 2005;**16**(2):121-125. DOI: 10.1111/j.1399-3038.2005.00227.x

[35] Daabis R. Allergic rhinitis and asthma: The united airways disease. Pulmonary Research and Respiratory Medicine. 2016;**3**(2):e3-e4. DOI: 10.17140/PRRMOJ-3-e005

[36] Laprise C, Boulet LP. Asymptomatic airway Hyperresponsiveness: A three-year follow-up. American Journal of Respiratory and Critical Care Medicine. 1997;**156**(2 Pt 1):403-409. DOI: 10.1164/ajrccm.156.2.9606053

[37] Jacobs TS, Forno E, Brehm JM, Acosta-Perez E, Han YY, Blatter J, et al. Underdiagnosis of allergic rhinitis in underserved children. The Journal of Allergy and Clinical Immunology. 2014;**134**(3):737-739. DOI: 10.1016/j.jaci.2014.03.028

[38] Wright AL, Holberg CJ, Martinez FD, Halonen M, Morgan W, Taussig LM. Epidemiology of physician-diagnosed allergic rhinitis in childhood. Pediatrics. 1994;**94**(6):895-901

[39] Settipane RJ, Settipane GA. IgE and the allergy-asthma connection in the 23-year follow-up of Brown University students. Allergy and Asthma Proceedings. 2000;**21**(4):221-225. DOI: 10.2500/108854100778248890

[40] Hon KL, Wang SS, Leung TF. The atopic march: From skin to the airways. Iranian Journal of Allergy, Asthma, and Immunology. 2012;**11**(1):73-77. DOI: 1011.01/ijaai.7377

[41] Bantz SK, Zhu Z, Zheng T. The atopic march: Progression from atopic dermatitis to allergic rhinitis and asthma. Journal of Clinical and Cellular Immunology. 2014;**5**(2):202. DOI: 10.4172/2155-9899.1000202

[42] Akdis CA, Akdis M, Bieber T, Bindslev-Jensen C, Boguniewicz M. Asthma and immunology/PRACTALL consensus group, et al. diagnosis and treatment of atopic dermatitis in children and adults: European academy of Allergology and clinical immunology/American Academy of allergy, asthma and immunology/PRACTALL consensus report. Allergy. 2006;**61**(8):969-987. DOI: 10.1111/j.1398-9995.2006.01153.x

[43] Goksör E, Loid P, Alm B, Åberg N, Wennergren G. The allergic march comprises the coexistence of related patterns of allergic disease not just the progressive development of one disease. Acta Paediatrica. 2016;**105**(12):1472-1479. DOI: 10.1111/apa.13515

[44] Gillman A, Douglass JA. Asthma in the elderly. Asia Pacific Allergy. 2012;**2**:101-108. DOI: 10.5415/apallergy.2012.2.2.101

[45] Schneider L, Hanifin J, Boguniewicz M, Eichenfield LF, Spergel JM, Dakovic R, et al. Study of the atopic march: Development of atopic comorbidities. Pediatric Dermatology. 2016;**33**(4):388-398. DOI: 10.1111/pde.12867

[46] van der Hulst AE, Klip H, Brand PL. Risk of developing asthma in young children with atopic eczema: A systematic review. The Journal of Allergy and Clinical Immunology. 2007;**120**:565-569. DOI: 10.1016/j.jaci.2007.05.042

[47] Kapoor R, Menon C, Hoffstad O, Bilker W, Leclerc P, Margolis DJ. The prevalence of atopic triad in children with physician-confirmed atopic dermatitis. Journal of the American Academy of Dermatology. 2008;**58**:68-73. DOI: 10.1016/j.jaad.2007.06.041

[48] Burgess JA, Dharmage SC, Byrnes GB, Matheson MC, Gurrin LC, Wharton CL, et al. Childhood eczema and asthma incidence and persistence: A cohort study from childhood to middle age. The Journal of Allergy and Clinical Immunology. 2008;**122**:280-285. DOI: 10.1016/j.jaci.2008.05.018

[49] Alduraywish SA, Standl M, Lodge CJ, Abramson MJ, Allen KJ, Erbas B, et al. Is there a march from early food sensitization to later childhood allergic airway disease? Results from two prospective birth cohort studies. Pediatric Allergy and Immunology. 2017 Feb;**28**(1):30-37. DOI: 10.1111/pai.12651

[50] Yu J. Allergic march model. In: Proceedings of the KAPARD-KAAACI & West Pacific Allergy Symposium Joint International Congress; 10 May 2013; Seoul, Korea. Seoul: KAAACI; 2013. pp. 123-126

[51] Illi S, von Mutius E, Lau S, Nickel R, Grüber C, Niggemann B, et al. The natural course of atopic dermatitis from birth to age 7 years and the association with asthma. The Journal of Allergy and Clinical Immunology. 2004;**113**:925-931. DOI: 10.1016/j.jaci.2004.01.778

[52] Ker J, Hartert TV. The atopic march: What's the evidence? Annals of Allergy, Asthma & Immunology. 2009 Oct;**103**(4):282-289. DOI: 10.1016/S1081-1206(10)60526-1

[53] Amat F, Saint-Pierre P, Bourrat E, Nemni A, Couderc R, Boutmy-Deslandes E, et al. Early-onset atopic dermatitis in children: Which are the phenotypes at risk of asthma?

Results from the ORCA cohort. PLoS One. 2015 Jun 24;**10**(6):e0131369. DOI: 10.1371/journal.pone.0131369

[54] Wüthrich B, Schmid-Grendelmeier P. Natural course of AEDS. Allergy. 2002;**57**:267-268. DOI: 10.1034/j.1398-9995.2002.1n3572.x

[55] Gray CL, Levin ME, Du Toit G. Respiratory comorbidity in south African children with atopic dermatitis. South African Medical Journal. 2017 Sep 22;**107**(10):904-909. DOI: 10.7196/SAMJ.2017.v107i10.12418

[56] Dharmage SC, Lowe AJ, Matheson MC, Burgess JA, Allen KJ, Abramson MJ. Atopic dermatitis and the atopic march revisited. Allergy. 2014 Jan;**69**(1):17-27. DOI: 10.1111/all.12268

[57] Thomsen SF. Epidemiology and natural history of atopic diseases. European Clinical Respiratory Journal. 2015;**2**:24642. DOI: 10.3402/ecrj.v2.24642

5

Meaning of Endotype-Phenotype in Pediatric Respiratory Pathology

Francisco Muñoz-López

Abstract

Respiratory processes that take place in childhood (preschool and adolescence) have a predominant frequency, especially rhinitis and asthma. Family predisposition and the environment define the characteristics of the endotype and the phenotype. Heritage, both of the genes related to bronchial hyperresponsiveness and those related to atopy (production of specific IgE against allergens and hypereosinophilia) are the fundamental basis of those processes that begin at preschool age and continue into adulthood if they do not receive early and etiological treatment. The physiological vagal hyperresponsiveness of the infant; the environment in which it develops, even from the prenatal phase (pregnant smoker); and viral infections are responsible for frequent bronchial processes in the early years that, sometimes, also extend into adolescence. In summary, the coordination of the endotype and the phenotype has led to the acknowledgement and acceptance of these three tracheobronchial processes: transient early wheezing, non-atopic wheezing, and atopic wheezing/asthma.

Keywords: children, phenotype, endotype, bronchospasm, wheezing, asthma

1. Introduction

The phenotype is defined as "observable characteristic with no direct relationship to a disease process, including physiology, triggers and inflammatory parameters" and the endotype as "distinct disease entities which may be present in cluster of phenotypes, but each defined by a specific biological mechanisms." [1, 2].

The variability of bronchopulmonary processes that take place in childhood makes it difficult to establish the criteria for the definition of asthma and, therefore, the phenotype. Age is one of the most important determinants of the phenotype in early childhood and adolescence, including determinants from genetics to the environment. In early childhood, airway development, the environment (especially pregnant smoker), and frequent viral infections, without a doubt, have a decisive influence to establish the phenotype. Symptomatology and lung function (especially the specific airway resistance, atopy, and airway hyperresponsiveness (AHR) at age of 3–5 years) identify several groups of variants: only wheeze, wheeze with irritants, chest congestion and cough, wheeze with allergens that correlate to atopy, and AHR. Asthma that began at those ages, usually preceded by rhinitis, usually lasts until adolescence, if an adequate treatment was not carried out, especially based on the etiology (immunotherapy). In some cases, at that age, the causality may be different, environment and acquired habits (especially smoking) that lead to inflammation of the airways, similar to what occurs in adults (occupational asthma). Three variants have been proposed based on the endotypes: mild to intermittent asthma, asthma with severe exacerbations and multiple allergens, and severe obstructive asthma with neutrophilia [2, 3].

Allergic diseases can be predicted taking into account the key factor in their onset, genetic predisposition, since it is inherited as autosomal dominant trait. Knowledge that at least one of the parents suffers from an allergic disease is a factor to consider. In fact, it is the most reliable indicator for predicting predisposition, although not sufficient to predict it accurately. If both parents are allergic, and even more if they are asthmatic, the risk of allergic respiratory disease can be predicted even better. Although the existence of first-degree relatives suffering from allergic disease is considered the most valuable data, among many others that have been studied, the degree of reliability can be specified as 50% of cases.

2. Genetic predisposition: chromosomes and genes involved

The allergic predisposition (atopic) is of a polygenic nature, that is to say, the genes that support the polymorphisms that give rise to the body's abnormal response to substances (allergens) that are well tolerated by most people and which originate the production of specific IgE antibodies (reagins) against proteins with antigenic capacity contained therein. Even with no atopic predisposition, at any age, excessive exposure to allergens equally can cause specific IgE production, with consequent clinical translation.

The genetic basis of asthma is not unique, but depends on a complex polymorphism, and it is not strange that the involvement of the various genes that are supposed to be implicated is not yet known. The allergic reaction is linked to the predominance of Th2 lymphocyte activity and the subsequent increase in specific IgE. Chromosome 11 (11q13) was the first to identify genes involved in its production; in it lies the synthesis of the β chain of the high-affinity IgE receptor.

It is estimated that at least 100 genes are involved in the pathogenesis of atopy and asthma. Some 30 loci on various chromosomes have been linked on the one hand with the function of the airways and another on the production of IgE [4, 5]. Chromosome 5 (5q31-q33) contains the genes that modulate the production of interleukins secreted by Th2 lymphocytes, such as IL-4 and IL-13, responsible for the atopic response when involved in the secretion of IgE by

B lymphocytes (plasma cells), as well as other interleukins (IL-3, IL-5, IL-9) which also intervene. In addition, in the same gene, the protocadherin-1 (PCDH1) that could alter the integrity of the bronchial epithelium, the first line of defense against inhalation of environmental substances, has been identified [6]. On the other hand, the onset of asthma in the pediatric age has linked to chromosome 17q21, the main genetic determinant of the ORMDL3 gene that encodes endoplasmic reticulum proteins, and has also been associated with poor outcome in children exposed to environmental irritants, especially tobacco smoke [7, 8].

Logically, genes related to the allergic reaction are common to other allergic processes, such as those caused by food or drugs mainly, which may be the cause of dermatological (eczema, urticaria), digestive, or anaphylactic processes. Sometimes, because of the same, there is allergic rhinitis, but it must be taken into account that it is not always an exclusive manifestation of the allergy but at the same time, the genes involved in the pulmonary function (airway hyperresponsiveness) can intervene. In these cases, rhinitis precedes asthma, as in many cases eczema manifests itself early in infants who later suffer from asthma.

Based on these data, the respiratory processes of allergy cause are rhinitis, tracheobronchitis, and asthma.

3. Respiratory processes

3.1. Rhinitis

The respiratory mucosa shows structural and functional homogeneity in all areas where it is found with the exception of greater vascularization in the nasal area. Its specific function lies in providing a defense against the noxious agents that so abundantly penetrate through the airways. The entire inner layer of the airway participates in the ciliary defense system with which the epithelial cells are endowed, in addition to the various mucosal glands and cells of the immune system, present in the subepithelial layer throughout the mucous membrane. Likewise, it can present a unified response, although in different ways, against allergens in individuals with an atopic disposition. For this reason, allergic disease is commonly manifested by symptoms that affect the entire mucosa (rhinitis, asthma, rhinosinusitis, rhinoconjunctivitis), although frequently only a partial stretch is affected, with symptoms exclusive to the upper airway.

In most asthma cases, children display rhinitis or rhinopharyngitis during some time prior to symptoms at lower levels of the respiratory tract. Even at birth or in the first months of life, children can display symptoms of allergic rhinitis, although at that age specific sensitization can hardly be demonstrated. The symptoms that can precede the onset of asthma are hydrorrhea, nasal congestion, and sneezing. Later, when asthma is treated correctly and symptoms disappear, rhinitis symptoms—albeit mild—tend to remain as an aftermath.

3.2. Tracheobronchitis

If the concept of asthma is based on the occurrence of dyspnea (shortness of breath is preponderant), episodes of coughing and breathing noises can also lead to an asthma diagnosis.

In many cases (at any age) coughing is productive, and low wheezing is detected by auscultation, sometimes due to tracheobronchial obstruction by mucus secretion or by some degree of constriction of the smooth bronchial muscle. Asthmatic children sometimes display these same symptoms, alternating with dyspnea episodes (**Table 1**).

3.3. Asthma

Even under proper treatment conditions, asthma is usually persistent. Patients experience unexpected relapses, although most children experience clear and progressive improvement, both in terms of seizure frequency and intensity. The speed of improvement largely depends on the prognostic outlook. Many children stop having attacks shortly after starting hyposensitization treatment, and in these cases, a positive prognosis is highly likely. However, another non-negligible group in the framework of undeniable improvement displays a greater tendency to relapse, sometimes as a result of seemingly banal respiratory processes caused by epidemic viral infections or nonspecific triggers, such as change in the weather, overexertion, or exposure to environmental contaminants. In general terms, without a solid underlying statistical basis, it has been estimated that in 75% of cases, childhood asthma is benign and subject to good prognosis, 20% of asthmatic children suffer from a mild form, and the remaining 5% suffer from severe asthma. Children in this 25% group are therefore most likely to suffer from asthma in adulthood [4, 5]. In any case, we must bear in mind that wheezing is a common symptom in other processes which should be considered (**Table 2**).

Cough	Whistling rales	Dyspnea	Expectoration
Rhinopharyngitis	Tracheobronchitis	Wheezing bronchitis	Chronic bronchitis
Sinusitis	Foreign body	Bronchiolitis	Bronchiectasis
Adenoiditis	Mucoviscidosis	Gastro-oesophageal reflux	Pneumonia
Whooping cough	Bronchiectasis	Extrinsic allergic alveolitis	Mucoviscidosis
Tracheobronchitis	Hemosiderosis	Extra-tracheobronchial:	Hemosiderosis
Laryngitis	Lymphadenopathy	• Pleuritis	COPD
Bronchitis	Pulmonary cysts	• Pneumonia	
Bronchiectasis	Immotile cilia syndrome	• Tuberculosis	
Foreign body	Lobular emphysema	• Pulmonary edema	
Gastrooesophageal reflux	Tracheoesophageal fistula	• Etc.	
Inhalation of irritating gases	Eosinophilic bronchitis		
Eosinophilic bronchitis			
COPD			
Psychogenic			

Table 1. Common tracheobronchial symptoms and more frequent processes (other than asthma).

Common	Asthma Gastroesophageal reflux Infections: bronchiolitis, bronchitis, pneumonia, upper respiratory
Uncommon	Bronchopulmonary dysplasia Foreign body aspiration
Rare	Bronchiolitis obliterans Congenital vascular abnormalities Cystic fibrosis Immunodeficiency diseases Mediastinal masses Primary ciliary dyskinesia Tracheobronchial anomalies Vocal cord dysfunction

Table 2. Causes of wheezing in children.

Several follow-up studies over several years reach different conclusions in the numbers of asthma persisting in adulthood. These differences can be explained by the different criteria taken into account for estimating the persistence of the disease, in addition to the different conditions of patients' lives, such as the workplace, smoking, climate, urban or rural living, etc. It is known that broncholability (airway hyperresponsiveness) persists indefinitely, although with proper and early treatment it can decrease significantly. This weakness can be displayed in unfavorable situations, such as a viral infection and excessive exposure to environmental pollutants, with the onset of sporadic respiratory symptoms (wheezing) which should not be labeled as asthma and much less be interpreted as asthma relapse.

It is difficult to establish a prognosis beforehand, although some data are available to evaluate it. The immune system matures throughout childhood, so most infections occur in the early years of life. Depending on their environment, children may experience up to a hundred infections in their first 8 or 10 years of life, i.e., an average of one infection per month, so that the immune system receives sufficient stimuli for maturation. While they do not always appear with a very striking clinical picture, these respiratory tract infections can trigger bronchial obstructions of varying intensity. This can result in the false diagnosis of asthma, without the existence of a hypersensitivity reaction or inflammation that leaves permanent side effects. As the defense system matures when a child is between 6 and 8, the child stops experiencing bronchial obstruction, and these "false asthma patients" will be the ones who heal spontaneously.

Some endocrine system maturational factors (still undetermined) in some children boost an improvement around puberty, more evident in boys than in girls. But this improvement is only apparent. In most cases it is not uncommon for more or less mild symptoms to appear sporadically, sometimes during physical exercise, in addition to other minor symptoms such as rhinitis or eczema, when present. The typical physical and psychological changes during this age make asthma patients often underestimate their symptoms and abandon treatment. However, spirometry tests often reveal impaired respiratory function, to varying degrees, predominantly affecting peripheral bronchi ("small airways"), evidenced by the reduced mid-expiratory flow.

To make a prognosis, the location of bronchial obstruction must be determined, and it is not detectable when the respiratory function is checked only by measuring the peak expiratory flow (PEF). The obstruction of peripheral bronchi is an indicator of poor outcome. It has even become established that this data may have prognostic value, so that 7-year-old children without asthma are more likely to develop asthma in the following 6 years if their average expiratory flow is lower than normal. Expanding on this concept, the reduction of mean flow at that age also predicts the persistence of asthma in adults, 25 years later.

3.3.1. Pathogenesis

Asthma is a disease whose onset in childhood has, in most cases, a genetic factor of not only allergic predisposition (production of specific IgE against allergens and eosinophilia) but also factors responsible for airway hyperresponsiveness (AHR). In other cases, especially of later onset, bronchial inflammation, with initial involvement of the respiratory mucosa, asthma is a consequence of environmental irritants or viral infection, in which case neutrophilic is the dominant.

In the pathogenesis of asthma, bronchospasm occurs first aided by the AHR, and it is what characterizes the initial phase of asthma attack. Airway smooth muscle contraction involves the formation of actin-myosin cross bridges with the rate of formation dependent upon the activity of myosin light chain kinase and myosin light chain phosphatase. Subsequently, the release of various proteolytic enzymes of eosinophils (ECP, MBP, EPO, EPX) and phospholipid metabolites (LT, PG, TX) triggers the inflammatory reaction, which is responsible of the prolongation of the crisis as well as the chronicity of the process. Congenital AHR is the consequence of several mutations in the genes encoding β_2-adrenergic receptors of the bronchial smooth muscle, related to the greater sensitivity of the same in the people affects due to the mutation. The consequence of this mutation is the α-adrenergic (constrictor)/β-adrenergic (relaxant) imbalance. In addition, mast cells have been demonstrated in the bronchial smooth muscle of these patients, which undoubtedly have a predominant role in the hyperresponsiveness when the mediators responsible for bronchial smooth muscle constriction and the attraction of eosinophils and neutrophils (histamine, tryptase, chymase) and later those involved in the inflammatory reaction (leukotrienes, prostaglandins, thromboxanes) are relapsed [1, 2].

Genetic predisposition (endotype) can be based either in the mutation that leads to congenital AHR or the multiple factors affecting atopic. The coincidence to both genetic backgrounds determines the early onset of rhinitis/asthma which has led to the conception of different phenotypes. Family atopy is a key factor for the onset of allergic disease in infancy, but the absence of AHR, sometimes, is manifested by skin, digestive, or anaphylactic (food, drug) reactions. If the family atopic predisposition is absent, the AHR that can be secondary to environmental factors will also be basic in the pathogenesis of asthma that in these cases, the onset will be later.

The AHR is responsible for acute and sporadic bronchospasm (episodes of dyspnea). The other symptoms, not sporadic, but habitual of greater or less intensity depending of the gravity, environment, and treatment, are mainly due to the inflammation that accompanies the process, whose cause differs in different circumstances [5–10].

Dominant symptoms, age of onset, persistence, and causes (viruses, allergens, environmental irritants) are the factors that influence the variability of phenotypes, not always persistent from childhood to adulthood, which undoubtedly differentiate the process at the different stages of life.

3.3.2. *Prognostic criteria*

The beforehand assessment of disease progression can be established based on the following data: family history, child-dependent factors, environment, disease characteristics, and early and correct treatment. The sum of unfavorable data worsens prognosis.

Family genetics, especially parental, increases the risk proportionally to the acuteness of the allergic process (asthma, eczema). Moreover, immunodeficiencies must be taken into account. They favor respiratory infections, especially selective IgA deficiency, which is present very often due to hypersensitivity reactions, perhaps due to an immune compensation mechanism. Within the environment, both the location of the home and the atmosphere within the home may have a significant influence. In terms of age of onset, it should be noted that in the first 2 or 3 years of life, episodes of shortness of breath may occur due to various anatomical-physiological causes (immune immaturity, bronchial constriction, vagal tone) which result in narrowing of the bronchial lumen in various circumstances. This should not be labeled as asthma. Thus, it is estimated that between 45 and 85% of these children in a few years will no longer exhibit symptoms. They are considered "false asthma patients" who will heal spontaneously. The possibility exists for the child to suffer from rhinovirus-induced bronchiolitis leading to significant desquamation of bronchial epithelium and inflammatory reaction which facilitates the passage of pneumo-allergens leading to sensitization, even in the absence of prior atopic predisposition.

Sensitization to multiple allergens is another cause of poor outcome, especially if these involve a fungus. These microorganisms result in a type of asthma which is more difficult to control. With regard to an atopic predisposition, suffering from several allergic diseases is another cause of poor outcome. Atopic eczema is the most influential, in direct proportion to how extensive and stubborn it is.

3.3.3. *Evolutionary criteria*

Not all children with wheeze at early age will have asthma later; the sex also influences the natural evolution of the process with a shift in severity and prevalence biased toward women after puberty (**Table 3**).

In summary, the evolution of the process can be summarized as follows:

Good evolution: decrease in the number of asthma attacks in 1 year to half or less than the previous year, respiratory function within normal limits.

	Age (year)		
	<5	5–11	12–18
Prevalence by sex	M > F	M > F	Before puberty: M > F After puberty: F > M
Predominant effector cell	Neutrophil Eosinophil	Eosinophil	Eosinophil
Reticular basement membrane	Begins after the first birthday	Not as thick as adults	Thickening approaches that are seen in adults
Lung function	Measures difficult to obtain	Changes associated with duration of asthma symptoms	Deficits present in those patients who began wheezing before age 3 but might not present in those who began wheezing in later childhood
Incidence of exacerbations	++++	+++	++
Taken from Szefler et al. [11].			

Table 3. Pathophysiologic changes of asthma by age.

Moderate evolution: decrease in the number of attacks in 2 years to at least half of the previous year at the start of treatment, improving the intensity of attacks and maintaining an acceptable respiratory function.

Poor evolution: the number and intensity of attacks do not change, and the respiratory function does not improve but actually tends to worsen, with FEF_1 between 70 and 80% of predicted and $FMF_{25–75}$ between 40 and 60% of forecast.

Deterioration: aggravation of the crisis in frequency and/or intensity, with impaired respiratory function: FEV_1 < 80% and $FMF_{25–75}$ < 60% of forecast.

3.3.4. Healing criteria

Atopic genetic predisposition is not modified by any therapeutic measure, but clinical signs can be suppressed in a large number of patients with appropriate preventive measures and early treatment, targeting primarily causal aspects (immunotherapy can partly correct the altered immune response).

The clinical criterion is possibly the most valuable with regard to how long the child must be free of symptoms, particularly dyspnea, since sometimes children unexpectedly relapse after a long time of being symptom-free. A widely accepted period of time is 2 years without an attack.

In parallel to the absence of subjective clinical symptoms, the objective assessment of the respiratory function (spirometry tests) is another data factor that must unavoidably be taken into account. This is because children cannot be considered asthma-free if bronchial obstruction persists, although they may be free from obvious symptoms. Certainly, a child with alterations in spirometric values cannot be considered risk-free.

Chronological	2 years without crisis
Functional	Absence of signs of bronchial obstruction (large and small airways)
Airway hyperresponsiveness	Decreased response to allergen inhalation
	Decreased response to methacholine or histamine inhalation
	Decreased response to physical exercise
Immunoallergics	Decreased response to prick test
	Decrease of total IgE
	Increase of IgG (IgG_1–IgG_4)
	Increase of Th1 lymphocytes
	Decrease of basophil degranulation (decrease of histamine release)

Table 4. Asthma healing criteria.

Table 4 shows the different data to be assessed after the etiological treatment (immunotherapy), the results of which will depend on the asthma cure criteria. This brings changes in the immune response (reduction of IgE, increase in IgG_1-IgG_4, and increase in Th1 lymphocytes), together with the decrease in histamine. Bronchial hyperresponsiveness, however, is maintained, although reduced by elimination or reduction of bronchial inflammation, which in itself does not represent a risk of relapse, as it is verified after an average of 10 years after the medical discharge [12].

4. Preschool children

Some anatomo-physiological characteristics of the airways of infants and young children predispose to the occurrence of processes that lead to narrowing or bronchial obstruction, which are manifested by common symptoms, such as cough, dyspnea, and noise or wheezing.

The smaller bronchial caliber is a basic fact that facilitates the obstruction, as a consequence of the inflammation of the mucosa, of the constriction of the smooth muscle or of the increase of the secretion of the tracheobronchial mucous glands. Also known is the physiological vagal tone of the infant, which lasts during the first years of life. Pathologically, bronchial hyperresponsiveness is a fundamental fact in the pathogenesis of asthma. This AHB, by stimulation of the bronchial smooth muscle, is usually secondary to the inflammatory reaction that takes place in various circumstances in the bronchial mucosa, but it is also a characteristic of individuals with atopic predisposition, since there are certain abnormalities in the protein chain of the β-receptors of the smooth muscle.

In relation to the infectious bronchopulmonary disease, so frequent in the first years of life, there is the well-known immaturity of the immune system, which in some children last for several years (transient immunodeficiency of the infant), facilitating the appearance of bronchial inflammatory processes, which they manifest with symptoms partly common to other tracheobronchial processes. The inflammation of the small airways is correlated with the existence of exhaled nitric oxide (FeNO) whose values have been proposed for the diagnostic confirmation of asthma, even up to school age because it is considered as a potential biomarker to distinguish endotypes. However, despite its strong correlation with atopy, it seems that it can only be considered as a biomarker for transient wheezing but not for persistent wheezing phenotypes.

Viral infections (respiratory syncytial virus (RSV) and rhinovirus (RV)) are a frequent cause of respiratory processes in young children, often transient (bronchiolitis), although in some cases the persistence of chronic inflammation, disrupted epithelium, and airway remodeling can condition the major bronchoconstrictor response to environmental irritants and, especially, to allergens, causing asthma [13].

With this background, it is not uncommon for processes of different causality to manifest clinically with similar symptoms, which can lead to erroneous diagnoses, if the knowledge of differential signs is not in-depth, such as genetic background, habits, and family environment, among others (**Table 5**).

Dominant symptom: cough	Maxillary sinusitis
	Adenoid vegetations
	Rhinopharyngitis
	Whooping cough
	Primary ciliary dyskinesia
Pseudoasmatic symptoms	Infectious pathology
	• Immunodeficiencies
	• Bronchiolitis
	• Bronchitis obliterans
	Tracheobronchial foreign body
	Cystic fibrosis of the pancreas
	Gastroesophageal reflux
	Mediastinal tumors and adenopathies
Less frequent processes	Congenital anomalies
	• Laringo and tracheomalacia
	• Vascular rings
	Alpha-1 antitrypsin deficiency
	Hypersensitivity pneumonitis
	Pulmonary hemosiderosis
	Alveolar proteinosis
	Eosinophilic lung

Table 5. Most outstanding processes for differential diagnosis.

In a large study (8310 mothers) in which the presence of respiratory symptoms that took place between 6 and 81 months after birth was investigated, the authors reached this conclusion:

1. Sixty-eight percent of the children never had episodes of wheezing .
2. Ten percent had them sporadically, with a prevalence between 18 and 42 months.
3. Eight percent presented them for a long time, between 30 and 69 months.
4. In 2% the prevalence was low until 19 months, increasing after 18 months.
5. Late onset in 5% of the children, in which the prevalence of sibilance lasted up to 42 months in 50% of them.
6. Persistent wheezy (7%) with 65% prevalence at 6 months and approximately 90% prevalence thereafter [14].

In a more recent study, the same authors analyze the need to assess the exhaled nitric oxide fraction (FeNO) together with the respiratory function, family history, and environment in which the child lives, in addition to the treatment received, facts that may condition the persistence of the process for a longer time [15].

A study carried with the purpose of knowing if the different respiratory processes in young children could be related to breastfeeding and its duration finds above all a possible protection against viral infections, but it has not been possible to establish its participation in the establishment of phenotypes related to other respiratory processes.

It is really difficult to establish a certain diagnosis of asthma in the first years of life, since in many cases it is the evolution of symptoms over the years that allows confirming the diagnosis with support of the appropriate immuno-allergological study. The diagnosis of asthma will be reached by previously excluding other possible causes of dyspnea or wheezing. As a more frequent diagnostic alternative, "wheezing bronchitis" would be characterized by single or repeated episodes of dyspnea or wheezing and/or noisy breathing, of variable intensity, which may be febrile, which begin in the first year of life and do not continue more than the third year. In summary, in preschool children this respiratory episodes can be classified as (a) occasional, one episode every 4–6 weeks or less; (b) frequents, more of one episode in 4–6 weeks, isolated intercrisis symptoms, mild; (c) moderate persistence, very frequent exacerbations, symptoms that interfere with daily activities and sleep; and (d) severe persistent, daily or almost daily symptoms, with frequent episodes of dyspnea.

Coinciding with these concepts, different phenotypes of bronchospasm pathology in children have been differentiated, distinguishing asthma and transient bronchitis (wheezy bronchitis) that encompassed various processes suffered by a group of children that after preschool age do not have bronchospasm, a consequence of the predisposing factors. However, it is not always easy to determine the phenotype of a certain patient, and it may even be that over time, as it evolves, there is a need to change the criteria. Hence the need to pay attention to the characteristics of the symptoms and their evolution, in addition to a whole series of circumstances, such as the suffering other allergic processes by the same child (eczema, milk protein allergy), early onset of the clinic, or the existence of similar pathology among siblings, parents, or other close relatives, environmental contaminants, climate, etc. The lack of family history in approximately 20% of cases adds another obstacle to the diagnosis.

In most children, asthma begins in the first 5 years of life. Different studies indicate that between 15 and 35% of preschool children have had some episode of respiratory difficulty, accompanied or not by wheezing or other respiratory sounds (wheezing bronchitis); however, 60–65% of those children will not suffer a crisis after the third year.

Apart from asthma and wheezing bronchitis, many other bronchopulmonary diseases have an early start, with a symptomatology that may recall those processes, as more frequent, sinusitis, adenoiditis, mucoviscidosis, ciliary dyskinesia, various malformations, gastroesophageal reflux, etc., to be taken into account in all cases.

Physiological factors (reduced bronchial caliber, physiological vagal tone, immune immaturity) tend toward normalization, while pathological factors (familial atopy, congenital or acquired bronchial hyperresponsiveness) depend on their incidence and decrease or increase depending on the circumstance.

5. School age and teenagers

The asthmatic adolescent presents particular characteristics, in part conditioned by the teenager's personality but also, possibly, because this illness has a different expression than in other ages. It is a fact that an undetermined percentage of children improve when reaching adolescence, even being free from symptoms in some asthma cases qualified as mild or moderate. Nevertheless no cases of severe asthma disappear totally at this age. Some undetermined factors, possibly hormone-related, might influence this improvement in males. It should be clarified if this improvement is real and *definitive. Many* children at this age, with sporadic and mild symptoms more or less frequent (coughing, mild dyspnea after exercise), get used to their illness and say they feel well, although it is not rare listen to whistling of different intensity. Even in asymptomatic cases, with normal auscultation, the spirometry presents disturbances that show bronchial obstruction.

The persistence of respiratory processes that begin at preschool age can occur if the phenotype corresponds to the existence of atopic predisposition or, also, in some children infected by rhinovirus (RV) [16]. At these ages, asthma derives predominantly from atopy in relation to Th2 lymphocytes (IgE), eosinophilia, and airway inflammation. Early initiation of adequate treatment avoids the persistence and/or severity of asthma at these ages, especially in cases in which asthma was considered mild or moderate. However, no case of severe asthma stops manifesting at this stage of life and may become chronic due to the persistence of obstruction of the airways, manifesting recurrently serious or episodic, when predisposing factors are scarce. The persistence of asthma in these ages may be due to the intensity of the atopy (association of atopic eczema) and the AHR; the process self-control, failure to comply or the abandon treatment and inadequate medication in the crisis; and family or work environment, smoking, powder, animals, etc.

Some undetermined factors, possibly hormonal, must influence the improvement and also the inversion that occurs at this age, in terms of frequency by sex, with predominance in the female, predominant in adulthood. In some cases in which the symptomatology is very sporadic, however, spirometry can show alterations that reveal bronchial obstruction that will condition the subsequent evolution. However, in milder cases, it is possible that spirometry remains within normal limits, so the methacholine or histamine test can help demonstrate the hyperresponsiveness.

Four phenotypes related to responsible allergens (especially fungi) and AHR have been distinguished: [1] later sensitization to indoor allergens, [2] multiple early sensitization, [3] early sensitization to outdoor allergens (especially *Alternaria*) and later sensitization to indoor (including *Aspergillus*), and [4] early sensitization to indoor allergens and later sensitization to outdoor allergens [17, 18]. In some cases, asthma begins in adolescence, possibly due to the low familial predisposition of atopy (only uncles or grandparents) and only slight bronchial hyperresponsiveness, which is why it is possible that the environment or the beginning of smoking is responsible for its start [19].

At these ages, coming from the smallest ones or beginning in them, the following phenotypes and endotypes of asthma can be distinguished that usually extend until the adult age:

1. Eosinophilic: allergic, by aspirin, severe hypereosinophilic of late onset, and allergic bronchopulmonary mycosis
2. Prone to exacerbations: allergic, by aspirin, severe hypereosinophilic of late onset, wheezing from a younger age, exacerbation by virus, and premenstrual syndrome
3. Related to obesity: obstruction of air flow, severe steroid dependence, severe hypereosinophilic of late onset
4. Overexertion: athletes, wheezing from preschool age.
5. Fixed airflow limitation: noneosinophilic (neutrophilic)
6. Scarce response to steroids: neutrophilic, eosinophilic, obesity—airflow obstruction [1]

In cases of severe asthma, different clinical pictures can be distinguished, conditioned by the phenotype: [1] persistent chronic symptoms, [2] recurrent severe asthma exacerbations, [3] persistent airflow obstruction, and [4] brittle asthma: type 1 (persistent wild swing in peak flow) and type 2 (sudden acute deteriorations). In some of these variants, the aforementioned viruses (RSV) may be responsible.

One of the main problems at this age in the no compliance of medication. This feeling of well-being makes the adolescent to stop it, using the drugs only when not feeling well and, frequently, in an uncontrolled way and not using the proper medication. Mortality in teenager asthma has been related to self-management of severe crisis, with insufficient or inappropriate medication.

6. Resulting processes

Summarizing the concepts presented, the coordination of the endotype and the phenotype are the basis for the establishment of these currently accepted tracheobronchial processes:

1. Transient early wheezing: no family or analytical history of atopy; early onset and disappearance between 3 and 5 years; decreased lung function, but recovered before 6 years of age; no bronchial hyperreactivity (normal methacholine test); and eosinophilia or high levels of IgE. Possible predispositions: prematurity, genetic (congenital reduction of functional residual capacity (V_{max} FRC)), or environmental (smoking mother, irritants).
2. Non-atopic wheezing: beginning before 3 years of age, the majority (73% of cases) after viral infections (RSV, para-influenza, others), although infection by RSV before 3 years of age has been associated with the risk of persisting wheezing episode till 10 years of age. In general, there is no family history of atopy or clinical or analytical signs of it in the same patient: decreased lung function after infection and progressive normalization with maximum persistence of the process up to 13 years of age.
3. Atopic wheezing/asthma: in which there is no lack of familial atopic predisposition, it starts before 6 years (80%); early sensitization to pneumo-allergens; positive specific IgE and skin tests; frequent coincidence with associated allergic processes (rhinitis, eczema, urticaria); progressive deterioration of lung function and bronchial hyperreactivity; persistence that may reach adulthood, if adequate treatment is not carried out at an early stage (especially immunotherapy when indicated, anti-inflammatory, bronchodilators); and environmental measures [4, 20–23].

7. Controversies

Despite the evidence of the different ways of presenting the bronchospastic processes in the pediatric age, the evidence of the aforementioned predisposing factors has been questioned because there are several respiratory processes with similar symptoms but varying in the age of onset, persistence, family history, and coexistence or not with other processes of allergic cause (cutaneous, digestive). Likewise, the different coincidence of wheezing, atopy, or AHR can condition the different respiratory processes, based on the different uses of the term phenotype, such as:

1. Any observable trait (partial phenotype) includes signs, symptoms, measurements, and biological markers.
2. Clinically useful grouping defines groups that differ with respect to features of interest, e.g., risk factors, response to treatment, and prognosis.
3. Hypothesized disease entity defines a condition that is thought to represent a distinct disease entity.

These factors are the basis for doubting the reality of the phenotypes whose definition is also debatable, requiring a better definition of the term and its possible relationship with the aforementioned respiratory processes. "In the meantime, we should treat phenotypes as exactly that the best current working hypothesis" how the authors of the work finish [24].

Author details

Francisco Muñoz-López

Address all correspondence to: 5314fml@comb.cat

Department of Pediatric Immunoallergology, Faculty of Medicine, University of Barcelona, Clínic Hospital-Sant Joan de Déu Hospital, Spain

References

[1] Lötvall J, Akdis CA, Bacharier LB, Bjerrmer L, Casale TB, Custovic A, et al. Asthma endotypes; a new approach to classification of disease entities within the asthma. The Journal of Allergy and Clinical Immunology. 2011;**127**:355-360

[2] Lin C-Y. Endotypes of asthma in children. Journal of Pediatric Respiratory Disease. 2014;**10**:51-58

[3] Lødrup Carlsen KC, Pijnenburg M. Identification of asthma phenotypes in children. Educational aims. Breathe. 2011;**8**(1):39-44

[4] Bacharier LB, Boner A, Carlsen KH, Eigenmann PA, Frischer T, Götz M, et al. Diagnosis and treatment of asthma in children: A PRACTALL consensus report. Allergy. 2008;**63**:5-34

[5] Papadopoulos NG, Arakawa H, Carlsen KH, Custovic A, Gern J, Lemarke R, et al. International consensus on (ICON) pediatric asthma. Allergy. 2012:976-997

[6] Alkhouri H, Hollins F, Moir LM, Brightling CE, Armour CL, Hughes JM. Human lung must cells modulate the functions of airway smooth muscle cells in asthma. Allergy. 2011;**66**:1231-1241

[7] Chapman DG, Irvin CG. Mechanisms of airway hyper-responsiveness in asthma: The past, present and yet to come. Clinical et Experimental Allergy. 2015;**45**:706-719

[8] Henderson AJ. Childhood asthma phenotypes in the twenty-first century. Breathe. 2014;**10**(2):101-108

[9] Agache I, Akdis C, Jutel M, Virchow JC. Untangling asthma phenotypes and endotypes. Allergy. 2012;**67**:835-846

[10] Muñoz-López F. Etiopatogenic mechanisms of bronchial asthma. Journal of Translational Science. 2017;**3**(4):1-3

[11] Szefler SJ et al. Asthma across the ages. Journal of Allergy and Clinical Immunology. 2014;**133**:3-13

[12] Muñoz-López F. Intensity of bronchial hyperresponsiveness and asthma relapse risk in the young adult. Allergologia et Immunopathologia. 2007;**35**(2):62-70

[13] Jartti T, Gern JE. Roke of viral infections in the development and exacerbation of asthma in children. The Journal of Allergy and Clinical Immunology. 2017;**140**:895-906

[14] Granell R, Sterne JAC, Henderson J. Associations of different phenotypes of wheezing illness in early childhood with environmental variables implicated in the aetiology of asthma. PLoS One. 2012;**7**(10). DOI: 10.1371/journal.pone.0048359

[15] Duijts L, Granell R, Sterne JAC, Henderson AJ. Childhood wheezing phenotypes influence asthma, lung function and exhaled nitric oxide fraction in adolescence. The European Respiratory Journal. 2016;**47**:510-519

[16] Lukkarinen M, Koistinen A, Turunen R, Lehtinen P, Vourinen T, Jastti T. Rhinovirus-induced first wheezing episode predicts atopic but not noatopic asthma at school age. The Journal of Allergy and Clinical Immunology. 2017;**140**:988-995

[17] Bush A, Menzies-Gow A. Phenotypic differences between pediatric and adult asthma. Proceedings of the American Thoracic Society. 2009;**6**:712-719

[18] Eun Lee MD, Si Hyeon Lee BS, Kin Y-H, Cho H-J, Yoon J, Yang S-I, et al. Association of atopy phenotypes with new development of asthma and bronchial hyperresponsiveness in school-aged children. Annals of Allergy, Asthma & Immunology. 2017;**118**:542-550

[19] Muñoz-López F. Bronchial hyperresponsiveness and asthma in the pediatric population. Allergologia et Immunopathologia. 2014;**42**(3):230-234

[20] Martínez FD, Wright AL, Taussig LM, Holberg CJ, Jalonen M, Morgan W. Asthma and wheezing in the first six year of life. The New England Journal of Medicine. 1995;**332**:133-138

[21] Stein RT, Martinez FD. Asthma phenotypes in childhood: Lessons from an epidemiological approach. Pediatric Respiratory Reviews. 2004;**5**:155-161

[22] Taussig LM, Wright AL, Holberg CJ, Jalonen M, Morgan WJ, Martínez FD. Tucson children's respiratory study: 1980 to present. The Journal of Allergy and Clinical Immunology. 2003;**111**:661-675

[23] Calderón MA, Gerth van Wijk R, Eichler I, M atricardi PM, Varga EM, Kopp MV, et al. Perspectives on allergen-specific immunotherapy in childhood: An EAACI position statement. Pediatric Allergy and Immunology. 2012;**23**(4):300-306

[24] Spycher BD, Silverman M, Kuehni CE. Phenotypes in childhood asthma: Are they real? Clinical and Experimental Allergy. 2010;**40**:1130-1141

6

Functional Lung Examination in Diagnostics of Asthma and its Phenotypes

Frantisek Lopot, Vaclav Koucky, Daniel Hadraba,
David Skalicky and Karel Jelen

Abstract

In this chapter, we review the diagnostic approach to asthma phenotypes in children using lung function testing. Various methods are reviewed and their advantages and disadvantages are discussed. Medical history and physical examination including lung auscultation is the first line examination, which may raise the suspicion on asthma. Besides the simple lung auscultation, more advanced approaches (computer analysis of breath sounds) are described. Spirometry and other classical lung function testing methods (body plethysmography, dilution techniques) are discussed with respect to their contribution to asthma diagnostics and phenotype classification. Afterward, impulse oscillometry and methods intended for patients with insufficient cooperation follows. We highlight their potential in diagnostics of early asthma stages. Measurement of exhaled nitric oxide is discussed and its potential for allergic asthma (eosinophilic inflammation) detection is assessed. In conclusion, various lung function testing methods may contribute to both setting the diagnosis of asthma itself and classification of asthma phenotypes. Their smart combination allows for more precise diagnostics and treatment of young patient with bronchial asthma.

Keywords: asthma in children, wheezing, diagnostics, phenotype, endotype classification, lung function testing, spirometry, impulse oscillometry, FeNO, lung auscultation, harmonic analysis, Fourier transform

1. Asthma phenotypes and endotypes in children

Asthma is a heterogeneous disease, usually characterized by chronic airway inflammation. It is defined by the history of respiratory symptoms such as wheeze, shortness of breath, chest tightness, and cough that vary over time and in intensity, together with variable expiratory airflow limitation [1]. Currently, asthma is considered to be a syndrome rather than one disease with common etiopathogenesis. There have been various attempts to subclassify asthma into more homogeneous groups with similar pathophysiology and clinical presentation. Such subclassification will help to improve the therapeutic approach to our patients and will offer a possibility of individualized therapy, which will increase the safety and efficacy of asthma treatment. Moreover, research in more homogeneous groups of patient will offer better insight into the pathogenesis of bronchial asthma with.

Recently, the terms asthma phenotype and endotype have been introduced. "Phenotype" is defined as a recognizable cluster of demographic, etiologic, and clinical characteristics. These are generally regarded to arise from interactions between the genotype and environmental influences. It may be described by clinical characteristics including physical, biochemical, and other variables that can be objectively measured. There is no reference to an underlying pathophysiological process. The term "endotype" is used to describe a disease subtype based on distinct pathological mechanisms [2].

A number of phenotypes and endotypes in children have been proposed, unfortunately up to now, there is no clear consensus in this field. Martinez et al. categorized wheezing during the first 6 years of childhood into three distinct groups—transient early, persistent, and late-onset wheeze. This classification is based on the presence or absence of wheezing before the age of 3 years and its persistence or incidence to age 6 years. The limitation of this approach comes from the fact that it can be set only retrospectively and thus it is of little clinical impact. Later, another classification of early wheeze has been suggested by a European Respiratory Society task force—a dichotomy based on trigger factors: episodic viral wheeze and multiple-trigger wheeze [3]. Besides the time- and symptom-based approaches, there exist many other phenotypes, which have been adopted from adults: allergic asthma, nonallergic asthma, asthma with fixed airflow limitation, asthma with obesity, and so on. They have some importance in older children (adolescents).

Although phenotype- and endotype-based approaches to asthma are of an extreme importance for research purposes and for understanding asthma itself, to date, no strong relationship has been found between specific pathological features and particular clinical patterns or treatment responses. More research is needed to understand the clinical utility of phenotypic classification in asthma.

2. Functional lung examination in asthma diagnostics

Setting a diagnosis of asthma is difficult and requires a complex approach. There exists no single test capable of setting the diagnosis without other concomitant examinations. Particular difficulties occur when conducting a confident diagnosis in children younger than 5 years. Symptoms of cough and wheeze are very common in this age and the assessment of airflow limitation is also age-restricted, all leading to difficulties with setting up the diagnosis. A probability-based approach, based on the pattern of symptoms during and between viral respiratory infections, may be helpful [1]. It allows to individually decide about the trial of controller treatment (usually inhaled corticosteroids—ICS), which may further underpin the diagnosis.

Besides the evaluation of clinical symptoms (wheeze, cough, breathlessness, activity, and social behaviour), adjunct tests may be employed as well [1]. Because of the scope of our chapter, we focus on lung function testing and exhaled nitric oxide levels.

The evaluation of airflow limitation and its reversibility is a key question in asthma-diagnostic approach. However, it must be noted that the presence of airflow limitation (even reversible after beta-agonists) does not confirm the diagnosis. Other aspects need to be taken into account when making conclusions. All the limitations of the functional examination may be deduced from this fact. A similar situation occurs in phenotype classification. In case of time-based classification of wheezing phenotypes, the early functional lung examination may assist to objectify the presence of airflow limitation and its development in time. In case of symptom-based classification, the functional examination is of smaller importance; however, it may assist in clinically uncertain situations. Endotype classification is usually based on invasive tests (e.g. endobronchial biopsies, bronchoalveolar lavage cytology, etc.). However, some tests such as exhaled nitric oxide measurement may indicate the allergic (eosinophilic) asthma endotype. To sum up, functional examination informs about the presence of airflow limitation and its reversibility, but with the exception of fractional exhaled nitric oxide (FeNO), it will only assist in phenotype classification.

3. Evaluation of bronchial obstruction by different lung function-testing methods

In this subchapter, various methods for detection of bronchial obstruction will be reviewed. We focus on tests that are routinely used in clinical settings. In addition, we discuss less available methods, which have the potential to enrich the spectrum of diagnostic tools in future. However, their clinical impact needs to be further studied.

The choice of diagnostic tool is influenced by several factors:

- sensitivity of the method with regard to bronchial obstruction, respectively asthma itself,
- specificity of the method with regard to bronchial obstruction, respectively asthma itself,
- invasiveness of the method and patient burden (e.g., need of sedation/anesthesia, radiation, etc.),
- age of the patient—depending on the ability of the child to follow up the instructions and coordinate breathing, some methods (e.g., spirometry) are available only in older children,
- availability of the method,
- time and financial demands.

When indicating an optimal diagnostic test, one should bear in mind its different characteristics and potential limitations in asthma diagnostics and phenotype classification. In a clinical setting, a combination of several methods is employed to reach a confident diagnosis.

3.1. Lung auscultation

Because of its simplicity, noninvasiveness, and wide applicability, lung auscultation is the first-line method in lung examination. This method is a part of the physical examination and is usually accompanied by aspection, palpation, and percussion. The subject of the examination is the sound effect of the air flow passing from and to the alveoli. A sit does not require special patient cooperation. This method can be applied to the whole-age spectrum of the patients. On the other hand, it has also several disadvantages. Taking the principle of the method into account, it is not possible to completely eliminate the contamination of the tracked sound signal by artifacts from the internal and external surroundings of the patient. Those signal artifacts may be of such intensity that important information gets lost. Moreover, the sensitivity of lung auscultation in the detection of bronchial obstruction is relatively low. The bronchial obstruction is not reliably recognizable if the airway lumen is reduced less than by 30–50% as compared to the healthy state. These problems can be solved in part by appropriate frequency tuning of the phonendoscope, or by processing the captured record by one of the advanced audio signal-processing methods—see subsequent subchapter. The first-mentioned adjustment is applicable in general but has only a limited effect with respect to the range of commonly observed frequencies. The second adjustment is bound to the possibility of making any record of the listening examination. Several phonendoscopes, which enable to make audio recordings, are currently available on the market. These recordings can then be played back and processed using specific software on a common PC.

Another disadvantage of lung auscultation is the considerable level of subjectivity in its evaluation. The Working Group of the European Respiratory Society and the American Thoracic Society (ERS/ATS task force) drew up a paper on the standardization of the lung sound nomenclature [4]. A library of reference auscultation findings has been created, including their interpretation [5]. Typical findings for bronchial obstruction include "wheezing" and non-constantly "prolonged expiration" (i.e., expiration phase more than two times longer than inspiration). The finding of these sound phenomena indicates the presence of bronchial obstruction with a high probability and is an indication for the beta-mimetic therapeutic test (salbutamol/albuterol). Positivity of this therapeutic test further supports the diagnosis of bronchial obstruction and indicates its reversibility. In order to obtain valid results of this test, several rules need to be followed—the application of sufficient dose of beta-mimetic (400 mg of salbutamol in the form of a "metered dose inhaler"), the correct way of application—via a "spacer" ("aerochamber"), and last but not the least, sufficient interval between the applications of beta-mimetics and the lung auscultation (15–20 min).

To conclude, lung auscultation and the detection of obstructive phenomena (wheezing, prolonged expiration) together with positive beta-mimetic test are the basic and most available diagnostic tools for bronchial obstruction.

3.2. Spirometry

Spirometry is a test that measures how an individual inhales or exhales volumes of air as a function of time. The primary signal measured in spirometry may be volume or flow. Spirometry is highly valuable as a screening test of general respiratory health. However, on its own, spirometry does not lead clinicians directly to an etiological diagnosis. Spirometry requires cooperation between the subject and the examiner, and the results obtained will depend on technical as well as personal factors. In children, the spirometry is recommended to be performed from the age of 3–5 years depending on the child's psychomotor development (ability to follow instructions and coordinate breathing) and experiences and skills of the examiner. Naturally, the success rate of spirometry in the preschoolers is much lower than in older children.

During spirometry, several maneuvers may be performed, which will answer various clinical questions:

- forced vital capacity (FVC) and forced expiratory volume in 1-s (FEV1);maneuver—derivation of maximum effort flow-volume curve;
- slow vital capacity (sVC) and inspiratory capacity (IC) maneuver;
- peak expiratory flow (PEF);
- maximum voluntary ventilation (MVV).

Details of the previously mentioned examinations may be found in ERS/ATS document [6]. Technical demands for the devices, guidelines for quality control and reporting may be found also in previously mentioned ATS/ERS document.

3.2.1. Diagnostic use of results

In principle, there are two main types of lung diseases, the so-called obstructive and restrictive ones. Both types lead to changes in ventilation and are reflected by specific spirometric parameters.

Figure 1 shows the usual shape of the expiratory limb of the maximum effort flow-volume curve (MEFV) as well as the physiologic time-volume tracing found in healthy individuals.

In case of a restrictive disorder, the velocity of expiration is usually normal, but there is a reduction in pulmonary volumes (**Figure 2**). Both the FVC and FEV1 parameters are reduced, and their reduction is proportional leading to normal FEV1/FVC index (the so-called Tiffeneau index is within the norm for the patient's age).

Contrarily, the obstructive disorder (**Figure 3**) is characterized by a decreased expiratory velocity, and lung volumes are usually preserved. In case of severe or complicated obstruction, air trapping and hyperinflation may occur, both leading to a secondary decrease in FVC. The typical finding of obstructive ventilation disorder is therefore a reduced FEV1, FVC is normal or decreased disproportionately to FEV1, resulting in a reduction of the Tiffeneau index mentioned earlier.

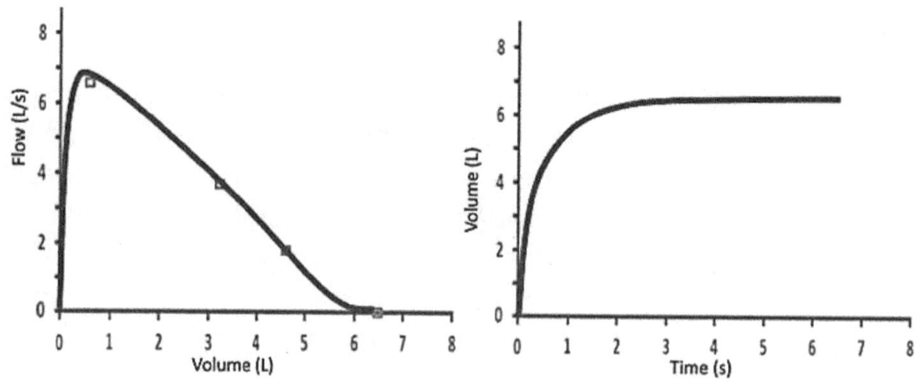

Figure 1. Typical shapes and values of breathing curves (taken from [7]).

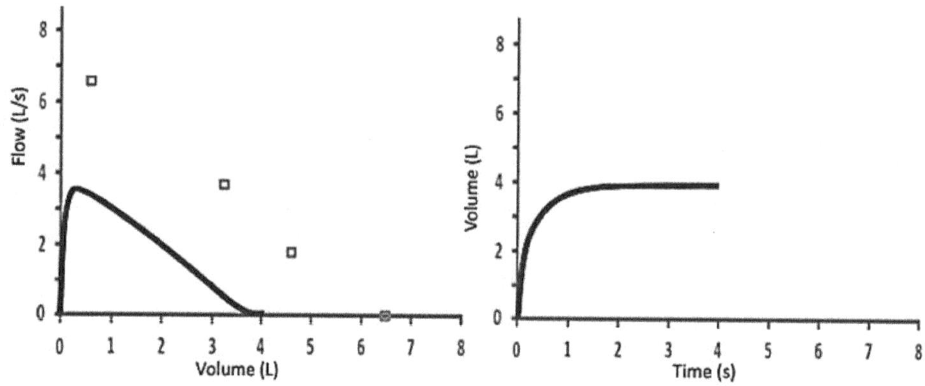

Figure 2. The effect of restriction disorder (taken from [7]).

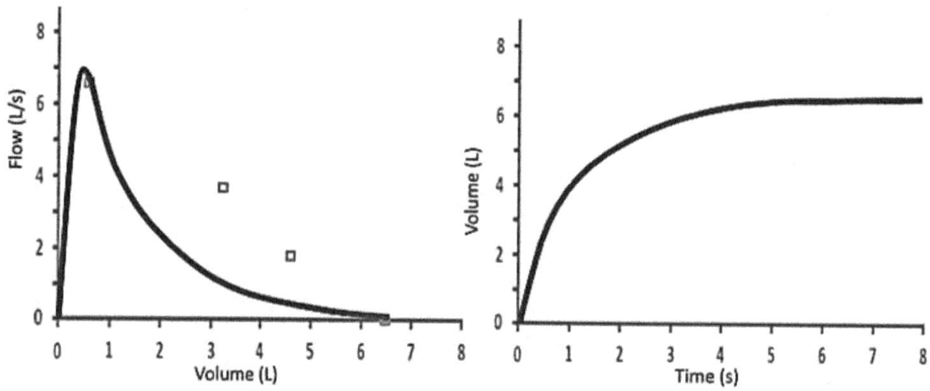

Figure 3. The effect of obstructive disorder (taken from [7]).

When interpreting the spirometry results, one should bear in mind that the complete assessment of pulmonary volumes is possible only using body plethysmography (or dilution techniques). After that, obstructive and restrictive ventilation disorders can be reliably distinguished. The optimal lung function interpretation strategy proposed by ATS/ERS task force is shown in **Figure 4**.

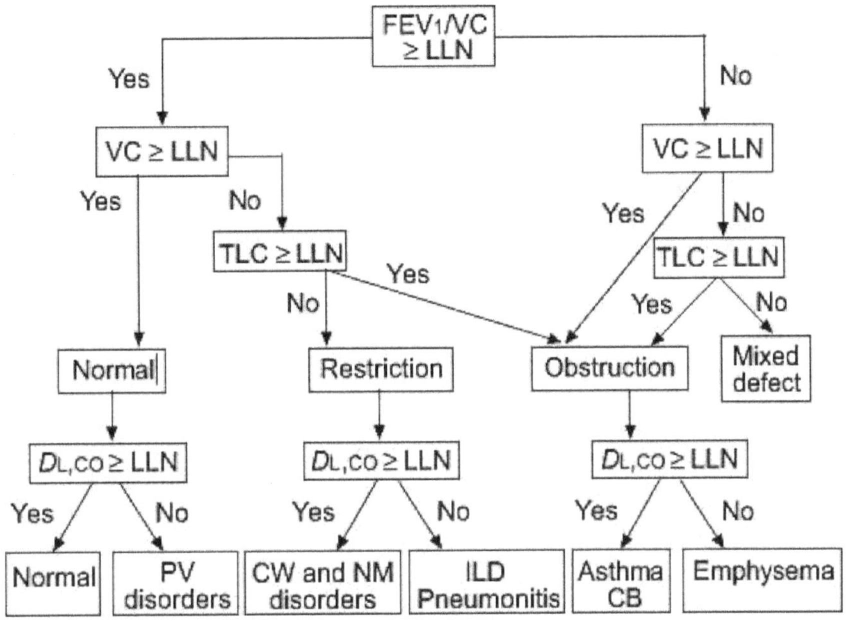

Figure 4. Algorithm for diagnostic evaluation of spirometry (taken from [8]). VC, vital capacity; LLN, lower limits of normal; FEV1, expiratory volume in 1 s; TLC, total lung capacity; $D_{L,CO}$, diffusing capacity for carbon monoxide; CW, chest wall; NM, neuromuscular; ILD, interstitial lung diseases; CB, chronic bronchitis.

As mentioned earlier, the information obtained from the simple spirometry is sufficient to raise only suspicion on the disease. The final diagnosis always needs to be confirmed by other methods (see subsequent subchapters) or by spirometry performed under specific conditions —the so-called bronchomotoric tests. They include bronchodilating test—that is, evaluation of airway obstruction after bronchodilator administration—usually beta-2-mimetics. If bronchial hyperresponsiveness needs to be evaluated, bronchoconstrictive test with direct or indirect stimuli capable of induction of bronchospasm may be used. The most commonly used bronchoprovocative stimuli include methacholine, histamine, mannitol, dry and cold cough, or physical activity.

3.3. Whole-body plethysmography

According to the definition, the whole-body plethysmography is a diagnostic method based on the measurement of volume changes of the patient's body during respiration. Applied to pulmonary function testing, it allows to determine the total pulmonary capacity (TLC) and all its components including indirectly measurable volumes. Similar to the spirometry, the results are significantly affected by conditions of measurement and their history before it. That is why it is generally not allowed to smoke, to eat heavy foods, to drink alcohol, to have an excessive physical activity, and so on, before this examination. The examination takes place in an airtight box. The patient stands or sits inside and breathes through the mouthpiece and the nose is closed by a pin. The examination proceeds in two phases (specific airway resistance measurement—performed with opened shutter and FRC measurement—inspiration and expiration against the closed shutter). A schematic derivation of the respective parameters is shown in **Figure 5**.

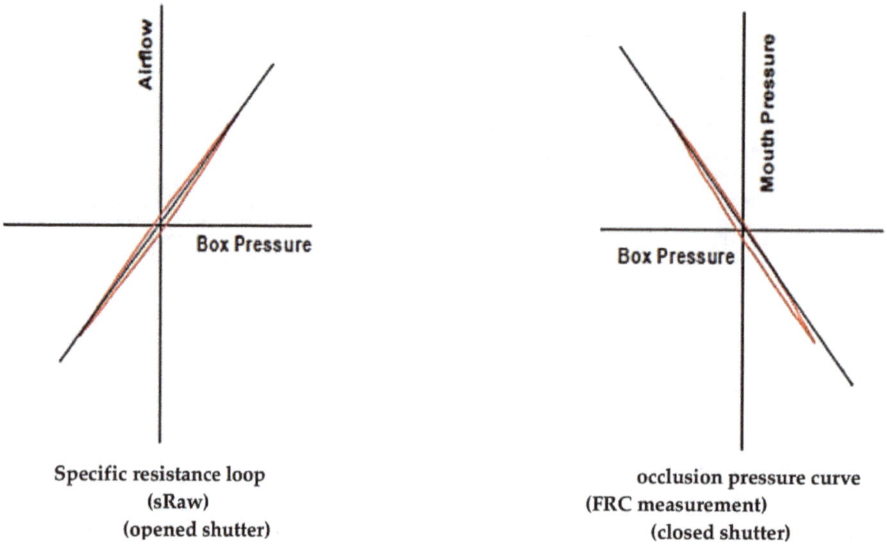

Figure 5. Output curves of plethysmography (taken from [9]).

3.3.1. *Diagnostic use of results*

As mentioned earlier, body plethysmography allows the evaluation of indirectly measurable pulmonary volumes and capacities—that is, residual volume (RV), functional residual capacity (FRC), and total lung capacity (TLC). They allow conducting a definitive diagnosis of restrictive lung disorder. In addition, it is possible to assess respiratory tract resistance (Raw) —important for airway obstruction assessment.

The quantification of the given parameter is performed using the inclination of the given curve/loop. The shape of specific resistance loop is also of a significant diagnostic value—it can indicate the localization of the obstruction within air passages (**Figure 6**).

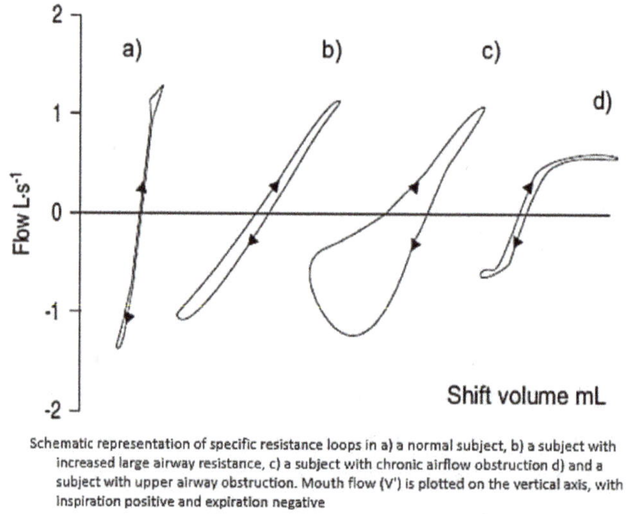

Figure 6. Typical shapes of specific resistance loops (taken from [9]). Note: the pressure in the box on the horizontal axis is replaced by the corresponding volume change of the air in the box.

Figure 7 shows a typical finding in a healthy individual, a patient with obstructive and restrictive disorder, respectively.

3.4. Dilution techniques

Dilution techniques represent complementary method to the abovementioned functional examinations. Similar to the body plethysmography, they enable to evaluate indirectly measured volumes and pulmonary capacities (RV, FRC, and TLC). In principle, two modifications of this method are available—the closed variant using Fick's principle and the opened method (e.g., multiple-breath inert gas washout test). In the diagnostics of bronchial obstruction and asthma, these methods give only complementary information.

3.5. Impulse oscillometry

Impulse oscillometry (IOS) is one of the modifications of forced oscillation techniques (FOTs). It is a noninvasive diagnostic method which is performed during tidal breathing and is based on the superimposition of external pressure signals on the patient's tidal breathing. In a simplified way, we can say that the whole respiratory tract including air in the airway is forced by external pulses of different course in time to oscillate. The behaviour of the respiratory tract is then described by several variables (resistance, reactance, inertance, and elastance) which allow assessing mechanical properties of the respiratory tract and its components (airways, lung parenchyma, and chest wall). To get reliable results, it is necessary only to ensure a regular breath pattern (no specific breathing maneuvers are required). The examination can thus be performed in all age categories of patients.

The following parameters are evaluated when interpreting IOS results:

- respiratory tract resistance (R_{rs}) and its frequency dependence,
- respiratory tract reactivity (X_{rs}) and its frequency dependence,
- auxiliary parameters (resonant frequency—F_{res}, volume dependence of Z_{rs} impedance, and others).

The outcome of the examination gives information about the resistance of the central and peripheral airways. Further, it also gives an overview of the mechanical properties of the respiratory tract. It should be noted that basic IOS examination (i.e., without specific breathing maneuvers) does not provide any information on lung volumes.

In conclusion, IOS is a suitable method for the diagnostics of bronchial obstruction in noncooperative and poorly cooperative patients.

3.6. Fractional exhaled nitric oxide (FeNO)

Measuring the fraction of nitric oxide in exhaled breath is relatively new and promising tool assisting conventional lung function testing in asthma diagnostics and phenol/endotype classification. Nitric oxide is an important mediator with plenty of different functions; when

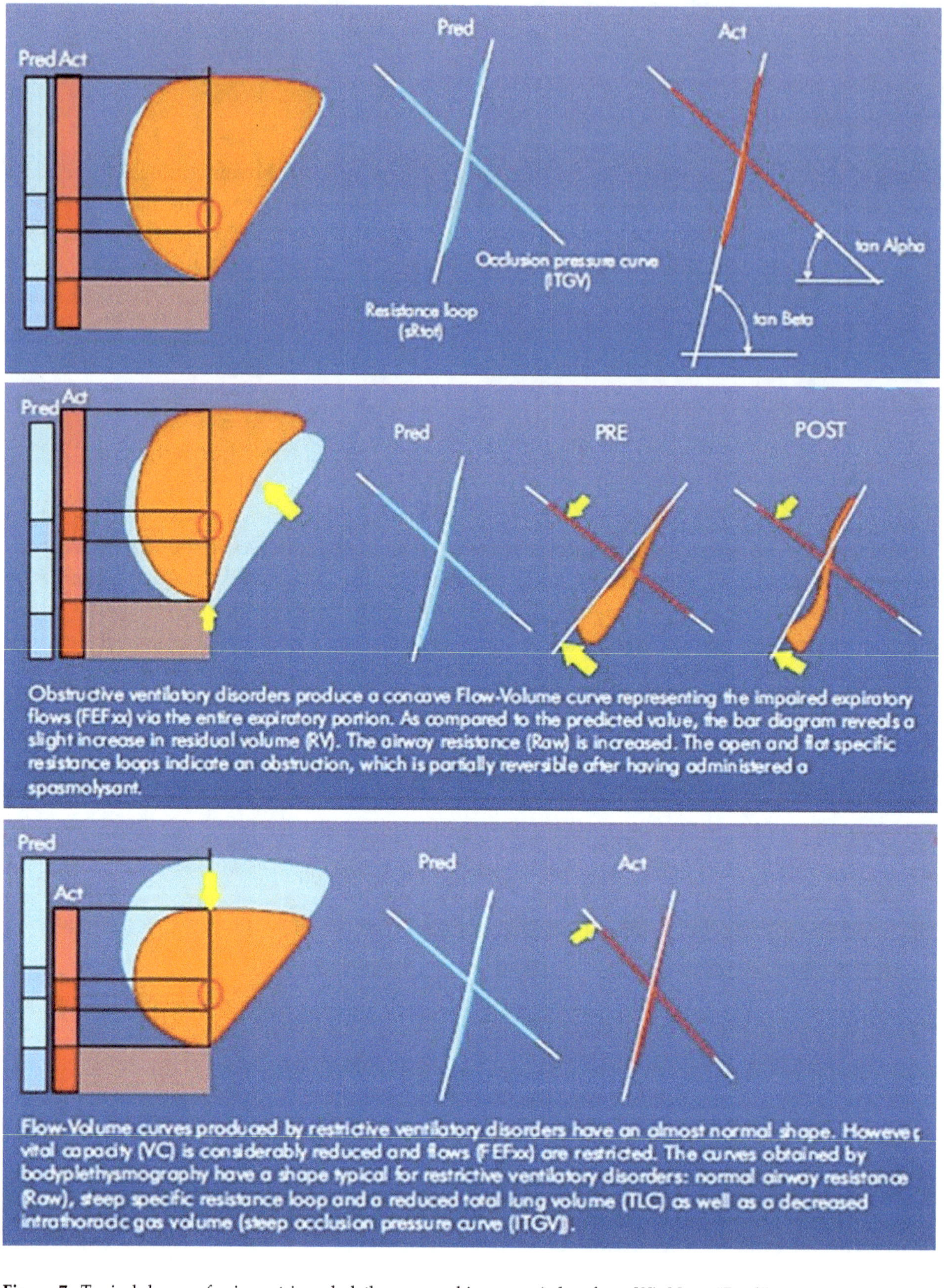

Figure 7. Typical shapes of spirometric and plethysmographic curves (taken from [9]). Note: "Pred" means predicted and "Act" means actual value or shape of the followed-up parameter.

assessed in exhaled air, it reflects the allergic airway disease, more precisely the activity of eosinophilic inflammation. While symptoms and lung function assess the pathogenetical mechanisms of allergic asthma indirectly, FeNO measurement reflects directly the activity of this inflammation. It is strongly and positively correlated with eosinophils in airway wall, bronchoalveolar lavage fluid, and induced sputum. As a noninvasive tool, it may greatly contribute to the diagnostics of allergic/eosinophilic phenotype of asthma [10].

Currently, there exist various modifications of FeNO-measuring systems including online and offline variants. Principally, there exist single- and multiple-breath approaches, both having its advantages and disadvantages. Technical aspects of these methods have been reviewed elsewhere [11]. FeNO measurements may be successfully performed in young children as well [12]. Modifications for infants are also available.

There is sufficient evidence about the usefulness of FeNO in clinical setting—especially in patients with asthma. FeNO measurements are highly correlated with eosinophilic airway inflammation, and as this type of inflammation positively responds to steroid treatment, it can guide the therapy. High levels of FeNO predict steroid responsiveness. Moreover, it can predict the relapse of asthma symptoms after steroid treatment withdrawal [13].

To conclude, we highlight the role of FeNO measurement in both asthma diagnostics and phenol/endotype classification. It may be regarded as an "inflamometer," as though this tool should be available to the pulmonologist managing asthma patients.

3.7. Lung function testing in infants, toddlers, and preschoolers

According to GINA 2017 [1], lung function testing (spirometry) is recommended for patients older than 4–5 years when setting the diagnosis of asthma and for long-time follow-up. As children younger than 3–4 years are usually not capable of performing acceptable trials of maximum effort flow-volume curve, alternative methods are used to objectify their lung function. These methods (infant pulmonary function testing—IPF) are not widely available, and their clinical impact remains unclear [14, 15]. However, based on the authors' experiences, IPF may be of a clinical benefit in the management of infants with recurrent wheeze.

Currently, there exist a number of commercially available methods assessing different aspects of lung function (**Table 1**). These methods require tidal breathing and face-mask tolerance; consequently, they are performed under light sedation (chloral hydrate). Generally, they are considered to be safe and well tolerated. Principally, it is also possible to perform bronchomotoric test in infants using various methods of IPF. Their limitations include the need of prolonged sedation (at least 30 min of quite sleep) to conclude the subsequent testing, various technical problems (no commercially available equipment for such testing), and the need of knowledge of the short-term variability of the respective parameters. In author's lung function laboratory, bronchodilator test with salbutamol is routinely performed with valuable clinical implications. To our knowledge, there is no laboratory performing bronchoconstrictive tests in infants on regular basis.

Method	Outcome	Parameter
1. Bodypletysmography	Lung volume	Functional residual capacity (FRC)
	Central airway obstruction	Airway resistance (Reff)
2. TidalBreathAnalysis	Ventilation	Minute ventilation
	Peripheral airway obstruction	Shape of the FV curve, tPTEF/tE
3. Resistance-Compliance	Mechanic properties of respiratory tract	Compliance (Crs)
		Resistance (Rrs)
4. Thoracoabdominal compression	Peripheral airway obstruction	Maximal flow at the FRC level
	Ventilatory reserve, airway collapse	Shape of the FV curve
5. Raised volume thoracoabdominal compression	Additionally to 4.: Lung volumes	Total lung capacity (TLC), vital capacity (VC)
6. Multiple breath washout test	Lung volume	Functional residual capacity (FRC)
	Ventilation inhomogeneity (most peripheral airway obstruction)	Lung clearance index (LCI)

Table 1. Summary of lung function methods intended for patients with limited cooperation and their outcome parameters.

The contribution of IPF in asthma diagnostics includes the detection of airway obstruction, its localization (peripheral or central airways), its quantification (mild, moderate, and severe) and reversibility (reaction on salbutamol). In addition, consequences of bronchial obstruction such as hyperinflation, ventilation inhomogeneity, and changes in breathing pattern may be detected as well.

4. Utilization of advanced methods for processing of audio signals

Together with the development of possibilities and availability of computer technology, the possibilities of using exact computational methods of signal processing grow both in basic research and in the field of practical problems. From a number of methods available, we prefer the harmonic analysis. The outcomes of all available methods are similar likely due to the demand for easy interpretation of results to physicians or patients. We describe the given approach on the basis of the Fourier transform analysis, where we have achieved the most convincing results so far.

4.1. Background

The validity and reliability of outputs of the advanced sound analysis significantly increases with the quality of the input data. It is also advantageous to know what frequencies are important to look for and what their presence means from both diagnostic and technical point of view.

The most specific issue is created by pediatric patients, where the quality of respiratory sound can also be affected by the size of the patient body. Children have a distinct quality of lung sounds, which is generally attributed to acoustic transmission through smaller lungs and thinner chest walls. Acoustic measurements have shown higher median frequencies of normal lung sounds in infants than in older children and adults [16]. Scientific studies show that higher median frequencies in infants were explained by lower power at low frequencies, while the decrease in power toward higher frequencies was similar at all ages (infants, children, and adults) [17].

4.2. Physical principle of sound in the airways

The harmonic analysis is a mathematical apparatus for processing the oscillating periodic signal, which the sound also is. Sound is an oscillation of acoustic pressure, which propagates by space. The oscillation of acoustic pressure is composed of many sine oscillations characterized by various frequencies. A timbre and character of sound detectable by human ear originates from the number of oscillated frequencies. The sound composed of the integer multiples of the base frequency (the lowest frequency) with a clearly defined period is perceived as a musical tone. On the contrary, the sound including the noninteger multiples of the base frequency and without a clearly defined period is perceived as noise [18].

The respiratory sound, which is caused by airflow in airways, is sound in a frequency range from 20 to 2000 Hz and higher. However, it can still be detected at or above 2000 Hz with proper sensitive microphones in a quiet room according to our experience [16, 17, 19]. The normal lung sound spectrum is devoid of discrete peaks and is not musical [18].

One of the manifestations of asthma and other respiratory diseases is bronchial obstruction. Such a narrowing of the air passages causes a vibration and turbulence of the airflow, which results in the change of the sound manifestation of breath. This change of sound, which is manifested by the presence of wheezing and crackles, can be detected by listening using the phonendoscope. For wheezing, the frequencies in the range of 300–1000 Hz with higher amplitudes in comparison with neighboring areas are typical [20]. The duration of these areas is normally from 0.5 to 0.75 s. These searched phenomena in the respiratory sound could be emphasized using an intensive respiration caused, for example, by physical activity [20–23].

4.3. Harmonic analysis and Fourier transform

Using harmonic analysis, such a sound can be decomposed and particular frequencies of mentioned sine oscillation can be searched. Thus, the important frequencies of wheezes can be discovered too. The visualized result of the Fourier transform is called the frequency spectrum [18] and its example is shown in **Figure 8**.

Figure 8 shows the frequency spectrum of analyzed music sound in a defined time range—the horizontal axis is a frequency scale and it indicates harmonic frequencies in this sound; the vertical axis indicates an amplitude level of every frequency in the sound. The frequencies can be clearly defined in this case because the analyzed sound is a mentioned musical sound.

For illustrative interpretation of the outputs of harmonic analyzes, we have developed our own software. The software operates on the principle of mentioned Fast Fourier Transform using Matlab background and creates frequency spectra throughout the length of the analyzed recording, working with defined time intervals [22]. The length of the time intervals corresponds to the duration of wheezing approximately. For better clarity of outcomes of performed analysis, a specific suitable color scaling for frequencies in the obtained frequency spectra was applied [21, 22]. Then, every level of amplitude is defined by one concrete color (**Figure 9**).

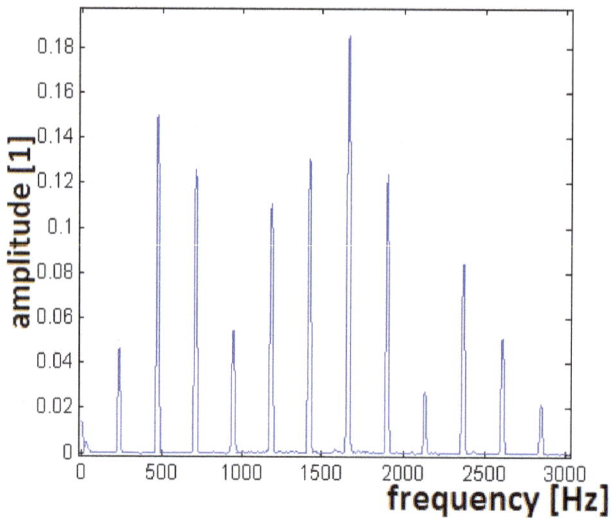

Figure 8. Illustration of frequency spectrum.

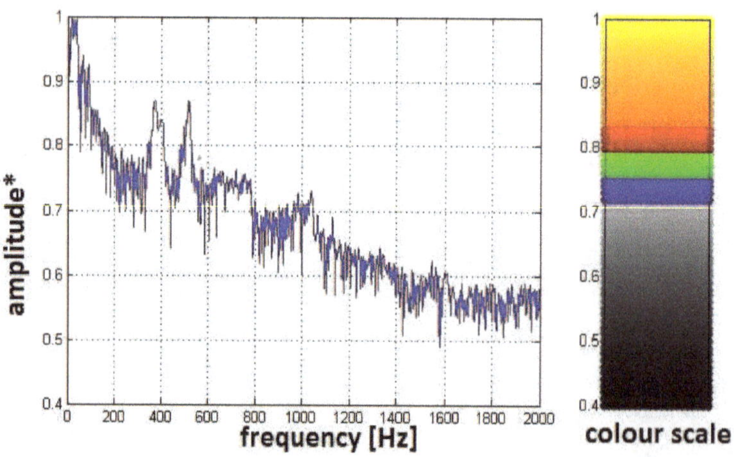

Figure 9. Color scaling of obtained frequencies. The color scale matches special colors according to values of all amplitudes.

Finally, the colored data were rearranged back to the time line of original recording (**Figure 10**).

By this approach, the oscillations of acoustic pressure are presented by the progression of the frequency spectra of the sound recording in time (**Figure 10**). Such a method of sound-recording acquisition of patients' breath, which is required for frequency spectrum creation and for the detection of wheezing in this spectrum, is completely noninvasive and without the need of cooperation of patient.

4.4. Our experimental work

While looking for a way of how to utilize the harmonic analysis in auscultation examinations most effectively, we have performed relatively large set of experiments. The main part of the work includes data collection. Based on these data, we have verified and modified the properties of our method to best suit our purpose. All audio recordings of respiratory sounds were obtained in collaboration with the Department of Pneumology in UH Motol.

The following text is focused on the part of our study, which was attended by nine volunteer patients with asthma aged from 9 to 18 years. It is a relatively homogeneous group in terms of diagnosis and clinical manifestations. In this group, it was also possible to perform the generally respected spirometric examination for subsequent result comparison.

4.4.1. Instrumentation

The usual commercially available electronic phonendoscope Littmann 3200 recording the heard respiratory sound was utilized in the study. The instrument digitizes the recording with a sampling frequency of 4000 Hz and allows the application of a specific input filtration. The

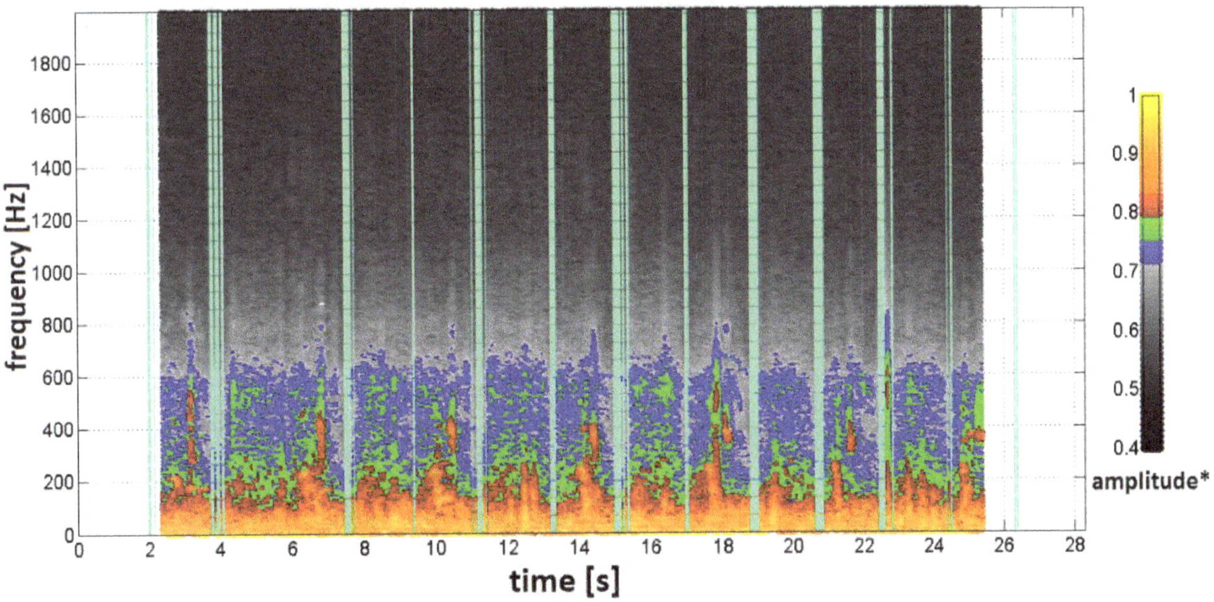

Figure 10. The frequency spectrum of sound recording of patient's breath. The pale blue vertical lines indicate moment of transitions between inspiration and expiration phase. The lines repeat in 2-s time interval. It corresponds to the length of respiratory cycle (inspiration + expiration) for ordinary human in defined age [21].

manufacturer does not provide any information about the sensitivity of the device, but guarantees that the limiting factor in the evaluation of the recordings will always be the auditory organ of the listener and not the sensitivity of the instrument.

4.4.2. Measurement protocol

The quality of respiratory sound recording is affected by location, where the sound was recorded [20, 22–24]. Probably, the best location for respiratory sound recording is on the back on paravertebral line on the right and left side (lung lobes in **Figure 11a** and **b**) and on jugulum (**Figure 11c**). The sound with frequencies up to 600 Hz goes through lung parenchyma better than the sound with frequencies over 600 Hz. These frequencies could be detected better on jugulum.

The recordings were acquired in the examination of patients during restful and deep breathing, which was induced by light physical load (10–15 squats) according to instructions and under the supervision of the attending physician.

4.5. Results

Data processing followed the procedure described in Chapter 4.3. In all patients included in our study, specific artifacts (**Figure 12**, black-circled areas) appeared in the expiration phases. In two of those cases, these artifacts were not listened by experienced physicians just as a result of their extinction within the other recorded noise. Data processed so far indicated that in asthmatic patients, there are clearly visible manifestations of the obstruction in the expiration phases in the frequency ranging from approximately 400 to 600 Hz, regardless of whether they are identifiable by listening or only through our analysis.

Even the control records of healthy volunteers are not without interest. From **Figure 13**, it is well seen that they show significantly lower level of noise compared to the asthmatic patients in all of the breathing phases.

It is worth noting that there are vertical pale blue lines indicating the transitions between inspiration and expiration. These lines were also determined automatically by applying a harmonic analysis with the use of the fact that the airflow stops at that moment [21].

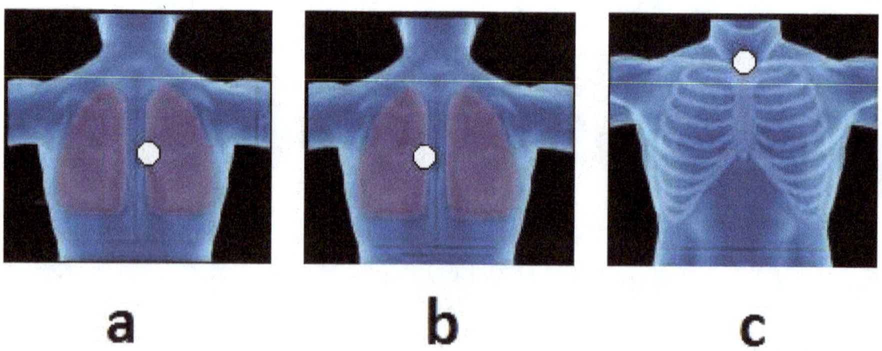

Figure 11. Locations for sound recording.

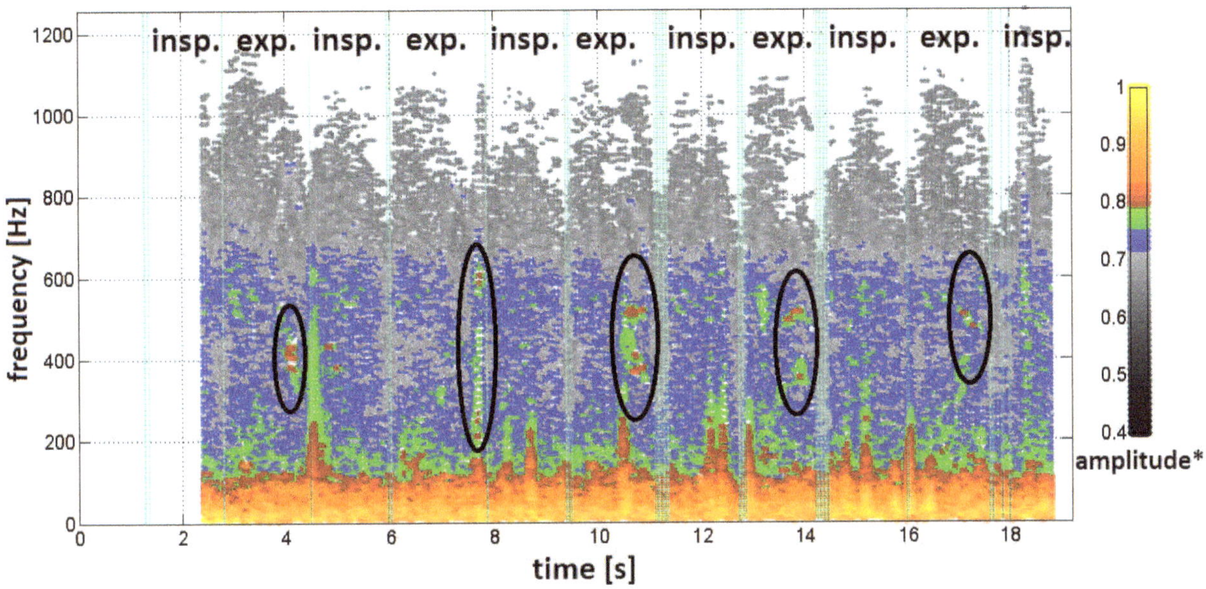

Figure 12. Development of amplitude and frequency spectrum of an asthmatic patient.

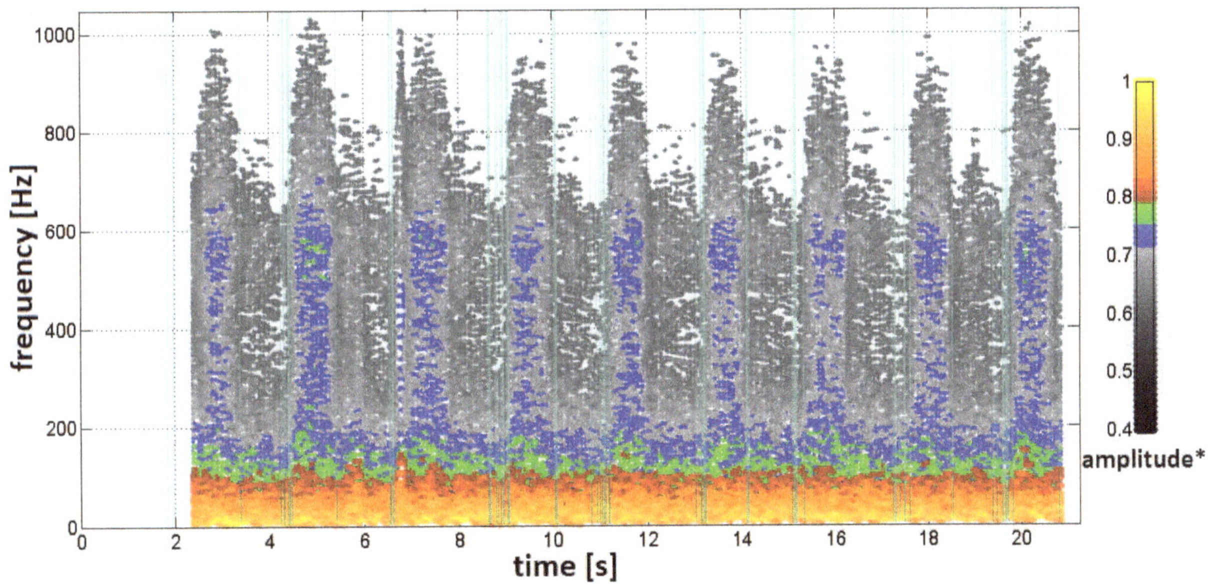

Figure 13. Development of amplitude and frequency spectrum of a healthy volunteer.

5. Conclusion

Data processed so far show that—despite the relatively simple technique used—the audio display provides valuable diagnostic information. Furthermore, using a suitable method, this information can easily be detected in the record through specific sound phenomena despite other sounds in the record. Therefore, we believe that research focused on alternative complementary methods has its importance—it can provide solutions in cases where other commonly observed methods fail or are complicated to be applied.

Acknowledgements

This text is supported by Progres Q41 grant.

Author details

Frantisek Lopot[1,4], Vaclav Koucky[2,4], Daniel Hadraba[1,3,4], David Skalicky[1,4]* and Karel Jelen[1,4]

*Address all correspondence to: skalickydavid@seznam.cz

1 Department of Anatomy and Biomechanics, Faculty of Sports and Physical Education, Charles University, Praha, Czech Republic

2 Second Faculty of Medicine, Charles University, Praha, Czech Republic

3 Department of Paediatrics, University Hospital Motol, Praha, Czech Republic

4 Department of Biomathematics, Institute of Physiology, Czech Academy of Sciences, Praha, Czech Republic

References

[1] Global Initiative for Asthma. Global Strategy for Asthma Management and Prevention. 2017. Available from: www.ginasthma.org

[2] Henderson JA. Childhood asthma phenotypes in the twenty-first century. Breathe. 2014; **10**:100-108. DOI: 10.1183/20734735.014613

[3] Brand PL, Baraldi E, Bisgaard H, Boner AL, Castro-Rodriguez JA, Custovic A, de Blic J, de Jongste JC, Eber E, Everard ML, Frey U, Gappa M, Garcia-Marcos L, Grigg J, Lenney W, Le Souëf P, McKenzie S, Merkus PJ, Midulla F, Paton JY, Piacentini G, Pohunek P, Rossi GA, Seddon P, Silverman M, Sly PD, Stick S, Valiulis A, van Aalderen WM, Wildhaber JH, Wennergren G, Wilson N, Zivkovic Z, Bush A. Definition, assessment and treatment of wheezing disorders in preschool children: An evidence-based approach. The European Respiratory Journal. Oct 2008;**32**(4):1096-1110. DOI: 10.1183/09031936.00002108

[4] Pasterkamp H, Brand PL, Everard M, Garcia-Marcos L, Melbye H, Priftis KN. Towards the standardisation of lung sound nomenclature. The European Respiratory Journal. Mar 2016;**47**(3):724-732. DOI: 10.1183/13993003.01132-2015. Epub Dec 2, 2015

[5] Reference Database of Respiratory Sounds—Wheezes. European Respiratory Society [online]. Available from: http://www.ers-education.org/e-learning/reference-database-of-respiratory-sounds.aspx [Accessed: 2017-01-10]

[6] Miller MR, Hankinson J, Brusasco V, Burgos F, Casaburi R, Coates A, Crapo R, Enright P, van der Grinten CP, Gustafsson P, Jensen R, Johnson DC, MacIntyre N, McKay R, Navajas D, Pedersen OF, Pellegrino R, Viegi G, Wanger J. ATS/ERS task force. Standardisation of spirometry. The European Respiratory Journal. Aug 2005;**26**(2):319-338

[7] Burgos F, Giner J. Spirometry Course, SIBELMED Barcelona [online]. 2015. Available from: http://slideplayer.com/slide/8897191/ [cit: 2017-01-014]

[8] Pellegrino R, Viegi G, Brusasco V, Crapo RO, Burgos F, Casaburi R, Coates A, van der Grinten CP, Gustafsson P, Hankinson J, Jensen R, Johnson DC, MacIntyre N, McKay R, Miller MR, Navajas D, Pedersen OF, Wanger J. Interpretative strategies for lung function tests. The European Respiratory Journal. Nov 2005;**26**(5):948-968

[9] Hossam EM. Body Plethysmography, AinShams University [online]. Available from: http://slideplayer.com/slide/6664818/ [cit: 2017-01-014]

[10] Taylor DR, Pijnenburg MW, Smith AD, De Jongste JC. Exhaled nitric oxide measurements: Clinical application and interpretation. Thorax. Sep 2006;**61**(9):817-827

[11] American Thoracic Society; European Respiratory Society. ATS/ERS recommendations for standardized procedures for the online and offline measurement of exhaled lower respiratory nitric oxide and nasal nitric oxide, 2005. American Journal of Respiratory and Critical Care Medicine. Apr 15, 2005;**171**(8):912-930

[12] Baraldi E, de Jongste JC, Gaston B, Alving K, Barnes PJ, Bisgaard H, Bush A, Gaultier C, Grasemann H, Hunt JF, Kissoon N, Piacentini GL, Ratjen F, Silkoff P, Stick S, European Respiratory Society/American Thoracic Society (ERS/ATS) Task Force. Measurement of exhaled nitric oxide in children, 2001. The European Respiratory Journal. Jul 2002;**20**(1): 223-237

[13] Pijnenburg MW, Hofhuis W, Hop WC, De Jongste JC. Exhaled nitric oxide predicts asthma relapse in children with clinical asthma remission. Thorax. Mar 2005;**60**(3):215-218

[14] Godfrey S, Bar-Yishay E, Avital A, Springer C, Peterson-Carmichael SL, Rosenfeld M, Ascher SB, Hornik CP, Arets HG, Davis SD, Hall GL. Survey of clinical infant lung function testing practices. Pediatric Pulmonology. Feb 2014;**49**(2):126-131

[15] Rosenfeld M, Allen J, Arets BH, Aurora P, Beydon N, Calogero C, et al. An official American Thoracic Society workshop report: Optimal lung function tests for monitoring cystic fibrosis, bronchopulmonary dysplasia, and recurrent wheezing in children less than 6 years of age. Annals of the American Thoracic Society. 2013;**10**:S1-S11

[16] Beck R, Elias N, Shoval S, Tov N, Talmon G, Godfrey S, Bentur L. Computerized acoustic assessment of treatment efficacy of nebulized epinephrine and albuterol in RSV bronchiolitis. BMC Pediatrics. **7**(1):22. DOI: 10.1186/1471-2431-7-22. ISSN 14712431 [online]. Available from: http://bmcpediatr.biomedcentral.com/articles/10.1186/1471-2431-7-22 [cit: 2016-05-01]

[17] Pasterkamp H, Kraman SS, Wodicka GR. Respiratory sounds. American Journal of Respiratory and Critical Care Medicine. 1997;**156**(3):974-987. DOI: 10.1164/ajrccm.156.3.9701115. ISSN 1073-449x [online]. Available from: http://www.atsjournals.org/doi/abs/10.1164/ajrccm.156.3.9701115 [cit: 2016-05-01]

[18] Syrový V. Hudební akustika. 3rd ed. Praze: Akademie múzických umění; 2013. Akustická knihovna Hudební fakulty AMU. ISBN 978-80-7331-297-8

[19] Kraman SS, Wodicka GR, Pressler GA, Pasterkamp H. Comparison of lung sound transducers using a bioacoustics transducer testing system. Journal of Applied Physiology. 2006; **101**(2):469-476. DOI: 10.1152/japplphysiol.00273.2006. ISSN 8750-7587 [online]. Available from: http://jap.physiology.org/cgi/doi/10.1152/japplphysiol.00273.2006 [cit: 2016-05-01]

[20] Ayres JG. Astma. Praha: Grada; 2001. Informace a rady lékaře. ISBN 80-247-0091-3

[21] Skalický D, Lopot F, Koucký V, Kubový P, Pohunek P, Zoul V. Respiratory sounds as a source of information in asthma diagnosis. Lekar a technika – Clinician and Technology. 2017;**47**(2):56-59. ISSN 0301-5491 (Print), 2336-5552 (Online). Available from: https://ojs.cvut.cz/ojs/index.php/CTJ/article/view/4419

[22] Skalický D. Využití elektronického fonendoskopu v diagnostice astmatu. Praha. Diplomová práce. ČESKÉ VYSOKÉ UČENÍ TECHNICKÉ v Praze; 2016

[23] Teřl M, Pohunek P, editors. Strategie diagnostiky, prevence a léčby astmatu: uvedení globální strategie do praxe v ČR. 1st ed. Praha: Jalna; 2012. ISBN 978-80-86396-67-5

[24] Silbernagl S, Despopoulos A. Atlas fyziologie člověka. 6th ed. Praha: Grada; 2004. ISBN 978-80-247-0630-6

7

Asthma in the Disadvantaged: A Phenotype in Need of a Personalized, Multidisciplinary Approach to Therapy

Drew A. Harris, Caitlin Welch, Morgan Soper and Yun Michael Shim

Abstract

Most patients with asthma can be managed with standardized, traditional therapies; however, 5–10% of patients suffer from disease that is difficult to control. Uncontrolled asthma disproportionally affects low income and racial minority patients. The disadvantaged asthma phenotype is defined by the presence of overlapping social, economic and environmental factors. These factors, such as environmental exposures in substandard housing or suboptimal adherence to controller therapy due to impaired health literacy are challenging to address in the clinic or inpatient setting. Personalized management of the disadvantaged asthma phenotype must target these interconnected factors through a multidisciplinary approach that includes longitudinal collaboration with community-based organizations, social workers and legal aid.

Keywords: asthma phenotypes, vulnerable populations, asthma disparities, health equity, social determinants of health

1. Introduction

1.1. Health disparities in asthma

Asthma is a heterogeneous clinical syndrome centered on symptoms of dyspnea, cough, wheezing or chest tightness, along with reversible expiratory airway obstruction or bronchial hyperresponsiveness. Although asthma affects 5–10% of the world's population, asthma disproportionally impacts communities of color and the socioeconomically disadvantaged.

In adults, asthma is more common in non-Hispanic blacks (8.7%) and Puerto Ricans (13.3%) than in whites (7.6%), and asthma-specific mortality is significantly higher in non-Hispanic blacks (25.4 per million, annually) compared to whites (8.8 per million, annually) [1]. In children, the prevalence of asthma is much higher in Puerto Rican Hispanics (19.2%) and non-Hispanic blacks (12.7%) than in whites (8%) or Mexican Americans (6.4%) [2]. Asthma-specific mortality in children is nearly eight times higher in non-Hispanic blacks than in whites [3]. In addition to racial disparities, socioeconomic disparities in asthma outcomes are widespread, with socioeconomically disadvantaged asthmatics less likely to utilize preventative care for asthma and more likely to rely on urgent and emergent health care for asthma [4]. Asthma outcomes are substantially worse for racial minorities with lower socioeconomic status [5].

1.2. The disadvantaged asthma phenotype

The term "asthma" envelops multiple phenotypes of disease. A phenotype is defined by the observable properties produced by the interactions of a genotype and the environment. In recent years, multiple asthma phenotypes have been defined by natural history, clinical and physiological features, biology and biomarkers and response to therapy [6]. Specific asthma phenotypes are important to consider in order to identify a targeted, personalized approach to asthma therapies.

1.3. Social and environmental factors relevant in the disadvantaged asthma phenotype

Numerous social and environmental factors can influence the underlying immunologic and inflammatory processes that define an asthma phenotype. In this chapter, we introduce the disadvantaged asthma patient phenotype, defined by specific genetic, socioeconomic and environmental factors commonly experienced by the disadvantaged asthma patient.

Although genetics play an important role in the susceptibility of African American and Puerto Ricans to poor asthma outcomes [7, 8], race and ethnicity are complex social concepts that are informed by genetic, cultural and historical factors [9]. As such, it is challenging to separate genetic factors from social, cultural and environmental factors driving asthma disparities. Racial and ethnic disparities in asthma are likely due to a combination of genetic factors as well as socioeconomic and environmental determinants of health (see **Figure 1**).

These socioeconomic and environmental factors, such as environmental exposures in substandard housing or suboptimal adherence to controller therapy due to impaired health literacy are challenging to address in the clinic or inpatient setting. Personalized management of the disadvantaged asthma phenotype must target these interconnected factors through a multidisciplinary approach that includes longitudinal collaboration with community-based organizations, social workers and legal aid. This chapter will start with a description of specific socioeconomic and environmental challenges most relevant to identify in the disadvantaged asthma phenotype. Following this, recommendations for a multidisciplinary approach to address modifiable factors and improve asthma outcomes in the disadvantaged asthma patient will be presented.

1.4. Indoor allergens in the disadvantaged patient's home

Racial disparities in allergic sensitization are an important contributor to racial disparities in asthma outcomes. Given the epidemic of allergy that has emerged over the last few decades,

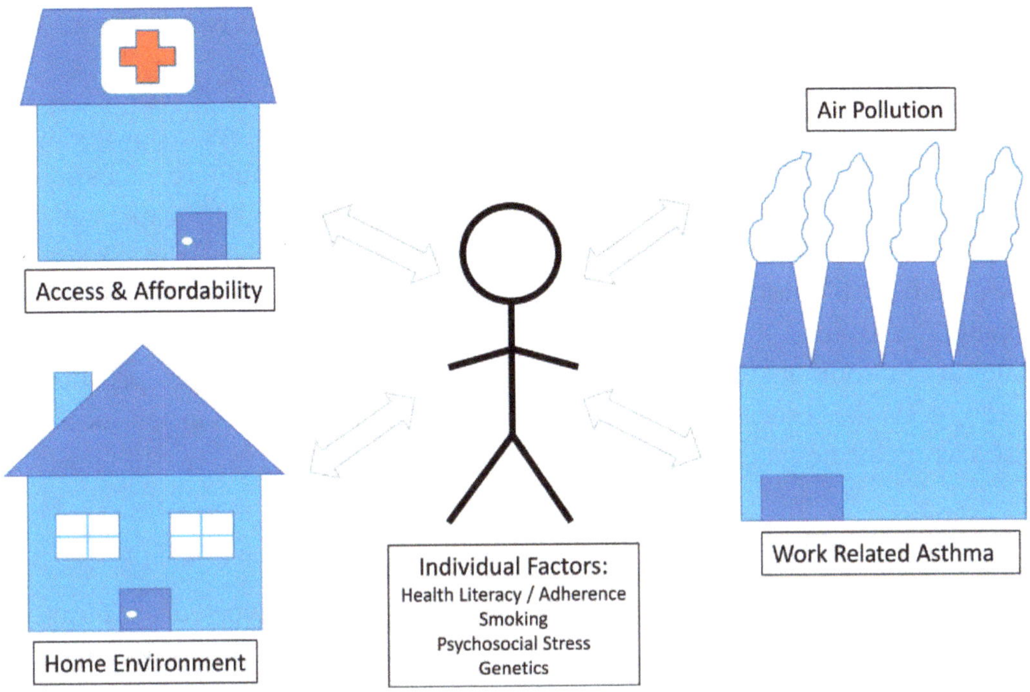

Figure 1. Multiple interconnected factors relevant to the disadvantaged asthma phenotype.

disparities in allergic sensitization are unlikely entirely explained by genetics alone. A combination of environmental exposures and host-susceptibility, such as epigenetic changes and gene-environment interactions, are important mechanisms to consider [10]. Within this context, the home environment is important to consider.

In the US, Black and Hispanic households are more than twice as likely as White households to live in substandard housing [11]. Living in substandard housing leads to increased exposure to indoor allergic asthma triggers such as cockroaches and mice. The increased exposures that racial minorities experience in substandard housing likely contributes to disparities in sensitization [12]. This has been demonstrated in multiple studies including: (1) The National Health and Nutrition Examination Surveys (NHANES) III study of 10,508 individuals, in which non-Hispanic black individuals were more likely than non-Hispanic white individuals to be atopic (62% versus 51.3%, OR = 1.6 95% confidence interval 1.2–1.8) [13]; (2) The Boston Epidemiology of Home Allergens and Asthma study, in which black women were 2.5 times more likely than white women to be sensitized to more than 3 allergens, including dust mite, dog, cat, cockroach, alternaria and aspergillus species [14]; and (3) A study in Hartford Connecticut in which Puerto Rican children with asthma were more likely than white children to be sensitized to indoor allergens such as cockroaches (OR 3.3 95%CI (1.7–6.4) and dust mites (OR 1.7 CI 1.2–2.4) [15].

Sensitization to indoor allergens such as cockroaches [15–17], dust mites [18], animals and the number of positive skin tests to allergens [19] has been associated with increased asthma morbidity and severity. Thus although the interplay between individual genetics and susceptibility to home environmental exposures is not yet fully understood, it is important to consider the exposure to high levels of indoor allergens as well as indoor allergy sensitization in identifying a treatment strategy for patients with a disadvantaged asthma phenotype.

1.5. Considerations for the disadvantaged patient living in a rural environment

Although asthma disparities have traditionally been associated with urban environments, there is increasing recognition that in the US, rural residents suffer from greater poverty and have less medical insurance than those living in urban areas [20]. Rural asthma patients are more likely to have to travel greater distances to travel to health care, which leads to increased asthma morbidity and mortality [21]. Within a month after an emergency room visit for asthma, rural adults are less likely than urban adults to have a follow up office visit for asthma [22]. Given the interconnectedness between poverty, access to care and many of the social and environmental factors discussed in this chapter, it is not surprising that recent evidence suggests that poverty and race, rather than residence in an urban location, are the major risk factors for prevalent asthma [9].

1.6. Work related asthma in the disadvantaged patient

In addition to indoor allergen exposures at home, exposures at work are an important but largely unappreciated determinant of asthma within disadvantaged populations [23]. Work-related asthma occurs in 20–50% of employed asthmatics due to exposures to dusts, fumes, cleaning products, mold, construction debris and temperature extremes [24]. Those who experience work-related asthma are more likely to become unemployed and have lost work time. In the disadvantaged asthma patient, work related asthma can have devastating financial consequences: job insecurity from work-related asthma can lead to worsened asthma measures [25], loss of insurance and healthcare access, and subsequent widened inequities [26]. The economic stress due to the cessation of work or reduced work hours due to asthma symptoms, and subsequent lower incomes can further worsen asthma outcomes [27–31]. Despite the prevalence and importance of work related asthma in disadvantaged populations, work related asthma is often unrecognized by both patients and providers [32].

1.7. Smoking and environmental tobacco smoke in the disadvantaged

Although overall smoking rates of declined in US adults from 20.9% in 2005 to 16.8% in 2014, there remains significant racial and socioeconomic disparities in smoke exposure. Individuals living below poverty (26.3%) smoke more often than those above poverty (15.2%). Households in poverty (36%) are more likely than households above poverty (22%) to have an in-home smoker. African Americans (21.5%), Hispanics (16.2%) and mixed race individuals (24.8%) are much more likely to smoke than Asians (13.3%) or Whites (12.9%) [33].

Cigarette smoking is associated with increased asthma incidence, increased asthma severity, worse asthma related quality of life, and increased risk of asthma hospitalizations [34]. Cigarette smoking may also reduce the responsiveness to inhaled corticosteroids, the cornerstone of controller therapy for asthma [35]. Cigarette smoke can cause divergent inflammatory responses depending on host-factors. Although racial and ethnic differences in susceptibility to tobacco smoke is controversial, African Americans have been shown in several studies to have increased susceptibility to cigarette smoke with worsened lung function [36] and more rapidly progressing lung disease [37] compared to Caucasians.

Environmental tobacco smoke increases risk for new onset asthma, especially in those with a genetic predisposition [38]. Maternal environmental tobacco smoke exposure during pregnancy is associated with childhood asthma, even if the mother does not smoke actively during pregnancy [39]. When exposed in childhood, environmental tobacco smoke is associated with increased asthma symptoms, missed school days, and worsened lung function [40]. Environmental tobacco smoke is further known to increase asthma exacerbations and hospitalizations in both children and adults [41, 42].

1.8. Outdoor air pollution disparities

In numerous studies around the world, lower socioeconomic individuals live in areas with increased air pollution [43–45]. Lower socioeconomic individuals are more susceptible to poor health effects from air pollution; high socioeconomic individuals have access to more resources to protect themselves from exposure to air pollution such as private transportation (versus relying on public transit), indoor versus outdoor work environments, access to climate control, including filtration for indoor environments [45]. In addition, there are racial disparities to outdoor air pollution exposure: even after controlling for urban area size and socioeconomic status, racial minorities are more exposed to outdoor air pollution than whites [46].

Air pollutants, including particulate matter, gases (ozone, nitrogen dioxide and sulfur dioxide) and mixed traffic air pollution cause oxidative injury to airways that leads to inflammation and remodeling which can lead to incident asthma. Air pollution may also increase the risk of sensitization and subsequent inflammatory responses to inhaled outdoor allergens [47]. Asthma is widely accepted to be aggravated by air pollution [48] and more recent evidence suggests air pollution may also contribute to new onset asthma in children [49]. In a study of 10 European cities, 14% of the cases of incident asthma and 15% of all asthma exacerbations were attributed to air pollution near roadways [50].

Given the disparate exposure and susceptibility to outdoor air pollution within the poor and racial minorities, and given the known impact of this exposure on incident asthma and asthma morbidity, air pollution is an important factor to consider in the disadvantaged asthma patient.

1.9. Psychosocial stress: increased in the disadvantaged patient

In the US, racial minorities and the SES disadvantaged experience higher amounts of psychosocial stress [51]. Poor neighborhoods have less shops, banks, health care services and transportation. Residents in these communities must then spend expend a greater amount of time and effort to address basic tasks of living [52]. Lower SES communities have higher community violence and crime rates [53], and greater crowding and exposure to noise [54]. In disadvantaged neighborhoods, smaller social networks [54], and decreased "social capital" (which describes a community's investment in public goods and community services), leads to increased community stress, such as violence [55], and decreased community resilience to stress. Low SES neighborhoods are also less likely to foster facilities for stress outlets such as regular exercise, which may lead to health compromising efforts to cope with stress such as smoking and substance abuse [52].

Although psychosocial stress is commonly associated with disorders that cause significant respiratory distress, such as vocal cord dysfunction [56], stress can also affect individual biology, disease progression and management of asthma [57]. Stress has been linked to increased asthma expression [58]. An acute stress may increase the risk of asthma exacerbations through an enhanced Th2 immune response [59]. Chronic stress potentiates airway reactivity and inflammatory response to asthma triggers, such as allergens and infections [58, 60]. Increased inflammatory cytokines (IL4, IL5, IFN-Gamma) and increased asthma symptoms have been linked to acute stressful events in children who also have chronic stress [61]. Chronic stress increases susceptibility to environmental pollutants on incident asthma [62, 63]. Stress reduces expression of the B2-adrenergic receptor, and in turn reduces response to bronchodilators, a cornerstone of asthma management [64].

In some studies, stress has been an even stronger risk factor than environmental exposures for asthma morbidity [65]. Multiple sources of stress, commonplace in the disadvantaged asthma patient, have been associated with increased asthma morbidity.

Although housing stress can lead to increased environmental exposures, an often-overlooked health effect of living in substandard housing is the deprivation, disadvantage, and emotional toll experienced by asthmatics and their households [66].

Housing stressors, including housing insecurity, inability to pay rent, living without heat or electricity, or trouble with a landlord has been shown to worsen asthma morbidity [67, 68]. Stress related to immigration and acculturation factors has also shown to worsen asthma morbidity and increase emergency room utilization for asthma [69]. Intimate partner violence has been shown to increase asthma incidence in affected families [70]. Individuals who experience higher severity of food insecurity develop worse asthma symptoms [71]. Stress related to perceived discrimination has also been shown to affect asthma morbidity in racial and ethnic minorities [72].

1.10. Suboptimal adherence and medication use

Inhaled corticosteroids improve long-term outcomes in asthma patients, and current guidelines recommend inhaled corticosteroids as the backbone of inhaled regimens for those with persistent asthma [73]. Despite this recommendation, in a nationally representative population study in the US, less than 1/3 of those who meet guideline based recommendations for treatment with an inhaled steroid are using them [74]. This unfortunate reality of practice is further magnified in disadvantaged asthma patients. In a study of 1485 children, black and Hispanic children with persistent asthma had significantly decreased odds of using inhaled corticosteroids compared to white children. These undertreated minority children had more than twice the odds of being hospitalized for asthma in the past year compared to white children [75]. In another study of 190 African American or Hispanic adults recently hospitalized with asthma and the majority of which living in poverty, less than half were utilizing inhaled corticosteroids [76].

2. A multidisciplinary approach to personalize asthma therapy within the disadvantaged asthma phenotype

Phenotypic categorization of asthma patients is essential to individualize and optimize asthma therapy. Patients with a disadvantaged asthma phenotype are no exception. The social and environmental factors described above are essential to identify in order to individualize a treatment strategy that addresses the relevant social and environmental factors (**Table 1**).

With this in mind, how do we first identify these important factors in our disadvantaged asthma patients? Although there is an increasing trend in understanding social determinants of health in medical education [77], most medical providers are not trained or provided with sufficient resources to identify and address the social and environmental challenges faced by the disadvantaged asthma patient. Previous studies have suggested that many providers recognize the importance of social and environmental factors, but do not routinely screen for or identify them in their practice [78]. Time constraints and the perception that most social and environmental needs cannot be remedied are often cited by clinicians as reasons for not diagnosing social and environmental needs in their patients [79]. However, given the importance that these factors play in asthma control in the disadvantaged asthma patient, identifying these factors should be considered a cornerstone of the medical history in these patients.

Emerging evidence suggests screening for social needs and connecting patients to existing community organizations or services can significantly improve health outcomes [80]. There are many publically available tools accessible to providers to help identify social needs in clinical practice [81], including some that easily integrate into electronic health record systems [82]. These screening tools will help providers to identify patients with exposures in substandard housing, as well the presence of other social determinants of health known to impact asthma outcomes in the disadvantaged such as inadequate health literacy, the presence of interpersonal and community violence, housing, energy and food insecurity. Although work related asthma is not a focus of current social needs screening tools, a three-question survey tool has recently been endorsed by the American Thoracic Society and the National Institute of Occupational Safety and Health and should be considered in disadvantaged adults with new onset or newly worsening asthma [83].

A number of nonconventional interventions can be considered to address other factors discussed above that are known to exacerbate the burden and severity of asthma in patients with a disadvantaged asthma phenotype. A multidisciplinary team with unique expertise to personalize delivery of care and address the individual social, environmental, economic and medical care should be considered.

Management strategy summary for the disadvantaged asthma phenotype
Screen for modifiable social and environmental factors
Utilize a multidisciplinary approach to address identified social and environmental factors, including partnerships with social workers, legal aid and community resources
Ensure adherence to a guideline-based asthma medication regimen, including attention to access to care, cultural beliefs, inadequate health literacy, and disparities in prescribing patterns
Recognize work related asthma, assist patients with reducing workplace exposures and accessing benefits when unable to work due to asthma
Counsel and assist patients regarding smoking cessation

Table 1. Management summary.

First, many providers will recognize that social workers are often at the forefront of helping to ameliorate the social and environmental conditions that impact asthma. Social workers are indeed often able to connect patients to community, hospital or government resources to address the needs of disadvantaged patients. However, although social workers are vital in the care of many disadvantaged asthmatics, the complex factors described in this chapter will require active engagement by medical providers as well as collaboration with professionals outside of the traditional medical team.

As described above, ensuring adherence to a guideline-based asthma medication regimen, most often centered on an inhaled corticosteroid, is an additional critical component to treatment of the disadvantaged asthma patient. There are multiple explanations to the underuse of controller medications in disadvantaged asthma patients including limited access to care, cultural beliefs, inadequate health literacy, and disparities in prescribing patterns leading to suboptimal quality of care [75]. Despite these barriers, using a culturally sensitive approach through asthma education programs targeting disadvantaged asthma patients, multiple pediatric programs have successfully improved adherence to preventive therapies and improved asthma outcomes [84]. Identifying reasons for suboptimal adherence, such as fear of adverse effects, fear of addiction, cost, inconvenience or complexity of treatment regimens can lead to an individualized conversation, education and medication regimen changes that can improve adherence in the disadvantaged asthma patient [85].

In this context, ensuring access and affordability of prescribed asthma medication is essential. In the US, disadvantaged patients are challenged by the lack of currently available generic inhaled corticosteroids and bronchodilators. Although inhaled corticosteroids and bronchodilators have been the mainstay of asthma therapy for over five decades, most of these medications remain under active patents for specific device delivery mechanisms, as well as chemical formulations. For the uninsured patient, the cost of an inhaled corticosteroid and or any bronchodilators can be upwards of $4000 annually. Even for those with commercial insurance, the out of pocket deductible can approach $500 per year [86]. High cost of inhalers in general is due to at least two major historical events. First, when the Montreal Protocol entered into force in 1989 [87], chlorofluorocarbons (CFC) was phased out with fear that CFC in inhalers could contribute to destruction of the ozone layer. Even though the contribution from the CFC in inhaler was infinitesimal, the urgency based on an assumption that the ozone layer would repair itself within 50 years led to complete ban of CFC including CFC in inhalers. Subsequent development of hydrofluoroalkane (HFA) led to reformulated inhalers and disappearance of generic inhalers. Second, producing generic inhalers is a complex process unlike generic pills. Each inhaler carries multiple patents consisted of specific chemical formulation (including HFA) and the delivery system (protected under the FDA as an investigational device). Such challenge is highlighted by the recent difficulty in bringing out generic Advair to the U.S. by two pharmaceutical companies (Mylan and Hikma). Mylan and Hikma Pharmaceuticals were prepared to bring generic Advair to US marker in spring of 2017. However, the FDA extended complete response letters to both companies, in early 2017 which effectively put the possibility of generic Advair well into 2018. The details of why these companies failed to obtain FDA approval are still unclear.

Inadequate access and affordability of asthma treatments is not unique to the US. In a study of 24 countries, the median cost of an inhaled corticosteroid was 20% of average local monthly per capita income [88]. Inhaled steroids are not even available to be purchased in some developing countries. One example is in India, where low-income patients with asthma do not have access to any inhaled corticosteroid through the public health care sector [89].

Second, collaboration with lawyers is an unconventional approach that holds promise to address multiple social and environmental factors that drive asthma morbidity within the disadvantaged asthma patient [90]. Although there is evidence to support home environmental interventions such as carpet removal, air cleaners, allergen impermeable covering for bedding and pest control to improve asthma outcomes [91, 92], in many instances, these interventions are insufficient in the disadvantaged asthma patient. For example, patients living with leaky pipes, mold, pests, inadequate heat, or wrongful evictions are more challenging environmental problems to address using conventional environmental interventions. Lawyers can advocate through legal recourse including tenant-landlord law, housing code enforcement, eviction and utility shutoff prevention programs to improve factors known to exacerbate asthma in the disadvantaged patient. Often funded in part by Legal Services Corporation (an independent nonprofit established by Congress in 1974 to provide support for civil legal aid to low-income Americans), there are over 133 independent non-profit legal aid programs, at least one in every state [24]. Despite this funding, there remains a substantial gap between low-income Americans' civil legal needs and available resources to address them [93]. Increasingly health systems are recognizing the importance of legal solutions to many social and environmental problems [94] and future research is needed to study the effectiveness of legal interventions and partnerships to improve health outcomes, such as in asthma.

Third, work-exacerbated asthma, as described above, is often unrecognized by patients, clinicians and providers and contributes to worse clinical and socioeconomic outcomes in the disadvantaged asthma patient [24, 95]. Clinicians must assume an active role to connect workplace exposures to asthma symptoms. Recognizing the challenges disadvantaged asthmatic workers face provides opportunities to help. Work related asthma can frequently be managed by reducing workplace exposures and/or providing work accommodations. If unable to work to due to work related asthma, clinicians can help the disadvantaged asthma patient access available benefits.

Fourth, given the known socioeconomic and racial differences in smoking and environmental smoke exposure and given the effects of smoke exposure on asthma outcomes, smoking cessation is an important goal in the disadvantaged asthma patient. Smoking cessation is associated with improvements in lung function and reduction in asthma symptoms [96]. However, Black and Hispanic smokers are less likely to make successful quit attempts than whites [97], which is in part, because black and Hispanics are less likely than white smokers to have been screened for tobacco use and advised to quit by health care professionals [98]. With this in mind, it is essential to ensure smoking cessation counseling and resources are integrated into the management of the disadvantaged asthma patient who smokes. Smoking cessation programs that target disadvantaged smokers and include referrals to community resources that address the socio-contextual mediators of tobacco use (including referrals to community resources to help with job counseling, educational opportunities and physical activity) is highly effective at improving smoking cessation rates compared to a more traditional approach [99].

3. Conclusions

Most patients with asthma can be managed with standardized, traditional therapies; however, 5–10% of patients suffer from disease that is difficult to control. Uncontrolled asthma disproportionally affects low income and racial minority patients. The disadvantaged asthma phenotype is defined by the presence of overlapping social, economic and environmental factors. These factors, such as environmental exposures in substandard housing or suboptimal adherence to controller therapy due to impaired health literacy are challenging to address in the clinic or inpatient setting. Personalized management of the disadvantaged asthma phenotype must target these interconnected factors through a multidisciplinary approach that includes longitudinal collaboration with community-based organizations, social workers and legal aid.

Author details

Drew A. Harris*, Caitlin Welch, Morgan Soper and Yun Michael Shim

*Address all correspondence to: drew.harris@virginia.edu

Department of Medicine, Division of Pulmonary and Critical Care, Complex Airways Diseases Program, University of Virginia, Charlottesville, Virginia, USA

References

[1] McCracken JL et al. Diagnosis and management of asthma in adults: A review. JAMA. 2017;**318**(3):279-290

[2] Moorman JE et al. National surveillance for asthma—United States, 1980-2004. MMWR Surveillance Summaries. 2007;**56**(8):1-54

[3] Forno E, Celedon JC. Health disparities in asthma. American Journal of Respiratory and Critical Care Medicine. 2012;**185**(10):1033-1035

[4] Kim H et al. Health care utilization by children with asthma. Preventing Chronic Disease. 2009;**6**(1):A12

[5] Smith LA et al. Rethinking race/ethnicity, income, and childhood asthma: Racial/ethnic disparities concentrated among the very poor. Public Health Reports. 2005;**120**(2):109-116

[6] Wenzel SE. Asthma phenotypes: The evolution from clinical to molecular approaches. Nature Medicine. 2012;**18**(5):716-725

[7] Galanter JM et al. Genome-wide association study and admixture mapping identify different asthma-associated loci in Latinos: The genes-environments & admixture in Latino Americans study. The Journal of Allergy and Clinical Immunology. 2014;**134**(2):295-305

[8] Pino-Yanes M et al. Genetic ancestry influences asthma susceptibility and lung function among Latinos. The Journal of Allergy and Clinical Immunology. 2015;**135**(1):228-235

[9] Keet CA et al. Neighborhood poverty, urban residence, race/ethnicity, and asthma: Rethinking the inner-city asthma epidemic. The Journal of Allergy and Clinical Immunology. 2015;**135**(3):655-662

[10] Wegienka G et al. Racial differences in allergic sensitization: Recent findings and future directions. Current Allergy and Asthma Reports. 2013;**13**(3):255-261

[11] Jacobs DE. Environmental health disparities in housing. American Journal of Public Health. 2011;**101**(Suppl. 1):S115-S122

[12] Rauh VA, Chew GR, Garfinkel RS. Deteriorated housing contributes to high cockroach allergen levels in inner-city households. Environmental Health Perspectives. 2002;**110**(Suppl. 2):323-327

[13] Arbes SJ Jr et al. Prevalences of positive skin test responses to 10 common allergens in the US population: Results from the third National Health and Nutrition Examination Survey. The Journal of Allergy and Clinical Immunology. 2005;**116**(2):377-383

[14] Litonjua AA et al. Variation in total and specific IgE: Effects of ethnicity and socioeconomic status. The Journal of Allergy and Clinical Immunology. 2005;**115**(4):751-757

[15] Celedon JC et al. Ethnicity and skin test reactivity to aeroallergens among asthmatic children in Connecticut. Chest. 2004;**125**(1):85-92

[16] Kang BC, Wu CW, Johnson J. Characteristics and diagnoses of cockroach-sensitive bronchial asthma. Annals of Allergy. 1992;**68**(3):237-244

[17] Rosenstreich DL et al. The role of cockroach allergy and exposure to cockroach allergen in causing morbidity among inner-city children with asthma. The New England Journal of Medicine. 1997;**336**(19):1356-1363

[18] McNichol KN, Williams HE. Spectrum of asthma in children. II. Allergic components. British Medical Journal. 1973;**4**(5883):12-16

[19] Sarpong SB, Karrison T. Skin test reactivity to indoor allergens as a marker of asthma severity in children with asthma. Annals of Allergy, Asthma & Immunology. 1998;**80**(4):303-308

[20] Valet RS, Perry TT, Hartert TV. Rural health disparities in asthma care and outcomes. The Journal of Allergy and Clinical Immunology. 2009;**123**(6):1220-1225

[21] Jones AP, Bentham G, Horwell C. Health service accessibility and deaths from asthma. International Journal of Epidemiology. 1999;**28**(1):101-105

[22] Withy K, Davis J. Followup after an emergency department visit for asthma: Urban/rural patterns. Ethnicity & Disease. 2008;**18**(2 Suppl. 2):S2-247-S2-251

[23] Caldeira RD et al. Prevalence and risk factors for work related asthma in young adults. Occupational and Environmental Medicine. 2006;**63**(10):694-699

[24] Henneberger PK et al. An official american thoracic society statement: Work-exacerbated asthma. American Journal of Respiratory and Critical Care Medicine. 2011;**184**(3):368-378

[25] Loerbroks A et al. Job insecurity is associated with adult asthma in Germany during Europe's recent economic crisis: A prospective cohort study. Journal of Epidemiology and Community Health. 2014;**68**(12):1196-1199

[26] Landsbergis PA, Grzywacz JG, LaMontagne AD. Work organization, job insecurity, and occupational health disparities. American Journal of Industrial Medicine. 2014;**57**(5):495-515

[27] Blanc PD et al. The prevalence and predictors of respiratory-related work limitation and occupational disability in an international study. Chest. 2003;**124**(3):1153-1159

[28] Blanc PD et al. Asthma, employment status, and disability among adults treated by pulmonary and allergy specialists. Chest. 1996;**109**(3):688-696

[29] Blanc PD et al. Asthma-related work disability in Sweden. The impact of workplace exposures. American Journal of Respiratory and Critical Care Medicine. 1999;**160**(6):2028-2033

[30] Blanc PD et al. Work disability among adults with asthma. Chest. 1993;**104**(5):1371-1377

[31] Eisner MD et al. Risk factors for work disability in severe adult asthma. The American Journal of Medicine. 2006;**119**(10):884-891

[32] Harris DA et al. Improving the asthma disparity gap with legal advocacy? A qualitative study of patient-identified challenges to improve social and environmental factors that contribute to poorly controlled asthma. The Journal of Asthma. 2017 Oct, pp. 1-9

[33] Jamal A et al. Current cigarette smoking among adults—United States, 2005-2014. MMWR. Morbidity and Mortality Weekly Report. 2015;**64**(44):1233-1240

[34] Eisner MD, Iribarren C. The influence of cigarette smoking on adult asthma outcomes. Nicotine & Tobacco Research. 2007;**9**(1):53-56

[35] Thomson NC, Spears M. The influence of smoking on the treatment response in patients with asthma. Current Opinion in Allergy and Clinical Immunology. 2005;**5**(1):57-63

[36] Dransfield MT et al. Racial and gender differences in susceptibility to tobacco smoke among patients with chronic obstructive pulmonary disease. Respiratory Medicine. 2006;**100**(6):1110-1116

[37] Chatila WM et al. Smoking patterns in African Americans and whites with advanced COPD. Chest. 2004;**125**(1):15-21

[38] Lajunen TK, Jaakkola JJ, Jaakkola MS. The synergistic effect of heredity and exposure to second-hand smoke on adult-onset asthma. American Journal of Respiratory and Critical Care Medicine. 2013;**188**(7):776-782

[39] Simons E et al. Maternal second-hand smoke exposure in pregnancy is associated with childhood asthma development. The Journal of Allergy and Clinical Immunology. In Practice. 2014;**2**(2):201-207

[40] Mannino DM et al. Health effects related to environmental tobacco smoke exposure in children in the United States: Data from the Third National Health and Nutrition Examination Survey. Archives of Pediatrics & Adolescent Medicine. 2001;**155**(1):36-41

[41] California Environmental Protection Agency. Health effects of exposure to environmental tobacco smoke. Tobacco Control. 1997;**6**(4):346-353

[42] Eisner MD et al. Directly measured second hand smoke exposure and asthma health outcomes. Thorax. 2005;**60**(10):814-821

[43] Brochu PJ et al. Particulate air pollution and socioeconomic position in rural and urban areas of the Northeastern United States. American Journal of Public Health. 2011;**101**(Suppl. 1):S224-S230

[44] O'Neill MS et al. Health, wealth, and air pollution: Advancing theory and methods. Environmental Health Perspectives. 2003;**111**(16):1861-1870

[45] Hajat A, Hsia C, O'Neill MS. Socioeconomic disparities and air pollution exposure: A global review. Current Environmental Health Reports. 2015;**2**(4):440-450

[46] Clark LP, Millet DB, Marshall JD. National patterns in environmental injustice and inequality: Outdoor NO_2 air pollution in the United States. PLoS One. 2014;**9**(4):e94431

[47] Guarnieri M, Balmes JR. Outdoor air pollution and asthma. Lancet. 2014;**383**(9928): 1581-1592

[48] Norris G et al. Asthma aggravation, combustion, and stagnant air. Thorax. 2000;**55**(6): 466-470

[49] McConnell R et al. Asthma in exercising children exposed to ozone: A cohort study. Lancet. 2002;**359**(9304):386-391

[50] Perez L et al. Chronic burden of near-roadway traffic pollution in 10 European cities (APHEKOM network). The European Respiratory Journal. 2013;**42**(3):594-605

[51] Matthews KA, Gallo LC. Psychological perspectives on pathways linking socioeconomic status and physical health. Annual Review of Psychology. 2011;**62**:501-530

[52] Taylor SE, Repetti RL, Seeman T. Health psychology: What is an unhealthy environment and how does it get under the skin? Annual Review of Psychology. 1997;**48**:411-447

[53] Sampson RJ, Raudenbush SW, Earls F. Neighborhoods and violent crime: A multilevel study of collective efficacy. Science. 1997;**277**(5328):918-924

[54] Evans GW. The environment of childhood poverty. The American Psychologist. 2004;**59**(2):77-92

[55] Kennedy BP et al. Social capital, income inequality, and firearm violent crime. Social Science & Medicine. 1998;**47**(1):7-17

[56] Mobeireek A et al. Psychogenic vocal cord dysfunction simulating bronchial asthma. The European Respiratory Journal. 1995;**8**(11):1978-1981

[57] Yonas MA, Lange NE, Celedon JC. Psychosocial stress and asthma morbidity. Current Opinion in Allergy and Clinical Immunology. 2012;**12**(2):202-210

[58] Wright RJ, Cohen RT, Cohen S. The impact of stress on the development and expression of atopy. Current Opinion in Allergy and Clinical Immunology. 2005;**5**(1):23-29

[59] Kang DH, Weaver MT. Airway cytokine responses to acute and repeated stress in a murine model of allergic asthma. Biological Psychology. 2010;**84**(1):66-73

[60] Chen E, Miller GE. Stress and inflammation in exacerbations of asthma. Brain, Behavior, and Immunity. 2007;**21**(8):993-999

[61] Marin TJ et al. Double-exposure to acute stress and chronic family stress is associated with immune changes in children with asthma. Psychosomatic Medicine. 2009;**71**(4):378-384

[62] Shankardass K et al. Parental stress increases the effect of traffic-related air pollution on childhood asthma incidence. Proceedings of the National Academy of Sciences of the United States of America. 2009;**106**(30):12406-12411

[63] Clougherty JE et al. Synergistic effects of traffic-related air pollution and exposure to violence on urban asthma etiology. Environmental Health Perspectives. 2007;**115**(8): 1140-1146

[64] Brehm JM et al. Stress and bronchodilator response in children with asthma. American Journal of Respiratory and Critical Care Medicine. 2015;**192**(1):47-56

[65] Ritz T et al. Asthma trigger reports are associated with low quality of life, exacerbations, and emergency treatments. Annals of the American Thoracic Society. 2016 Feb;**13**(2):204-211

[66] Sandel M, Wright RJ. When home is where the stress is: Expanding the dimensions of housing that influence asthma morbidity. Archives of Disease in Childhood. 2006;**91**(11):942-948

[67] Quinn K et al. Stress and the city: Housing stressors are associated with respiratory health among low socioeconomic status Chicago children. Journal of Urban Health. 2010;**87**(4):688-702

[68] Archea C et al. Negative life events and quality of life in adults with asthma. Thorax. 2007;**62**(2):139-146

[69] Koinis-Mitchell D et al. Immigration and acculturation-related factors and asthma morbidity in Latino children. Journal of Pediatric Psychology. 2011;**36**(10):1130-1143

[70] Suglia SF et al. Maternal intimate partner violence and increased asthma incidence in children: Buffering effects of supportive caregiving. Archives of Pediatrics & Adolescent Medicine. 2009;**163**(3):244-250

[71] Ribeiro-Silva Rde C et al. Food and nutrition insecurity: A marker of vulnerability to asthma symptoms. Public Health Nutrition. 2014;**17**(1):14-19

[72] Thakur N et al. Perceived discrimination associated with asthma and related outcomes in minority youth: The GALA II and SAGE II Studies. Chest. 2017;**151**(4):804-812

[73] National Asthma Education and Prevention Program. Expert Panel Report 3 (EPR-3): Guidelines for the diagnosis and management of asthma-summary report 2007. The Journal of Allergy and Clinical Immunology. 2007;**120**(Suppl. 5):S94-138

[74] Adams RJ et al. Inadequate use of asthma medication in the United States: Results of the asthma in America national population survey. The Journal of Allergy and Clinical Immunology. 2002;**110**(1):58-64

[75] Crocker D et al. Racial and ethnic disparities in asthma medication usage and health-care utilization: Data from the National Asthma Survey. Chest. 2009;**136**(4):1063-1071

[76] Halm EA, Mora P, Leventhal H. No symptoms, no asthma: The acute episodic disease belief is associated with poor self-management among inner-city adults with persistent asthma. Chest. 2006;**129**(3):573-580

[77] Pettignano R et al. Interprofessional medical-legal education of medical students: Assessing the benefits for addressing social determinants of health. Academic Medicine. 2017 Sep;**92**(9):1254-1258

[78] Garg A et al. Screening for basic social needs at a medical home for low-income children. Clinical Pediatrics (Philadelphia). 2009;**48**(1):32-36

[79] Fleegler EW et al. Families' health-related social problems and missed referral opportunities. Pediatrics. 2007;**119**(6):e1332-e1341

[80] Gottlieb LM et al. Effects of social needs screening and in-person service navigation on child health: A randomized clinical trial. JAMA Pediatrics. 2016;**170**(11):e162521

[81] Health Leads Screening Toolkit. Health Leads Inc. 2016. Available from: http://www.healthleadsusa.org/

[82] National Association of Community Health Centers. PRAPARE Implementation and Action Toolkit. Available from: http://www.nachc.org/research-and-data/prapare/toolkit/

[83] Harber P et al. Recommendations for a clinical decision support system for work-related asthma in primary care settings. Journal of Occupational and Environmental Medicine. 2017;**59**(11):e231-e235

[84] McCallum GB et al. Culture-specific programs for children and adults from minority groups who have asthma. Cochrane Database of Systematic Reviews. 2017;**8**:CD006580

[85] Bender BG, Bender SE. Patient-identified barriers to asthma treatment adherence: Responses to interviews, focus groups, and questionnaires. Immunology and Allergy Clinics of North America. 2005;**25**(1):107-130

[86] Rosenthal E. The soaring cost of a simple breath. The New York Times. 2013;**12**(October):A1

[87] https://www.epa.gov/ozone-layer-protection/international-actions-montreal-protocol-substances-deplete-ozone-layer

[88] Watson JP, Lewis RA. Is asthma treatment affordable in developing countries? Thorax. 1997;**52**(7):605-607

[89] Kotwani A. Availability, price and affordability of asthma medicines in five Indian states. The International Journal of Tuberculosis and Lung Disease. 2009;**13**(5):574-579

[90] McCabe HA, Kinney ED. Medical legal partnerships: A key strategy for addressing social determinants of health. Journal of General Internal Medicine. 2010;**25**(Suppl. 2): S200-S201

[91] Carter MC et al. Home intervention in the treatment of asthma among inner-city children. The Journal of Allergy and Clinical Immunology. 2001;**108**(5):732-737

[92] Murray CS et al. Preventing severe asthma exacerbations in children. A randomized trial of mite-impermeable bedcovers. American Journal of Respiratory and Critical Care Medicine. 2017;**196**(2):150-158

[93] Legal Services Coporation. The Justice Gap: Measuring the Unmet Civil Legal Needs of Low-income Americans. 2017. Available from: http://www.lsc.gov/sites/default/files/images/TheJusticeGap-FullReport.pdf

[94] Cohen E et al. Medical-legal partnership: Collaborating with lawyers to identify and address health disparities. Journal of General Internal Medicine. 2010;**25**(Suppl. 2): S136-S139

[95] Vandenplas O, Toren K, Blanc PD. Health and socioeconomic impact of work-related asthma. The European Respiratory Journal. 2003;**22**(4):689-697

[96] McLeish AC, Zvolensky MJ. Asthma and cigarette smoking: A review of the empirical literature. The Journal of Asthma. 2010;**47**(4):345-361

[97] Kahende JW et al. Quit attempt correlates among smokers by race/ethnicity. International Journal of Environmental Research and Public Health. 2011;**8**(10):3871-3888

[98] Lopez-Quintero C, Crum RM, Neumark YD. Racial/ethnic disparities in report of physician-provided smoking cessation advice: Analysis of the 2000 National Health Interview Survey. American Journal of Public Health. 2006;**96**(12):2235-2239

[99] Haas JS et al. Proactive tobacco cessation outreach to smokers of low socioeconomic status: A randomized clinical trial. JAMA Internal Medicine. 2015;**175**(2):218-226

8

Phosphodiesterase 3 and 4 Inhibition: Facing a Bright Future in Asthma Control

Jan Beute, Vincent Manganiello and Alex KleinJan

Abstract

A recent status on asthmaticus multiple case report by Beute demonstrated the beneficial effects of phosphodiesterase III (PDE3) and phosphodiesterase IV (PDE4) inhibition. This chapter reviews the possible underlying mechanisms, beside the known effect, for the beneficial effects of a mixed PDE3/4 inhibitor in allergic airway inflammation. Structural cells of the lung and immune system express PDE3 and 4. PDE3 and 4 inhibition have a number of consequences related to physical function and cytokine production. The most direct effect of PDE3 inhibition being relaxation of smooth muscle cells results in bronchodilation. However, PDE3 inhibition appears to go further than a mere inhibitory activity in bronchial smooth muscle. It also affects structural cells, and more importantly, it creates an improved barrier function in endothelial cells. PDE3 and 4 inhibition therefore strengthens the immune barrier; but in addition, it modifies the cells of the immune system itself, as these also express PDE3 and 4 activity, thus changing their function. All aspects of asthma-related pathophysiology seem to be affected by PDE3 and 4 inhibition. Clinical use of a mixed PDE3/4 inhibitor in respiratory diseases is currently limited to a few studies, including life-threatening asthma in which mixed PDE3/4 inhibition has a beneficial effect.

Keywords: PDE3, PDE4, allergic airway inflammation

1. Introduction

Asthma is an obstructive airway disease characterized by inflamed airways, structural and physiological abnormalities in the airways, and shortness of breath [1]. Important primary air_ way cells are alveolar cells, endothelial cells, and smooth muscle cells; and secondary cells are involved in regulation of innate and adoptive immunology. Conventional treatment with inhaled corticosteroids combined with beta-adrenergic agonists supports and induces smooth muscle relaxation to reopen the inflamed airways, relieves symptoms, supports inspirational and expirational flow, and reduces inflammation [2]. These treatment regimens were also used in the extreme severe cases of asthma like status asthmaticus and patients with bronchospasm, in some cases with only minimal effect. The treatment goal in these severe cases of acute asthma is the prompt relief of respiratory distress. The great benefit of a mixed PDE3/4 inhibitor, in these severe cases, is the induction of acute as well as long-lasting bronchodilator effects [3].

At the moment, there is no effective treatment for these severe asthmatic patients [4] and there are no clear, effective guidelines. Moreover, treatment of these patients is multidisciplinary, involving first aid physicians, intensive care physicians, anesthetists, and pulmonary physicians, requiring golden standards and treatment regimens per hospital for optimal results. There are still too many asthma deaths; numbers in US are up to nine cases per day and in the UK are up to over three cases per day. Presently, in the Netherlands, there are annually more than 60.

This review discusses the PDE3 gene family and PDE3 inhibition, traditionally used in acute, refractory heart failure. We discuss the benefits of combined PDE3 and 4 inhibition in status asthmaticus [3], and the possible mechanisms which may be responsible for these beneficial effects of PDE3 and 4 inhibition.

2. The PDE superfamily: important regulators of cyclic nucleotide signaling pathways and networks

Intracellular signaling via complicated regulatory networks plays a critical role during physiological cellular responses. cAMP and cGMP were the first molecules described as intracellular second messengers [5]. They regulate multiple intracellular targets, including protein kinase A and protein kinase G, guanine nucleotide exchange proteins activated by cAMP (Epacs), cyclic nucleotide-gated ion channels, and PDE activities [6]. Intracellular concentrations of cAMP and cGMP are regulated through their synthesis by adenylyl cyclases (ACs) and guanylyl cyclases and their degradation via cyclic nucleotide PDEs. Ten different ACs have been identified and classified into two groups [7]. The first group consists of transmembrane enzymes which are activated by different hormones, neurotransmitters, chemokines, and cytokines in the G-protein-coupled receptor cascade [8]. Another group of cytosolic ACs is regulated by bicarbonate and calcium ions [8]. Whereas, cytosolic ACs are all encoded by one gene, transmembrane ACs represent a group encoded by nine different genes [9].

The large PDE superfamily is comprised of 11 PDE gene families (PDE1–PDE11). They specifically hydrolyze cyclic nucleotides, and can be classified according to their primary structures, tissue expression, biochemical properties, regulation, and their sensitivity to different pharmacological agents [10]. By catalyzing the hydrolysis of cAMP and cGMP, PDEs regulate the intracellular concentrations of these critical second messengers, and consequently, their downstream signaling pathways and networks. PDEs also function as important regulators in the compartmentation of cyclic nucleotide signaling pathways and networks. Individual PDEs are targeted/recruited to specific intracellular locations, where they are incorporated into specific multiprotein regulatory complexes ("signalosomes") through protein-protein interactions. By virtue of their localization to specific compartments, PDEs can thus regulate specific cyclic nucleotide signaling pathways [11].

3. PDE3 and PDE4

PDE3 is expressed in pulmonary structural cells and cells of the immune system. Lung structural cells, including smooth muscle cells, epithelial cells, and endothelial cells, express PDE3. PDE3A and B are encoded by two highly related and similarly organized genes on human chromosomes, 12p12 and 11p15 [12–14]. Both PDE3A and PDE3B hydrolyze cAMP and cGMP, with 4–10 times higher affinity (Vmax) for cAMP [15]. Biochemical and histochemical studies of the localization of PDE3 suggested that PDE3 was associated with the sarcoplasmic reticulum, Golgi endosome, and nuclear envelope in cardiac tissue [16]. PDE3 plays a major role in cardiac contraction by modulating cAMP-dependent phosphorylation of voltage-gated Ca^{2+} channels and Ca^{2+} entry [17]. In addition, recent studies with PDE3A and PDE3B KO mice indicate that PDE3A, not PDE3B, regulates basal contractility in mouse heart [18].

Kass et al. described one mechanism, whereby PDE3 might be functionally modulated by cGMP occupying the PDE3 catalytic site [19]. PDE3 binds both cAMP and cGMP at its catalytic site with high affinity, and endogenous cGMP, generated by NO-induced activation of guanyl cyclase, can function as a competitive inhibitor of hydrolysis of cAMP by PDE3 [20]. NO-induced cGMP/cAMP cross-talk, mediated via cGMP inhibition of cAMP hydrolysis by PDE3 which leads to increased levels of cAMP, is thought to mediate some of the effects of NO in inflammatory and lung structural cells. NO modulates pulmonary vascular tone, causing non-adrenergic-, non-cholinergic-mediated bronchodilation [21]. Overexpression of nitric oxide synthase in both endothelial and airway epithelial cells resulted in diminished airway inflammation [22]. Under normal conditions of NO/cGMP signaling, PDE4, with a high Km for cAMP, is thought to degrade cAMP because PDE3 with a lower Km for cAMP is inhibited by endogenous cGMP and thus can increase cAMP [23]. PDE3-induced vasorelaxation is potentiated when NO/cGMP is suppressed as PDE3 inhibition increases both cAMP and cGMP, in which cGMP inhibits cAMP degradation. PDE4 inhibition only increases cAMP and thus is unaffected by NO/cGMP suppression [23]. PDE3 seems to be more responsible for cAMP degradation at low intracellular cAMP concentrations, whereas PDE4 is more important for control of cAMP at higher concentrations [24]. This suggests a beneficial effect of NO in allergic airway inflammation and urges caution in the use of NOS inhibitors [22]. Since the first PDE3 inhibition papers in the 1990s, 11 PDE families have been identified, and presently at least four isoforms of PDE4 are known [25]. Also, the idea of signalosomes has been postulated and partly verified [26].

4. Modulation of structural cells and immune cells by PDE3 and 4 inhibition

Several structural cells express PDE3. Inhibition of PDEs has a number of consequences in the pathophysiology of asthma.

4.1. Smooth muscle cells and cardiomyocytes

Cardiac muscle tissue and smooth muscles are not under conscious control. The role of PDE3 in cardiac muscle and in vascular and bronchial smooth muscle slightly differs due to regulation by different modulators and inhibitors [19]. Vascular SMC and airway SMC are widely comparable [27]. Reducing cAMP by PDE3 modulates contraction; PDE3 inhibition (PDE3i) leads to relaxation of vascular and airway SMC which results in vasodilation and bronchodilation due to the elevated levels of cAMP. NO activates soluble- and membrane-bound guanylate cyclases, which synthesize cyclic guanylate monophosphate (cGMP), which subsequently can serve as a competitive inhibitor of PDE3 as well as activator of cGMP protein kinases [16]. The downstream effects of NO are limited, in part, by phosphodiesterase (PDE)-induced degradation of cGMP [28].

The primary mechanism behind the PDE3 regulation of myocardial physiology relates to its control of cAMP levels; inhibition of myocardial PDE3, especially PDE3A, leads to decreased cAMP breakdown, resulting in increased cAMP which mediates positive inotropic effects and increases in myocardial contractility [29]. Although PDE3 inhibitors increase myocardial contractility and vasodilation in heart failure patients [29], prolonged use of the PDE3 inhibitor milrinone in these patients increased mortality was observed, most likely due to arrhythmias and cardiac arrest [30]. Presently, milrinone has an approval for short term treatment of untreatable exacerbations of heart failure and as a chemical "bridge to transplant" [31]. The work of Chen Yan and her colleagues suggests that the untoward effects of chronic administration of relatively high dosis of milrinone may possibly be related to long term effects of cAMP on pathological remodeling and progression of heart failure [32], via upregulation of inducible cAMP early repressor (ICER) and subsequent increases in cardiomyocyte apoptosis [33]. According to this hypothesis, PDE3 inhibitors increase cAMP, leading to increased expression of ICER, which blocks transcription of PDE3. This cascade of events induced a pathological "feedback loop," with downregulation or inhibition of PDE3 leading to increased cAMP/PKA signaling, upregulation of ICER, continued downregulation of PDE3, and enhanced apoptosis in cardiaomyocytes [33].

In smooth muscle cells, increased cGMP levels induce vasorelaxation. Due to effects of PDEs on hydrolysis of cGMP, PDE inhibitors play a major role in the fine-tuned regulation of this function. In addition to PDEs, NO plays an important role in vasorelaxation, perhaps, in part, by its activation of cytosolic guanylate cyclases, leading to increased production of cGMP, and subsequent inhibition of PDE3. The PDE3 inhibitor, cilostazol (Pletal), is widely used to treat intermittent claudication (IC), a lower-extremity peripheral arterial disease characterized by exercise-/ischemia-induced leg pain. It is thought that cilostazol increases walking distance and alleviates IC symptoms by cAMP-mediated vasodilation and inhibition of both platelet activation and vascular wall inflammation [34].

Asthma can present itself with varying levels of severity, and a particular subgroup of patients, labeled as "severe asthmatics" is characterized by the persistence of symptoms despite therapy with corticosteroids [2, 35]. Examination of bronchial airways from patients with severe asthma shows a greater amount of ASM (Airway Smooth Muscle) cell mass and of subepithelial fibrosis compared to non-severe asthmatics [36, 37]. In ex-vivo studies, ASM cells from severe asthmatics demonstrated increased cell growth and proliferation [38] and an increase in proliferating cell nuclear antigen, a marker of proliferation [39]. Cultured ASM cells from mild-to-moderate asthmatics also proliferated faster than ASM cells from normal subjects [40]. Bhavsar et al. have previously demonstrated corticosteroid insensitivity in blood monocytes and alveolar macrophages from patients with severe asthma compared to those with non-severe asthma [41, 42]. Another feature of steroid insensitivity could be the ongoing ASM cell growth because the enhanced proliferation of ASM cells from patients with mild asthma is resistant to dexamethasone [43]. Given this perspective, it is of interest that studies with VSMC from PDE3A and PDE3B KO mice indicated that the absence of PDE3A, not PDE3B, diminished VSMC proliferation and indicated a G0 G1 cell cycle arrest [44]. PDE3 inhibition might reduce ASM proliferation in asthmatics.

4.2. Endothelial cells

Endothelial cells play an important role in the pathophysiology of asthma. Due to the expression of adhesion molecules, they enable cells to extravasate from the bloodstream into the inflamed tissue. Endothelial cells also possess a barrier function to prevent leakage of blood fluid in the tissue. Endothelial cells express PDE3 and 4, and inhibition of PDE3 and 4 of endothelial cells inhibited eosinophil and neutrophil adherence to monolayers of endothelial cells [45, 46]. PDE3 and 4 synergistically enhance the inhibition of VCAM1 expression and eosinophil adhesion to activated-human lung microvascular endothelial cells [45]. Inhibition of PDE3 leads to increases in cAMP which improves endothelial barrier functions and supports cell-cell junctions [47]. BW245c, a DP receptor antagonist, increases cAMP, and enhanced endothelial barrier function in a cAMP-dependent matter via the DP receptor, a G protein coupled receptor [48, 49]. Hyperpermeability of pulmonary endothelial monolayers, evoked by thrombin or *Escherichia coli* hemolysin, can be blocked by the simultaneous activation of adenylyl cyclase and inhibition of PDEs, especially PDE3 and PDE4 [50]. Sphingosine-1-phosphate (S1P1) induces endothelial cytoskeletal rearrangement and barrier enhancement by S1P1 receptor, PI3 kinase, Tiam1/Rac1, and alpha-actinin dependent mechanisms as well [51]. In vivo studies with asthma models indicate that compounds such as BW245c, sphingosine 1-phosphate receptor agonist (FTY720), and prostacyclin-2 analog (iloprost) impair Dendritic Cell (DC) migration [52–54]. This can be explained by a direct effect of these compounds on improving endothelial cell barrier function via elevated levels of cAMP [48, 55], which might affect DC migration from tissue to the draining lymph nodes.

PDE inhibition, a therapeutic approach to increase cAMP levels, was beneficial in treating capillary leakage and edema in a rat model of systemic inflammation induced by LPS [56]. Moreover, PDE3 inhibition was compared to dobutamine treatment (β-adrenoreceptor compounds); the former showed inotropic, lusitropic, and vasodilating properties which were not seen in patients treated with dobutamine [57, 58]. In bypass surgery patients, reduced inflammatory responses were observed during PDE3 inhibition compared to placebo treatment [59]. Furthermore, reduced TNF-α-levels, a cytokine which is increased in sepsis, were observed during PDE3 inhibition by enoximone compared to dobutamine-treated septic patients [58].

Hydrogen peroxide (H_2O_2), derived from neutrophils and other cells, supposedly is important in the development of vascular injury and thus of pulmonary edema. In a porcine pulmonary artery endothelial cell monolayer model, H2O2 increased hydraulic conductivity while selectivity was decreased. It is known that certain inhibitors of PDE isoenzymes 2, 3, and 4 could block H_2O_2-induced endothelial permeability [60]. The data suggest that adenylate cyclase activation/PDE inhibition is a powerful approach to block H_2O_2-induced increase in endothelial permeability. This concept appears especially valuable when endothelial PDE isoenzyme patterns and PDE inhibitor profiles are matched optimally [61].

4.3. Epithelial cells, pneumocyte type I and type II

Human epithelial cells express PDE3 [62]. NO and cAMP both modulate membrane water permeability via aquaporin5 expression in pneumocyte type I [63, 64]. Experimental lung edema can be attenuated by selective PDE3 and PDE4 inhibitors [50, 65–67]. In experimental pulmonary edema, PDE3 inhibition reduces the numbers of inflammatory cells in BAL [66]. In alveolar epithelial cells, LPS-induced biosynthesis of proinflammatory cytokines is regulated by cAMP and tightly controlled by PDEs, and can be reduced by PDE inhibitors [68].

Inhibition of PDE3 and elevation of cAMP improve epithelial and endothelial barrier function and reduce SMC proliferation, which are interesting therapeutic targets in the future for asthma.

5. Immune cells

Mechanisms for regulation of PDE3 activity in immune cells, including dendritic cells, monocytes, B-cells, NK cells $\gamma\delta$T cells, $\alpha\beta$T-cells, T-cells, macrophages, eosinophils, and neutrophils, all of which express PDE3 isoforms are largely unknown (immgen database http://www.immgen.org/databrowser/index.html). Theophylline is a nonspecific PDE inhibitor [69]. In asthmatic patients, the inflamed airway mucosa, characterized by the presence of eosinophils, IgE positive mast cells, T-cells and dendritic cells, exhibits dysregulated barrier immunity [70]. These various inflammatory cells each have their own position in the asthma cascade. PDE3 and PDE4 are the major isoenzymes regulating IgE-stimulated mediator release from rat peritoneal mast cells [71]. Alveolar macrophage activation can be inhibited by PDE3/PDE4 inhibitors [72]. DC cultures were treated with a PDE4 inhibitor and with combined inhibition of PDE3 and 4; the latter resulted in a two times stronger reduction in LPS-induced TNFα release in DC cultures [73]. *In vitro* inhibition of PDE4 in DCs resulted in reduced development of Th1 cells as measured in reduced capacity to produce IL-12p70 and TNFα upon LPS or CD40L stimulation [74]. Peripheral blood monocytes from atopic dermatitis patients and healthy controls show inhibition of LPS-induced TNFα release during treatment with PDE4 inhibitors [75].

Inhibition of PDE3 and PDE4 prevents immunogen-stimulated IL-2 release from CD4 and CD8 human T-cells. Human T-cells and B-cell express PDE3 [73, 76–78]. Knock down strategies or inhibitors of PDE4B or D inhibit IL-4, IL-5, and IFNγ expression or production [79–81]. Peripheral blood mononuclear cells from atopic dermatitis patients and healthy controls show inhibition of PMA-induced proliferation due to the treatment with PDE4 inhibitors. cAMP was found to inhibit T-cell proliferation and differentiation which was linked to IL-2 [82, 83]. IL-2 activation of CD25+ T cells (Treg cells) led to a drastic upregulation in AC activity and to cAMP accumulation; an opposite significant decrease in AC activity was seen in CD25− T cells [83]. The PDE activity remained unchanged in both cell subpopulations, suggesting that the mechanism of cAMP accumulation in stimulated Treg involves AC7 activation [83].

Cyclic AMP is a pleiotropic regulator of cell growth and function. In T-cells, cAMP suppresses TCR-triggered proliferation and cytokine production. cAMP is also a selective modulator of the actions of the proinflammatory transcription factor NF-κB. NF-κB plays a crucial role in switching on the gene expression of inflammatory and immune mediators and is therefore an important target for therapy [84]. cAMP is an important negative regulator of T cell activation, and increased levels of cAMP are associated with T cell hyporesponsiveness *in vitro* [85]. Stimulation of mouse CD4 T-cells by immature allogeneic DC combined with a PDE3 inhibitor resulted in functional Foxp3+ T-cells that delayed allograft rejection [86]. Moreover, PDE3 inhibition results in functional human Foxp3+ CD4+ T-cells which are driven by allogeneic APCs. The mechanism for these responses seems to be related to demethylation of FoxP3 gene [86]

Treatment with S-Petasin, an inhibitor of PDE3 and 4, reduced eosinophilic airway inflammation in an OVA model for asthma [87]. Although eosinophils do not express PDE3, reduced inflammation might be an indirect consequence of elevated levels of cAMP in endothelial cells that enhance endothelial barrier function and lowered the expression of adhesion molecules [45, 47]. PDE3 inhibitors sustained increased levels of cAMP in mast cells which are inhibitory to both basophils and human lung mast cells function [88]. Rat peritoneal mast cells showed reduced IgE-stimulated mediator release when treated with PDE3 inhibitors [71]. The conductive players in asthma, including T-cells and DC, and the central effector cells in asthma, including eosinophils, mast cells, basophils and neutrophils, can be targeted directly or indirectly with PDE3 inhibitors.

Recently, more and more interest is seen for the "old" theophylline which is a broad PDE inhibitor [69]. Theophylline [69] is a drug which targets PDE4 and, at high doses, also PDE3. However, it is a relatively weak bronchodilator at therapeutic concentrations. In patients, it is beneficial; and addition of theophylline can improve asthma control to a greater extent than beta2-agonist in patients with severe asthma [89]. Furthermore, in asthma patients poorly controlled by steroids, low dose theophylline added to inhaled corticosteroids improves asthma control [69]. The proposed mechanisms of action of theophylline include nonselective inhibition of PDE, antagonism of Adenosine receptors, inhibition of nuclear translocation of NF-κB, improved histone diacetylase 2, improved IL-10 secretion, induction of apoptosis of inflammatory cells (neutrophils and eosinophils) [90, 91], and inhibition of T-cell proliferation [85]. These features are of significant importance for severe asthma with poor steroid control, in which neutrophils are found and these patients were difficult to treat [4]. Theophylline exerted proapoptotic effects on monocyte-derived dendritic cells (DCs) and impaired DCs differentiation [90, 91].

6. PDE3 and 4 inhibition in the context of asthma

There is little literature available regarding enoximone in the context of airway disease. Bethke et al. showed that enoximone has inhibitory capacity on PDE3 and PDE4 [92]. Fujimura et al. researched cilostazol as a PDE3 inhibitor in asthma, showing its beneficial effect on bronchial hyper-responsiveness in elder asthmatics [93]. PDE4 inhibitors have been described in pre-clinical and clinical settings in the context of lung diseases like asthma and COPD [94, 95]. The PDE4 inhibitor roflumilast inhibits TGFβ-induced connective tissue growth factor (CTGF), collagen I and fibronectin in airway smooth muscle (ASM) cells of bronchial tissue rings [96].

Roflumilast is approved as part of the treatment regimen for Chronic Obstructive Pulmonary Disease (COPD) [97]. PDE3 inhibitors, including cilastozol, milrinone, and mixed PDE3/4 inhibitor enoximone, have mainly been used in the context of heart failure. Literature provides several cases with adverse effect and fatal outcome in the use of high dose PDE inhibitors for the chronic treatment of severe heart failure. A reason for this unfavorable outcome might have been that enoximone in heart failure was given in exceedingly high doses up to 2400 mg daily (31 mg/kg/dd) [98–100]; doses which were found to be extremely likely to cause severe side effects and a high mortality rate: after 6 months of treatment, at least half of the patients had died. Thus, the early research in pulmonary use has been abandoned and, since the late 90s, the sparse research into use of PDE3-inhibitors for pulmonary purposes has not led to the use of any of these drugs in the treatment of asthma. The first paper addressing actual clinical cases, in which enoximone treatment was given successfully in status asthmaticus and near fatal asthma was Beute [3], inspired by the resemblance between vascular and bronchial smooth muscle cell relaxation. In this paper, the doses used were considerably lower (1.15 mg/kg single dose) and the duration of administration was substantially shorter than in heart failure. Here, enoximone proved to be beneficial without side effects.

Enoximone is known as a PDE3 inhibitor that increases levels of cAMP as well as cGMP; however, in those cells where both compounds are present, cGMP will act as a competitive inhibitor on the breakdown of cAMP, thereby sustaining elevated levels of cAMP. cGMP can also be generated by nitric oxide (NO)-induced stimulation of guanylylcyclase (both abundantly present in smooth muscle cells), again impairing the breakdown of cAMP. The IC50 values of enoximone for PDE3 and PDE4 are 5.9 and 21.1 μM. The affinity of PDE3 for cAMP is 20 times higher than that of PDE4 [101].

These mechanisms probably allow for the favorable outcome of the relatively small doses of enoximone in Beute [3] and suggest an effect that exceeds its half-life.

Smooth muscle relaxation is more pronounced after administration of selective PDE3 inhibitors compared with PDE4 inhibitors. PDE3 inhibition leads to the enhancement of relaxation evoked by β2-receptor stimulation. Furthermore, simultaneous administration of siguazodan (PDE3 inhibitor) and rolipram (PDE4 inhibitor) enhances this relaxation, [102].

In **Figure 1**, both PDE3 and 4 are important in tailoring cyclic adenosine monophosphate signaling. PDE3/4 inhibitor increases intracellular cyclic adenosine monophosphate levels and has anti-inflammatory effects. Activation of a G-protein-coupled receptor (GPCR) activates adenylyl cyclase (AC) resulting in the induction of cAMP with the consequence of phosphokinase A (PKA) activation. Effect of PDE3/4 inhibition causes bronchodilation and improves endothelial and epithelial barrier function.

PDE4 is also present alongside the PDE3 isoenzyme in airway smooth muscle; the PDE3 isoenzyme is considered to predominate in airway smooth muscle, and inhibition of this enzyme leads to airway smooth muscle relaxation [103]. Moreover, PDE3 isoenzyme A is located in the cell membrane [25] and presumably easy to target, and could be involved in the rapid effects of therapy (minutes or earlier) seen during the intravenous emergency treatment in the studies of Beute [3].

Bringing to mind once again that all the cells and mechanisms mentioned in this chapter are regulated/influenced by either PDE3, PDE4, or both, and that all these cells and mechanisms

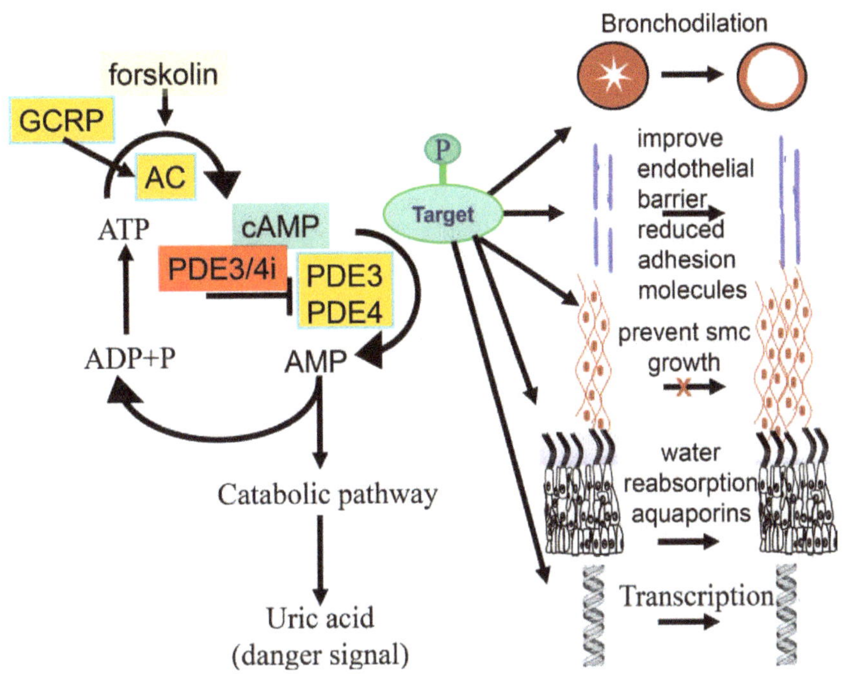

Figure 1. PDE3 and PDE4 inhibition improve harmful asthma-related processes.

are involved in the development, maintenance, or aggravation of asthma, there is a strong case for the assumption that enoximone may have a large impact on the acute treatment of severe asthma, on various separate levels. Additional safety studies will also be required.

As discussed above, further research in PDEs appears to be advisable in order to investigate their true potential.

Author details

Jan Beute[1], Vincent Manganiello[†2] and Alex KleinJan[1*]

*Address all correspondence to: a.kleinjan@erasmusmc.nl

1 Department of Pulmonary Medicine, Erasmus MC Rotterdam, Rotterdam, The Netherlands

2 Cardiovascular Pulmonary Branch, NHLBI, National Institutes of Health, Bethesda, Maryland

†VM was supported by the NHLBI Intramural Research Program. Dr. Manganiello died on January 10, 2016

References

[1] Barnes PJ. Immunology of asthma and chronic obstructive pulmonary disease. Nature Reviews. Immunology. 2008; :183-192
8

[2] Chung KF, Caramori G, Adcock IM. Inhaled corticosteroids as combination therapy with beta-adrenergic agonists in airways disease: Present and future. European Journal of Clinical Pharmacology. 2009;**65**:853-871

[3] Beute J. Emergency treatment of status asthmaticus with enoximone. British Journal of Anaesthesia. 2014. pp 1105-1108

[4] Wenzel SE. Asthma phenotypes: The evolution from clinical to molecular approaches. Nature Medicine. 2012;**18**:716-725

[5] Sutherland EW, Rall TW. Fractionation and characterization of a cyclic adenine ribonucleotide formed by tissue particles. The Journal of Biological Chemistry. 1958;**232**:1077-1091

[6] Francis SH, Blount MA, Corbin JD. mammalian cyclic nucleotide phosphodiesterases: Molecular mechanisms and physiological functions. Physiological Reviews. 2011;**91**: 651-690

[7] Sunahara RK, Taussig R. Isoforms of mammalian adenylyl cyclase: Multiplicities of signaling. Molecular Interventions. 2002;**2**:168-184

[8] Cooper DM, Crossthwaite AJ. Higher-order organization and regulation of adenylyl cyclases. Trends in Pharmacological Sciences. 2006;**27**:426-431

[9] Kamenetsky M, Middelhaufe S, Bank EM, Levin LR, Buck J, Steegborn C. Molecular details of cAMP generation in mammalian cells: A tale of two systems. Journal of Molecular Biology. 2006;**362**:623-639

[10] Beavo JA. Cyclic nucleotide phosphodiesterases: Functional implications of multiple isoforms. Physiological Reviews. 1995;**75**:725-748

[11] Maurice DH, Ke HM, Ahmad F, Wang YS, Chung J, Manganiello VC. Advances in targeting cyclic nucleotide phosphodiesterases. Nature Reviews Drug Discovery. 2014;**13**:290-314

[12] Willart MA, van Nimwegen M, Grefhorst A, Hammad H, Moons L, Hoogsteden HC, et al. Ursodeoxycholic acid suppresses eosinophilic airway inflammation by inhibiting the function of dendritic cells through the nuclear farnesoid X receptor. Allergy. 2012;**67**:1501-1510

[13] Miki T, Taira M, Hockman S, Shimada F, Lieman J, Napolitano M, et al. Characterization of the cDNA and gene encoding human PDE3B, the cGIP1 isoform of the human cyclic GMP-inhibited cyclic nucleotide phosphodiesterase family. Genomics. 1996;**36**:476-485

[14] Kasuya J, Liang SJ, Goko H, Park SH, Kato K, Xu ZD, et al. Cardiac type cGMP-inhibited phosphodiesterase (PDE3A) gene structure: Similarity and difference to adipocyte type PDE3B gene. Biochemical and Biophysical Research Communications. 2000;**268**: 827-834

[15] Degerman E, Belfrage P, Manganiello VC. Structure, localization, and regulation of cGMP-inhibited phosphodiesterase (PDE3). The Journal of Biological Chemistry. 1997;**272**: 6823-6826

[16] Lugnier C. Cyclic nucleotide phosphodiesterase (PDE) superfamily: A new target for the development of specific therapeutic agents. Pharmacology & Therapeutics. 2006;**109**: 366-398

[17] Fischmeister R, Hartzell HC. Regulation of calcium current by low-Km cyclic AMP phosphodiesterases in cardiac cells. Molecular Pharmacology. 1990;**38**:426-433

[18] Beca S, Ahmad F, Shen WX, Liu J, Makary S, Polidovitch N, et al. Phosphodiesterase Type 3A regulates basal myocardial contractility through interacting with sarcoplasmic reticulum calcium ATPase Type 2a signaling complexes in mouse heart. Circulation Research. 2013;**112**:289

[19] Kass DA, Takimoto E, Nagayama T, Champion HC. Phosphodiesterase regulation of nitric oxide signaling. Cardiovascular Research. 2007;**75**:303-314

[20] Leroy MJ, Degerman E, Taira M, Murata T, Wang LH, Movsesian MA, et al. Characterization of two recombinant PDE3 (cGMP-inhibited cyclic nucleotide phosphodiesterase) isoforms, RcGIP1 and HcGIP2, expressed in NIH 3006 murine fibroblasts and Sf9 insect cells. Biochemistry. 1996;**35**:10194-10202

[21] Bratt JM, Williams K, Rabowsky MF, Last MS, Franzi LM, Last JA, et al. Nitric oxide synthase enzymes in the airways of mice exposed to ovalbumin: NOS2 expression is NOS3 dependent. Mediators of Inflammation. 2010;**2010**. ID: 321061

[22] Kobayashi K, Nishimura Y, Yamashita T, Nishiuma T, Satouchi M, Yokoyama M. The effect of overexpression of endothelial nitric oxide synthase on eosinophilic lung inflammation in a murine model. International Immunopharmacology. 2006;**6**:1040-1052

[23] Yamazaki T, Anraku T, Matsuzawa S. Ibudilast, a mixed PDE3/4 inhibitor, causes a selective and nitric oxide/cGMP-independent relaxation of the intracranial vertebrobasilar artery. European Journal of Pharmacology. 2011;**650**:605-611

[24] Matthiesen K, Nielsen J. Cyclic AMP control measured in two compartments in HEK293 cells: phosphodiesterase K(M) is more important than phosphodiesterase localization. PLoS One. 2011;**6**:e24392

[25] Azevedo MF, Faucz FR, Bimpaki E, Horvath A, Levy I, de Alexandre RB, et al. Clinical and molecular genetics of the phosphodiesterases (PDEs). Endocrine Reviews. 2014;**35**:195-233

[26] Ahmad F, Degerman E, Manganiello VC. Cyclic nucleotide phosphodiesterase 3 signaling complexes. Hormone and Metabolic Research. 2012;**44**:930

[27] Berridge MJ. Introduction. Cell Signalling Biology. Module 2 Portland Press Limited. 2012:1-63

[28] Ghofrani HA, Pepke-Zaba J, Barbera JA, Channick R, Keogh AM, Gomez-Sanchez MA, et al. Nitric oxide pathway and phosphodiesterase inhibitors in pulmonary arterial hypertension. Journal of the American College of Cardiology. 2004;**43**:68S-72S

[29] Movsesian M, Wever-Pinzon O, Vandeput F. PDE3 inhibition in dilated cardiomyopathy. Current Opinion in Pharmacology. 2011;**11**:707-713

[30] Packer M, Carver JR, Rodeheffer RJ, Ivanhoe RJ, Dibianco R, Zeldis SM, et al. Effect of oral milrinone on mortality in severe chronic heart-failure. New England Journal of Medicine. 1991;**325**:1468-1475

[31] Movsesian M, Kukreja R. Phosphodiesterase inhibition in heart failure. In: Francis SH, Conti M, Houslay MD, editors. Phosphodiesterases as Drug Targets. Berlin, Heidelberg: Springer; 2011. pp. 237-249

[32] Yan C, Miller CL, Abe J. Regulation of phosphodiesterase 3 and inducible cAMP early repressor in the heart. Circulation Research. 2007;**100**:489-501

[33] Ding B, Abe J, Wei H, Xu HD, Che WY, Aizawa T, et al. A positive feedback loop of phosphodiesterase 3 (PDE3) and inducible cAMP early repressor (ICER) leads to cardiomyocyte apoptosis. Proceedings of the National Academy of Sciences of the United States of America. 2005;**102**:14771-14776

[34] Yasmin S, Yongge L, Junichi K. Bench to bedside. In: Cyclic Nucleotide Phosphodiesterases in Health and Disease. Boca Raton, London, New York: Taylor & Francis Group, CRC Press; 2006

[35] Chung KF, Godard P, Adelroth E, Ayres J, Barnes N, Barnes P, et al. Difficult/therapy-resistant asthma: the need for an integrated approach to define clinical phenotypes, evaluate risk factors, understand pathophysiology and find novel therapies. ERS Task Force on Difficult/Therapy-Resistant Asthma. European Respiratory Society. The European Respiratory Journal. 1999;**13**:1198-1208

[36] Benayoun L, Druilhe A, Dombret MC, Aubier M, Pretolani M. Airway structural alterations selectively associated with severe asthma. American Journal of Respiratory and Critical Care Medicine. 2003;**167**:1360-1368

[37] Macedo P, Hew M, Torrego A, Jouneau S, Oates T, Durham A, et al. Inflammatory biomarkers in airways of patients with severe asthma compared with non-severe asthma. Clinical and Experimental Allergy. 2009;**39**:1668-1676

[38] Trian T, Benard G, Begueret H, Rossignol R, Girodet PO, Ghosh D, et al. Bronchial smooth muscle remodeling involves calcium-dependent enhanced mitochondrial biogenesis in asthma. The Journal of Experimental Medicine. 2007;**204**:3173-3181

[39] Hassan M, Jo T, Risse PA, Tolloczko B, Lemiere C, Olivenstein R, et al. Airway smooth muscle remodeling is a dynamic process in severe long-standing asthma. The Journal of Allergy and Clinical Immunology. 2010;**125**:1037-1045. e3

[40] Johnson PR, Roth M, Tamm M, Hughes M, Ge Q, King G, et al. Airway smooth muscle cell proliferation is increased in asthma. American Journal of Respiratory and Critical Care Medicine. 2001;**164**:474-477

[41] Bhavsar P, Hew M, Khorasani N, Torrego A, Barnes PJ, Adcock I, et al. Relative corticosteroid insensitivity of alveolar macrophages in severe asthma compared with non-severe asthma. Thorax. 2008;**63**:784-790

[42] Hew M, Bhavsar P, Torrego A, Meah S, Khorasani N, Barnes PJ, et al. Relative corticosteroid insensitivity of peripheral blood mononuclear cells in severe asthma. American Journal of Respiratory and Critical Care Medicine. 2006;**174**:134-141

[43] Roth M, Johnson PR, Borger P, Bihl MP, Rudiger JJ, King GG, et al. Dysfunctional interaction of C/EBPalpha and the glucocorticoid receptor in asthmatic bronchial smooth-muscle cells. The New England Journal of Medicine. 2004;**351**:560-574

[44] Begum N, Hockman S, Manganiello VC. Phosphodiesterase 3A (PDE3A) deletion suppresses proliferation of cultured murine vascular smooth muscle cells (VSMCs) via inhibition of mitogen-activated protein kinase (MAPK) signaling and alterations in critical cell cycle regulatory proteins. The Journal of Biological Chemistry. 2011;**286**:26238-26249

[45] Blease K, Burke-Gaffney A, Hellewell PG. Modulation of cell adhesion molecule expression and function on human lung microvascular endothelial cells by inhibition of phosphodiesterases 3 and 4. British Journal of Pharmacology. 1998;**124**:229-237

[46] Wright LC, Seybold J, Robichaud A, Adcock IM, Barnes PJ. Phosphodiesterase expression in human epithelial cells. The American Journal of Physiology. 1998;**275**:L694-L700

[47] Noda K, Zhang J, Fukuhara S, Kunimoto S, Yoshimura M, Mochizuki N. Vascular endothelial-cadherin stabilizes at cell-cell junctions by anchoring to circumferential actin bundles through alpha- and beta-catenins in cyclic AMP-Epac-Rap1 signal-activated endothelial cells. Molecular Biology of the Cell. 2010;**21**:584-596

[48] Kobayashi K, Tsubosaka Y, Hori M, Narumiya S, Ozaki H, Murata T. Prostaglandin D2-DP signaling promotes endothelial barrier function via the cAMP/PKA/Tiam1/Rac1 pathway. Arteriosclerosis, Thrombosis, and Vascular Biology. 2013;**33**:565-571

[49] Polson JB, Strada SJ. Cyclic nucleotide phosphodiesterases and vascular smooth muscle. Annual Review of Pharmacology and Toxicology. 1996;**36**:403-427

[50] Suttorp N, Ehreiser P, Hippenstiel S, Fuhrmann M, Krull M, Tenor H, et al. Hyperpermeability of pulmonary endothelial monolayer: protective role of phosphodiesterase isoenzymes 3 and 4. Lung. 1996;**174**:181-194

[51] Singleton PA, Dudek SM, Chiang ET, Garcia JG. Regulation of sphingosine 1-phosphate-induced endothelial cytoskeletal rearrangement and barrier enhancement by S1P1 receptor, PI3 kinase, Tiam1/Rac1, and alpha-actinin. The FASEB Journal. 2005;**19**:1646-1656

[52] Hammad H, de Heer HJ, Soullie T, Hoogsteden HC, Trottein F, Lambrecht BN. Prostaglandin D2 inhibits airway dendritic cell migration and function in steady state conditions by selective activation of the D prostanoid receptor 1. Journal of Immunology. 2003;**171**:3936-3940

[53] Idzko M, Hammad H, van Nimwegen M, Kool M, Muller T, Soullie T, et al. Local application of FTY720 to the lung abrogates experimental asthma by altering dendritic cell function. The Journal of Clinical Investigation. 2006;**116**:2935-2944

[54] Idzko M, Hammad H, van Nimwegen M, Kool M, Vos N, Hoogsteden HC, et al. Inhaled iloprost suppresses the cardinal features of asthma via inhibition of airway dendritic cell function. The Journal of Clinical Investigation. 2007;**117**:464-472

[55] Konya V, Sturm EM, Schratl P, Beubler E, Marsche G, Schuligoi R, et al. Endothelium-derived prostaglandin I(2) controls the migration of eosinophils. The Journal of Allergy and Clinical Immunology. 2010;**125**:1105-1113

[56] Schick MA, Wunder C, Wollborn J, Roewer N, Waschke J, Germer CT, et al. Phosphodiesterase-4 inhibition as a therapeutic approach to treat capillary leakage in systemic inflammation. The Journal of Physiology. 2012;**590**:2693-2708

[57] Lehtonen LA, Antila S, Pentikainen PJ. Pharmacokinetics and pharmacodynamics of intravenous inotropic agents. Clinical Pharmacokinetics. 2004;**43**:187-203

[58] Kern H, Schroder T, Kaulfuss M, Martin M, Kox WJ, Spies CD. Enoximone in contrast to dobutamine improves hepatosplanchnic function in fluid-optimized septic shock patients. Critical Care Medicine. 2001;**29**:1519-1525

[59] Santarpino G, Caroleo S, Onorati F, Dimastromatteo G, Abdalla K, Amantea B, et al. Inflammatory response to cardiopulmonary bypass with enoximone or steroids in patients undergoing myocardial revascularization: A preliminary report study. International Journal of Clinical Pharmacology and Therapeutics. 2009;**47**:78-88

[60] Pearse DB, Shimoda LA, Verin AD, Bogatcheva N, Moon C, Ronnett GV, et al. Effect of cGMP on lung microvascular endothelial barrier dysfunction following hydrogen peroxide. Endothelium. 2003;**10**:309-317

[61] Suttorp N, Weber U, Welsch T, Schudt C. Role of phosphodiesterases in the regulation of endothelial permeability in vitro. The Journal of Clinical Investigation. 1993;**91**:1421-1428

[62] Fuhrmann M, Jahn HU, Seybold J, Neurohr C, Barnes PJ, Hippenstiel S, et al. Identification and function of cyclic nucleotide phosphodiesterase isoenzymes in airway epithelial cells. American Journal of Respiratory Cell and Molecular Biology. 1999;**20**:292-302

[63] Nagai K, Watanabe M, Seto M, Hisatsune A, Miyata T, Isohama Y. Nitric oxide decreases cell surface expression of aquaporin-5 and membrane water permeability in lung epithelial cells. Biochemical and Biophysical Research Communications. 2007;**354**:579-584

[64] Sidhaye V, Hoffert JD, King LS. cAMP has distinct acute and chronic effects on aquaporin-5 in lung epithelial cells. The Journal of Biological Chemistry. 2005;**280**:3590-3596

[65] Fanelli V, Puntorieri V, Assenzio B, Martin EL, Elia V, Bosco M, et al. Pulmonary-derived phosphoinositide 3-kinase gamma (PI3Kgamma) contributes to ventilator-induced lung injury and edema. Intensive Care Medicine. 2010;**36**:1935-1945

[66] Mokra D, Drgova A, Pullmann R Sr, Calkovska A. Selective phosphodiesterase 3 inhibitor olprinone attenuates meconium-induced oxidative lung injury. Pulmonary Pharmacology & Therapeutics. 2012;**25**:216-222

[67] Van der Mey M, Bommele KM, Boss H, Hatzelmann A, Van Slingerland M, Sterk GJ, et al. Synthesis and structure-activity relationships of cis-tetrahydrophthalazinone/pyridazinone hybrids: a novel series of potent dual PDE3/PDE4 inhibitory agents. Journal of Medicinal Chemistry. 2003;**46**:2008-2016

[68] Haddad JJ, Land SC, Tarnow-Mordi WO, Zembala M, Kowalczyk D, Lauterbach R. Immunopharmacological potential of selective phosphodiesterase inhibition. I. Differential regulation of lipopolysaccharide-mediated proinflammatory cytokine (interleukin-6 and tumor necrosis factor-alpha) biosynthesis in alveolar epithelial cells. The Journal of Pharmacology and Experimental Therapeutics. 2002;**300**:559-566

[69] Barnes PJ. Theophylline. American Journal of Respiratory and Critical Care Medicine. 2013;**188**:901-906

[70] Lambrecht BN, Hammad H. Asthma: The importance of dysregulated barrier immunity. European Journal of Immunology. 2013;**43**:3125-3137

[71] Lau HY, Kam MF. Inhibition of mast cell histamine release by specific phosphodiesterase inhibitors. Inflammation Research. 2005;**54**(Suppl. 1):S05-S06

[72] Milara J, Navarro A, Almudever P, Lluch J, Morcillo EJ, Cortijo J. Oxidative stress-induced glucocorticoid resistance is prevented by dual PDE3/PDE4 inhibition in human alveolar macrophages. Clinical and Experimental Allergy. 2011;**41**:535-546

[73] Gantner F, Schudt C, Wendel A, Hatzelmann A. Characterization of the phosphodiesterase (PDE) pattern of in vitro-generated human dendritic cells (DC) and the influence of PDE inhibitors on DC function. Pulmonary Pharmacology & Therapeutics. 1999;**12**:377-386

[74] Heystek HC, Thierry AC, Soulard P, Moulon C. Phosphodiesterase 4 inhibitors reduce human dendritic cell inflammatory cytokine production and Th1-polarizing capacity. International Immunology. 2003;**15**:827-835

[75] Gantner F, Tenor H, Gekeler V, Schudt C, Wendel A, Hatzelmann A. Phosphodiesterase profiles of highly purified human peripheral blood leukocyte populations from normal and atopic individuals: A comparative study. The Journal of Allergy and Clinical Immunology. 1997;**100**:527-535

[76] Barber R, Baillie GS, Bergmann R, Shepherd MC, Sepper R, Houslay MD, et al. Differential expression of PDE4 cAMP phosphodiesterase isoforms in inflammatory cells of smokers with COPD, smokers without COPD, and nonsmokers. American Journal of Physiology. Lung Cellular and Molecular Physiology. 2004;**287**:L332-L343

[77] Landells LJ, Spina D, Souness JE, O'Connor BJ, Page CP. A biochemical and functional assessment of monocyte phosphodiesterase activity in healthy and asthmatic subjects. Pulmonary Pharmacology & Therapeutics. 2000;**13**:231-239

[78] Giembycz MA, Corrigan CJ, Seybold J, Newton R, Barnes PJ. Identification of cyclic AMP phosphodiesterases 3, 4 and 7 in human CD4+ and CD8+ T-lymphocytes: role in regulating proliferation and the biosynthesis of interleukin-2. British Journal of Pharmacology. 1996;**118**:1945-1958

[79] Banner KH, Press NJ. Dual PDE3/4 inhibitors as therapeutic agents for chronic obstructive pulmonary disease. British Journal of Pharmacology. 2009;**157**:892-906

[80] Essayan DM, Kagey-Sobotka A, Lichtenstein LM, Huang SK. Differential regulation of human antigen-specific Th1 and Th2 lymphocyte responses by isozyme selective cyclic nucleotide phosphodiesterase inhibitors. The Journal of Pharmacology and Experimental Therapeutics. 1997;**282**:505-512

[81] Peter D, Jin SL, Conti M, Hatzelmann A, Zitt C. Differential expression and function of phosphodiesterase 4 (PDE4) subtypes in human primary CD4+ T cells: predominant role of PDE4D. Journal of Immunology. 2007;**178**:4820-4831

[82] Averill LE, Stein RL, Kammer GM. Control of human T-lymphocyte interleukin-2 production by a cAMP-dependent pathway. Cellular Immunology. 1988;**115**:88-99

[83] Bazhin AV, Kahnert S, Kimpfler S, Schadendorf D, Umansky V. Distinct metabolism of cyclic adenosine monophosphate in regulatory and helper CD4+ T cells. Molecular Immunology. 2010;**47**:678-684

[84] Gerlo S, Kooijman R, Beck IM, Kolmus K, Spooren A, Haegeman G. Cyclic AMP: A selective modulator of NF-kappaB action. Cellular and Molecular Life Sciences. 2011;**68**: 3823-3841

[85] Rodriguez G, Ross JA, Nagy ZS, Kirken RA. Forskolin-inducible cAMP pathway negatively regulates T-cell proliferation by uncoupling the interleukin-2 receptor complex. The Journal of Biological Chemistry. 2013;**288**:7137-7146

[86] Feng G, Nadig SN, Backdahl L, Beck S, Francis RS, Schiopu A, et al. Functional regulatory T cells produced by inhibiting cyclic nucleotide phosphodiesterase type 3 prevent allograft rejection. Science Translational Medicine. 2011;**3**:83ra40

[87] Shih CH, Huang TJ, Chen CM, Lin YL, Ko WC. S-petasin, the main sesquiterpene of petasites formosanus, inhibits phosphodiesterase activity and suppresses ovalbumin-induced airway hyperresponsiveness. Evidence-based Complementary and Alternative Medicine. 2011;**2011**:132374

[88] Weston MC, Peachell PT. Regulation of human mast cell and basophil function by cAMP. General Pharmacology. 1998;**31**:715-719

[89] Rivington RN, Boulet LP, Cote J, Kreisman H, Small DI, Alexander M, et al. Efficacy of Uniphyl, salbutamol, and their combination in asthmatic patients on high-dose inhaled steroids. American Journal of Respiratory and Critical Care Medicine. 1995;**151**:325-332

[90] Yasui K, Agematsu K, Shinozaki K, Hokibara S, Nagumo H, Yamada S, et al. Effects of theophylline on human eosinophil functions: comparative study with neutrophil functions. Journal of Leukocyte Biology. 2000;**68**:194-200

[91] Yasui K, Hu B, Nakazawa T, Agematsu K, Komiyama A. Theophylline accelerates human granulocyte apoptosis not via phosphodiesterase inhibition. The Journal of Clinical Investigation. 1997;**100**:1677-1684

[92] Bethke T, Eschenhagen T, Klimkiewicz A, Kohl C, von der Leyen H, Mehl H, et al. Phosphodiesterase inhibition by enoximone in preparations from nonfailing and failing human hearts. Arzneimittel-Forschung. 1992;**42**:437-445

[93] Fujimura M, Kamio Y, Saito M, Hashimoto T, Matsuda T. Bronchodilator and bronchoprotective effects of cilostazol in humans in vivo. American Journal of Respiratory and Critical Care Medicine. 1995;**151**:222-225

[94] Herbert C, Hettiaratchi A, Webb DC, Thomas PS, Foster PS, Kumar RK. Suppression of cytokine expression by roflumilast and dexamethasone in a model of chronic asthma. Clinical and Experimental Allergy. 2008;**38**:847-856

[95] Fabbri LM, Calverley PMA, Izquierdo-Alonso JL, Bundschuh DS, Brose M, Martinez FJ, et al. Roflumilast in moderate-to-severe chronic obstructive pulmonary disease treated with longacting bronchodilators: Two randomised clinical trials. Lancet. 2009;**374**:695-703

[96] Burgess JK, Oliver BG, Poniris MH, Ge Q, Boustany S, Cox N, et al. A phosphodiesterase 4 inhibitor inhibits matrix protein deposition in airways in vitro. The Journal of Allergy and Clinical Immunology. 2006;**118**:649-657

[97] Rabe KF. Update on roflumilast, a phosphodiesterase 4 inhibitor for the treatment of chronic obstructive pulmonary disease. British Journal of Pharmacology. 2011;**163**:53-67

[98] Kereiakes D, Chatterjee K, Parmley WW, Atherton B, Curran D, Kereiakes A, et al. Intravenous and oral Mdl-17043 (a new inotrope-vasodilator agent) in congestive heart-failure—Hemodynamic and clinical-evaluation in 38 patients. Journal of the American College of Cardiology. 1984;**4**:884-889

[99] Rubin SA, Tabak L. Mdl-17043—Short-term and long-term cardiopulmonary and clinical effects in patients with heart-failure. Journal of the American College of Cardiology. 1985;**5**:1422-1427

[100] Shah PK, Amin DK, Hulse S, Shellock F, Swan HJC. Inotropic therapy for refractory congestive heart-failure with oral fenoximone (Mdl-17,043)—Poor long-term results despite early hemodynamic and clinical improvement. Circulation. 1985;**71**:326-331

[101] Boswell-Smith V, Cazzola M, Page CP. Are phosphodiesterase 4 inhibitors just more theophylline? Journal of Allergy and Clinical Immunology. 2006;**117**:1237-1243

[102] Mokry J, Mokra D. Immunological aspects of phosphodiesterase inhibition in the respiratory system. Respiratory Physiology & Neurobiology. 2013;**187**:11-17

[103] Schudt C, Tenor H, Hatzelmann A. Pde isoenzymes as targets for antiasthma drugs. European Respiratory Journal. 1995;**8**:1179-1183

9

Subcellular Organelles in Immune Responses of Severe Asthma: The Roles of Mitochondria and Endoplasmic Reticulum

Yong Chul Lee and So Ri Kim

Abstract

Subcellular organelles including mitochondria and endoplasmic reticulum are now considered as one major target for many therapeutic approaches. In fact, recent evidence has uncovered the roles of mitochondria as a direct inflammatory and immune controller and contributor to the diseases by metabolic dysfunction and/or their abnormal dynamics. In addition, one of the important subcellular organelles, endoplasmic reticulum, also plays as an immune responder in several diseases including bronchial asthma. Recently, we have reported that the endoplasmic reticulum stress and mitochondrial reactive oxygen species (ROS) contribute to the pathogenesis of steroid-resistant severe bronchial asthma through the modulation of immune responses such as production of regulatory cytokines and NLRP3 inflammasome activation. These findings indicate that the subcellular organelles and their complex can be a promising target for the development of novel therapeutic strategies including medicines to cure severe asthma. This chapter is aimed to present the state-of-art information regarding the role of subcellular organelles in severe asthma.

Keywords: subcellular organelles, mitochondria, endoplasmic reticulum, inflammasome, severe asthma

1. Introduction

Subcellular organelle is a specialized subunit within a cell that has a specific function. Individual organelles are usually separately enclosed within their own lipid bilayers [1]. Specifically in eukaryotic cells, the organelles include nucleus, mitochondrion, endoplasmic reticulum (ER), Golgi apparatus, peroxisome, and lysosome which are found in the cytoplasm, a viscous liquid found within the cell membrane that houses the organelles and is the location of most of the action happening in a cell. Each organelle plays the specific functions such as DNA storage, energy production, production of lipid and proteins, export of the proteins from the cells, protein modification, and destruction of lipid and protein, respectively.

Among them, ER is the largest organelle in the cell and is a major site of protein synthesis and transport, protein folding, lipid and steroid synthesis, carbohydrate metabolism, and calcium storage [2–6]. One of the most prominent functions of the ER is protein synthesis. When ER is overloaded by increased demand in protein folding, cells initiate an adaptive response called unfolded protein response (UPR). In addition, the ER's secretory pathway of its products and the ER-associated degradation (ERAD) pathway try to keep the homeostasis with full activity [7, 8]. ER stress can be developed, if ER fails to overcome the overloads and UPR are not able to make the ER adapt to the stressful conditions, despite all ER's efforts and adaptive responses. Recent considerable studies have demonstrated that ER stress is associated with the pathogenesis of several diseases such as neurodegenerative disorders, metabolic disorders, cardiovascular diseases, malignancies, and respiratory disorders [9–12]. More specifically, in severe asthma or steroid-resistant asthma, the role of ER stress has been highlighted in terms of regulation and interaction of various signaling pathways linked to steroid resistance [13]. In addition, nowadays, changes of ER shapes and structure responded to ER stress are emerging as one of pathogenic mechanisms regarding several disorders [14].

Mitochondria are energy-producing organelles which are dynamic and possess mitochondrial own DNA distinct from nuclear genome [15]. Basically, they are in charge of the synthesis and catabolism of metabolites, generation and detoxification of reactive oxygen species (ROS), apoptosis, regulation of calcium, and generation of adenosine triphosphate (ATP) by oxidative phosphorylation [16]. Recently, a novel role for mitochondria has been revealed in various disorders such as infectious diseases, neurodegenerative diseases, cerebrovascular diseases, and metabolic diseases, especially in the association of innate immune and inflammatory responses [16–19]. In addition, our recent study has revealed that exceed generation of mitochondria ROS and alteration of mitochondrial DNA induced steroid-resistant neutrophilic asthmatic features through the activation of NLRP3 inflammasome in mice [20]. More interestingly, mitochondria are highly motile organelles. In fact, we know that mitochondria actively travel along the microtubule network in neurons and accumulate at sites of high-energy demands [21]. These mitochondrial dynamics and morphological changes are through constitutive cycles of fusion and fission [22]. Nowadays, impaired processes of mitochondrial dynamics have been accepted as a pathogenic contributor to various disorders, including lung diseases [23, 24].

The last decades have witnessed an explosion in the elucidation of the causative mechanisms implicated in bronchial asthma, especially severe or steroid-resistant asthma; however, the treatment of asthmatic patients is still challenging. One of the reasons can be that many newly developed therapeutic tools are single-targeted and linked to the shortage of broad clinical effect, although they might be effective in asthmatic patients with specific phenotypes. On the other hand, drugs with more widespread effects (e.g., kinase inhibitors) might be more effective pharmacologically, whereas the potential risk of side effects might increase [25].

Therefore, novel treatments should be considered to target the aspects of the multiple underlying allergic/immune/inflammatory processes and minimize the adverse effects on other systems. In terms of this point, targeting subcellular organelles, especially ER and mitochondria, has a strong competitive power for the development of future medications of asthma, especially steroid-resistant asthma, since restoration of their abnormal function to normal physiologic status of each subcellular organelle is going without serious adverse effects unlikely to the existing therapeutic approach of blocking or eliminating the pathogenic targets.

2. Severe asthma and its heterogeneity

For many years, the term severe asthma has been used interchangeably with other similar terms, and considerable effort has been concentrated to be uniform in the term and concept. Several academic societies and research groups have suggested the definition of severe asthma such as European Respiratory Society (ERS), American Thoracic Society (ATS), World Health Organization (WHO), and British Thoracic Society (BTS)/Scottish Intercollegiate Guideline Networks (SIGN) [26–30]. In various definitions of severe asthma with little differences, there is a common ground that severe asthma can be defined as a failure to achieve control with maximum doses of inhaled corticosteroid therapies [31]. Taken together, severe asthma contains the existing disease entities; steroid-insensitive asthma, steroid-resistant asthma, difficult asthma, and refractory asthma, and these subsets of asthmatics have been estimated up to 5–10% of all asthmatics.

Although there are still many different definitions for severe asthma available and difficulties in making an accurate definition for severe asthma, numerous data based on these definitions consistently demonstrate the heterogeneity of severe asthma in populations with asthma [32, 33]. In fact, in 2001, the National Heart, Lung, and Blood Institute initiated the Severe Asthma Research Program (SARP) to identify and characterize not only a large number of subjects with severe asthma but also to compare these subjects with those with mild to moderate asthma [34]. In the SARP adult clinical cluster analysis, five different groups of subjects with asthma were identified who differ in clinical and pathophysiologic parameters [33]. These five asthma phenotypes differ in lung function, age of asthma onset and duration, atopy, sex, symptom frequency, medication use, and health-care utilization. Clusters 1, 2, and 4 reflect the spectrum of allergic asthma from mild to severe airflow obstruction. The majority of these patients have early-onset disease, with history of atopy confirmed by skin prick testing and elevated total serum IgE. By contrast, Clusters 3 and 5 reflect the spectrum of adult-onset asthma characterized by older patients with less atopy, yet, high health-care utilization and poor quality of life [33]. The SARP clinical heterogeneity, even in severe asthma group, can provide a basis for the needs to investigate the different molecular and biological mechanisms and different therapeutic approaches for the patients with severe asthma. In addition, SARP cluster analysis revealed inflammatory heterogeneity through the evaluation of blood and sputum inflammatory cells. In addition, the data suggested that sputum eosinophils were increased in Cluster 4 subjects with severe allergic asthma, whereas both eosinophils and neutrophils were increased in subjects from Cluster 5 [33]. A sequential study has reported that grouping of subjects based on their sputum inflammatory cell profile identified four groups of subjects with distinguishing clinical characteristics [35]. For instance, patients showing both eosinophil (≥2%) and neutrophil (≥40%) predominant pattern, called as mixed granulocytic pattern, had the most severe asthma with severe chronic airflow obstruction and increased symptoms with high health-care utilization. In addition, according to this paradigm, all five clinical clusters of SARP showed all four patterns of sputum inflammatory profiles without a dominant pattern in any one cluster [34]. The lack of association between the clinical clusters and sputum inflammatory cell patterns does not only make the heterogeneity of severe asthma more complex but also emphasize that future analyses must incorporate clinical, physiologic, and inflammatory measures into one analysis [36].

Very recently, an interesting study of cluster analysis data has been released using U-BIOPRED (Unbiased BIOmarkers in PREDiction of respiratory disease outcomes) severe asthma cohort [37]. In this study, three transcriptome-associated clusters (TACs) were defined: TAC1 characterized by immune receptors IL33R, CCR3, and TSLPR, TAC2 characterized by interferon-, tumor necrosis factor (TNF)-α, and inflammasome-associated genes, and TAC3 characterized by genes of metabolic pathways, ubiquitination, and mitochondrial function. Subjects with severe asthma were classified into these three clusters based on their sputum transcriptomics data. Each TAC group exhibits their own differential clinical features: one Th2-high eosinophilic phenotype TAC1 and two non-Th2 phenotypes TAC2 and TAC3, characterized by inflammasome-associated and metabolic/mitochondrial pathways, respectively. This analytic approach is unlikely to previous ones such as SARP which showed the lack of association between the clinical clusters and sputum inflammatory cell patterns. Considering that clustering using clinical features alone has not yielded information on the underlying biology as similar inflammatory cell profiles have been seen between these clinical clusters [34], this study is worthy to approach with the unconventional direction from inflammatory or biologic clustering to clinical phenotyping. This approach provides a fresh framework on which to phenotype asthma and a more precise targeting of specific treatments [38]. Specifically, the development of novel medications has been poorer, targeting non-Th2 or non-type-2 severe asthma than Th2 or Type-2 severe asthma. In terms of this issue, this novel-clustering analysis data are expected to be helpful for the development of the medicines targeting non-type 2 asthmatics. In fact, two non-Th2 phenotypes TAC2 and TAC3 are associated with inflammasome and mitochondrial pathway, respectively. In addition, while the majority of subjects in TAC2 group show neutrophilic predominant inflammatory pattern, the subjects in TAC3 group can be further divided into paucigranulocytic, eosinophilic, and neutrophilic pattern subgroups. Interestingly, the differential characteristic of eosinophilic TAC3 subjects from Th2-type TAC1 subjects is the elevated levels of inflammasome, suggesting that non-Th2 type asthma can also have eosinophilic-dominant inflammation partly through the activation of inflammasome.

Considering nowadays the concept of severe asthma and heterogeneity, the improvement of the detailed characterization of the patients is required to achieve appropriate therapeutic responses for severe asthma. It is expected that the correct determination of phenotype and molecular endotype leads to more effective precision medicine for severe asthma.

3. ER stress in severe asthma

As introduced, ER is a specialized organelle that plays as an important regulator of protein homeostasis in cells of an organism. The ER is rich in chaperones and enzymes that help to fold the protein properly. ER chaperones and enzymes are fragile to various stresses; thus several stressful or pathologic conditions (e.g., disease situation) may lead to the impaired ER protein-folding capacity leading to the accumulation of misfolded and unfolded proteins in the ER lumen. This out-of-controlled state of ER is usually called as ER stress [13, 39, 40].

Three ER transmembrane sensors are inositol-requiring enzyme 1α (IRE1α), double-stranded RNA-dependent protein kinase (PKR)-like ER kinase (PERK), and activating transcription factor 6 (ATF6). The functions of the ER membranous proteins include monitoring protein homeostasis of ER lumen and activation of canonical UPR pathways to deliver the information on the ER status to cytoplasm [40, 41]. According to the classic model of the activation of UPR, in basal conditions, these three transmembrane proteins are bound by a chaperone, BiP/glucose-regulated protein 78 (GRP78) [42, 43]. The development of ER stress causes the separation of BiP from these UPR sensors bound. The activation of IRE1α and PERK is associated with the dimerization and auto-phosphorylation, while in case of ATF6, its translocation to the Golgi is required to get activated [7]. Activated forms of proteins mitigate ER stress through the reduction of protein synthesis, the enhancement of protein degradation, and the induction of production of ER chaperones. When the protective process fails to resolve ER stress, the cell is prepared for apoptosis which is also one of the biological protective mechanisms [44]. Recently, in addition to these canonical UPR, noncanonical aspects of UPR confer cells to interconnect protein homeostasis-related cellular apparatus to a wide array of cellular events including immunity and inflammation through various mechanisms, as substantially reviewed elsewhere [45, 46].

In addition, the complex roles of ER including protein synthesis and lipid synthesis, calcium regulation, and interactions with other organelles are reflected in an equally complex physical architecture. The ER is composed of a continuous membrane system that includes the nuclear envelope and the peripheral ER, defined by flat sheets and branching tubules [14]. While it is generally known how the basic shapes of ER sheets and tubules are determined, it is relatively unclear how changes in the shape or the ratio of sheets to tubules occur in response to specific cellular signals. In several conditions, increasing ER loads and ER stress such as mitosis, changes of ER structure, and shapes are noted. In fact, recent studies showed that splicing of XBP1 is activated during meiosis in both *Xenopus* and budding yeast [47, 48], suggesting that changes in ER structure during meiosis could be linked to the ER stress response. However, to date, it is remained unclear whether ER stress induces immediate restructuring of ER or not. In the same vein, it has not yet been determined whether the activation of ER stress-responsive-signaling pathways results in a modification of structural components of the ER [14].

Accumulating data have indicated that ER stress and UPR link to major inflammatory and stress-signaling networks including the nuclear factor kappa B (NF-κB) pathway and oxidative stress. Recent studies have unveiled the role of ER stress in the pathogenesis of various pulmonary disorders, including asthma, chronic obstructive pulmonary disease (COPD), idiopathic pulmonary fibrosis, and acute lung injury [9, 49–52].

As for bronchial asthma including severe form, the role of ER stress has been reviewed elsewhere [13, 40, 52]. In particular, neutrophilic steroid-resistant severe asthma animal model, which is similar to human TAC2 group, exhibited the significant increases in ER stress markers, GRP78 and CCAAT/enhancer binding protein-homologous protein (CHOP), as well as UPR-related proteins in lung tissues and BAL cells [9]. The mice showed typical asthmatic manifestations including bronchial hyperresponsiveness and airway inflammation which were not attenuated by the treatment with oral dexamethasone. Intriguingly, an ER stress regulator, 4-phenylbutyric acid (4-PBA), effectively attenuated steroid refractory asthmatic features as well as increases in ER stress linked to NF-κB activation which induces various severe inflammatory/immune responses in the lung. In addition, 4-PBA dramatically reduced the increased expression of IL-17, while it further enhanced the increase in IL-10 levels, leading to the attenuation of steroid-resistant asthmatic features. In another recent study using the same animal model [20], the activation of NLRP3 inflammasome was measured. The results revealed that NLRP3 inflammasome was significantly activated in lung tissues and BAL cells from neutrophilic-dominant severe asthma murine model and that the severe asthmatic symptoms were dramatically attenuated by the blockade of IL-1β which is one of major effector cytokines by NLRP3 inflammasome activation. A more recent study using another neutrophilic-dominant steroid-resistant asthma animal model and human data also has revealed the significant role of NLRP3 inflammasome in the pathogenesis of neutrophilic-dominant severe asthma [53]. These findings suggest that the neutrophilic-dominant steroid-resistant or severe asthma animal models can represent the TAC2 group of human severe asthma characterized by IFN, TNF-α, and inflammasome-associated genes and that ER stress can be more associated with this clustered asthma. A recent study has also demonstrated that ER stress inducer, tunicamycin, aggravates ER stress in mouse bronchial epithelial cells and increased the expression of inflammation indicators such as IL-6, IL-8, and TNF-α in lung tissues of neutrophilic severe asthmatic mice [54]. The double-stranded RNA (dsRNA)-activated serine/threonine kinase R (PKR) is well characterized as an essential component of the innate antiviral response. In view of the relation with ER stress, PKR phosphorylates e-IF2α, one of the branches for UPR, and at the same time, ER stress activates PKR which stimulates various inflammatory-signaling pathways [55, 56]. With this background, a recent interesting study showed that poly (I:C)-induced exacerbation of neutrophilic severe asthmatic mice was closely associated with PKR phosphorylation as well as increased ER stress in lung tissues including bronchial epithelial cells [56].

In addition to neutrophilic severe asthmatic phenotype, eosinophil-dominant severe asthma with fungal sensitization also showed the significant elevation of ER stress in mice [57]. In this study, *Aspergillus fumigatus* extract-inhaled mice showed typical asthmatic manifestations including eosinophilic airway inflammation and airway hyperresponsiveness which were not responded to treatment with oral steroid, while all asthmatic features and increased ER stress were very well controlled by 4-PBA, suggesting that ER stress is linked to the pathogenesis of eosinophilic-dominant severe asthma as well as neutrophilic-dominant one. Meanwhile, this animal model appeared to represent the TAC3 human severe asthma group. As described earlier, TAC3 is characterized by genes of metabolic pathways, ubiquitination, and mitochondrial function, and the subjects of TAC3 exhibit various inflammatory cell types including paucigranulocytic, eosinophilic, and neutrophilic pattern subgroups. Thus, this fungal extract-inhaled eosinophilic severe asthma murine model can be considered as an eosinophilic pattern TAC3, non-Th2 eosinophilic asthma. Actually, in this study, mitochondrial ROS was significantly increased in the lung from *A. fumigatus* extract-inhaled mice [57].

These observations suggest that ER stress plays a critical role in the pathogenesis of various phenotypes of severe asthma including neutrophilic, eosinophilic, and viral infection-related types, supporting that the ER stress-targeting strategy seems to be able to overcome the steroid resistance in severe asthma.

4. Mitochondria in severe asthma

Asthma is characterized by ongoing inflammation and accompanied by increased oxidative stress and subsequent lung injury. ROS production, which leads to oxidative stress, is one of critical features in chronic airway disorders [58]. Two major sources of ROS induced by external stimuli are mitochondria and the Nox family of nicotinamide adenine dinucleotide phosphate (NADPH) oxidase in vivo. Besides, the mitochondrial respiratory chain is considered to be an important part of ROS production within most cells [59]. In addition, the considerable interplay between mitochondria and ER in several respiratory disorders has been demonstrated [59, 60]. In fact, fungal extract-inhaled mice exhibiting features of eosinophilic severe asthma or representing eosinophilic TAC3 showed significant increases in the production of mitochondrial ROS in BAL cells [57]. *A. fumigatus* extract-stimulated tracheal epithelial cells from the mice also markedly more generated mitochondrial ROS compared to the control cells [57]. In addition, treatment with NecroX-5, a potent mitochondrial ROS inhibitor, effectively attenuated increases in mitochondrial ROS in BAL cells, reduced increases in GRP78 and CHOP in lung tissues from *A. fumigatus* extract-inhaled mice, and ameliorated pathophysiologic features of fungal extract-induced eosinophilic severe asthma. In addition to eosinophilic severe asthma, recent experimental data using ovalbumin (OVA) and lipopolysaccharide (LPS)-sensitized and OVA-challenged mice (OVA-LPS mice) representing TAC2 revealed that the increased generation of mitochondrial ROS and the alteration of mitochondrial DNA induced steroid-resistant neutrophilic asthmatic features through the activation of NLRP3 inflammasome in lung and that the restoration of mitochondrial ROS levels using mitochondrial-specific ROS scavenger dramatically attenuated steroid-resistant airway hyperresponsiveness and inflammation in mice [20]. These findings suggest that mitochondrial metabolic dysfunctions such as mitochondrial ROS generation and mitochondrial DNA damage are linked to other subcellular organelles (e.g., ER) and immunologic complex (e.g., inflammasome) in the pathogenesis of steroid-resistant asthma and that mitochondrial ROS plays a key role in the induction and maintenance of neutrophilic and eosinophilic steroid-resistant severe asthma. As supporting data, when N-acetylcysteine (NAC), which is a representative conventional antioxidant, was administered to both types of steroid-resistant severe asthma murine models, for example, eosinophilic and neutrophilic types, NAC did not affect steroid-resistant asthmatic features, mitochondrial ROS generation, and NLRP3 inflammasome activation (unpublished data), suggesting the importance of the role of mitochondrial ROS generation in the pathogenesis of steroid-resistant severe asthma as well as one of causes for the previous failures in the clinical trials for asthma patients to evaluate the effects of various conventional antioxidants.

Like this, mitochondria perform many roles beyond energy production, including the generation of ROS, redox molecules, and metabolites; regulation of cell signaling and cell death; and biosynthetic metabolism [61–63]. Thanks to these observations, mitochondria have recently become a promising target for the treatment of various inflammatory disorders, including bronchial asthma. However, most studies regarding mitochondria as a pathogenic contributor have dealt with mitochondrial metabolic dysfunction or mitochondrial genetic abnormality. As introduced, mitochondria are not static, highly dynamic in cells, and change the morphology.

Mitochondrial morphology is controlled by large guanosine triphosphatases in the dynamin family [64]. Among them, mitofusins 1 and 2 (MFN-1 and MFN-2) and optic atrophy protein 1 (OPA-1) are essential mediators of mitochondrial fusion [65]. By contrast, fission requires dynamin-related protein 1 (DRP-1) to be recruited from the cytosol to the mitochondrial surface [66]. Mitochondrial fission is known to be prevalent in diseased cells, with subsequent elimination of damaged mitochondria via mitophagy [67]. By contrast, mitochondrial fusion inhibits apoptotic cell death [22]. In fact, several reports have demonstrated that increased mitochondrial fission and decreased fusion are observed in cells from various lung diseases such as lung cancer [68, 69]. Interestingly, our preliminary data have revealed that mitochondrial dynamics were out of control in *A. fumigatus* extract-inhaled mice, and the restoration of abnormal mitochondrial dynamics could attenuate the steroid-resistant airway inflammation and airway hyperresponsiveness (unpublished data), providing the novel concept that a therapeutic strategy targeting mitochondrial dynamics can overcome steroid resistance in severe asthma. However, we are only beginning to evaluate and understand the related mechanisms and the role of mitochondrial dynamics in the pathogenesis of severe asthma. More future researches and studies are needed to support the role of mitochondria in the pathogenesis of severe asthma. In addition, the identification of the specific phenotype and/or endotype related to mitochondrial metabolic and morphologic dysfunction is eagerly required for the patient-oriented treatment or the precision medicine of severe asthma.

5. Potential clinical biomarkers and therapies related to mitochondria and ER

Biomarkers may facilitate the diagnosis and classification of severe asthma, predict efficacy of specific therapies, and assess medication response. Based on the data, to date, there are some potential biomarkers related to ER, mitochondria, and inflammasome in severe asthma. More specifically, the biomarker candidates are considered as the biomarkers for the prediction of efficacy of the subcellular organelle targeting therapies and for assessment therapeutic responses.

In fact, ER stress markers, GRP78 and CHOP, have been measured in BAL fluid from asthmatic patients [9]. Very interestingly, the levels were increased in BAL fluid from asthmatics compared to the levels from the healthy persons. The asthmatics were composed of patients who had been diagnosed and treated for asthma for more than 3 months with inhaled corticosteroid or combined inhaled corticosteroid and beta-β_2-agonist. In addition, the patients exhibited uncontrolled asthmatic symptoms scored below 19 points by asthma control test (ACT) scoring system despite the standard treatment including inhaled corticosteroid. Although the protein expression levels of GRP78 and CHOP were not correlated with the lung function, the protein expression reflected the asthmatic-controlled status in humans supported by the data from animal experiments, in which steroid-responded asthmatic mice showed the decrease in the expression levels of GRP78 and CHOP in lung tissues by the treatment of steroid, while the steroid-resistant asthmatic mice were refractory to the treatment with steroid in terms of the protein levels. When an ER stress inhibitor, 4-PBA, was administered to the steroid-resistant asthmatic mice, the levels of GRP78 and CHOP were substantially reduced in lung tissues and BAL cells with the attenuation of asthma symptoms [9]. These findings suggest the potential of the use of GRP78 and CHOP as biomarkers, classifying the patients into steroid-responsive group and steroid-resistant group after the standard treatment including inhaled corticosteroid as well as predicting or monitoring the therapeutic responses of ER stress inhibitor as a medication for severe asthma.

Mitochondrial ROS can be another biomarker candidate. In asthma, there is an elevated airway expression of products of oxidative stress. Actually, exhaled breath condensate levels of oxidative stress-related biomarkers, such as hydrogen peroxide (H_2O_2), nitrite/nitrate, 8-isoprostane, and others vary with asthma exacerbations, disease severity, and medication use [70]. As mentioned earlier, mitochondrial ROS may be a more critical player in the pathogenesis of severe asthma compared to general or total cellular ROS generation. Nowadays, several tools including simple detection kits and staining indicators have been introduced for measuring the specific mitochondrial ROS levels which distinct from the total cellular ROS generation in vivo. Thus, in addition to cellular ROS, mitochondrial ROS in various biological samples such as exhaled breath condensate, sputum, and BAL fluid can be expected to be one of biomarkers of the next generation for the diagnosis of severe or steroid-resistant asthma. Moreover, the studies using recently developed mitochondrial ROS inhibitor, NecroX compounds, have reported the excellent efficacy of this chemical as a potent and specific mitochondria-targeted antioxidant in several disease models [71–75]. Even in human studies, a phase II clinical trial is currently being performed to evaluate the efficacy, safety, and pharmacokinetics of intravenous injection of NecroX-7 immediately before percutaneous coronary intervention in patients with myocardial infarction (ClinicalTrials.gov; NCT02770664). Therefore, it can be hypothesized to consider that NecroX compounds may be developed as a novel therapeutic agent to control or cure the steroid-resistant severe asthma in future.

Furthermore, mitochondrial ROS is closely associated with the assembly of inflammasome, specifically NLRP3 inflammasome, which is formed by various stimuli in the inflammatory state. NLRP3, one of the cytosolic pattern recognition receptors, plays as one of the components of the inflammasome and recognizes a variety of inflammatory stimuli, pathogen-associated molecular pattern molecules (PAMPs), and damage-associated molecular pattern molecules (DAMPs) in cells. Subsequently, the assembled and activated NLRP3 inflammasome controls the production of important pro-inflammatory cytokines such as IL-1β and IL-18 [76]. Two common events that are required for these activators of the NLRP3 inflammasome are potassium efflux and ROS generation [77]. Recent interesting studies have revealed that steroid-resistant neutrophilic asthmatic manifestations were significantly controlled by the NLRP3 inflammasome activation, and the severe asthmatic symptoms were dramatically attenuated by the blockade of IL-1β or inflammasome inhibitor, MCC950 [20, 53]. Moreover, increased NLRP3 and IL-1β sputum gene expression were strongly associated with increasing asthma severity in humans, suggesting that the NLRP3 inflammasome is important in human disease as well [53]. In addition, the protein expression levels of NLRP3 and caspase-1 were more increased in BALF from uncontrolled asthmatics compared to healthy subjects [20]. Taken together, these data suggest the potential of NLRP3, IL-1β, or caspase-1 to use as diagnostic and therapeutic biomarkers in respiratory specimens and urge to perform the translational or clinical studies regarding this issue. In addition, until now, there are no interventional clinical data applying the agents targeting NLRP3 inflammasome such as MCC950 in steroid-refractory severe asthma; however, it can be a very promising target for the control of severe asthma.

Altogether, it is clear that there are huge needs for further researches and future translational and clinical studies to use the candidate markers and therapeutic agents related to subcellular organelles in clinical practice.

6. Conclusion and future directions

Severe asthma is characterized by uncontrolled symptoms and recurrent exacerbation with excessive chronic airway inflammation despite adequate and even maximum treatment with the current medications. Although multiple factors can cause poor responses and underlying pathogenic differences are being revealed explaining the various therapeutic responses including steroid insensitivity, effective therapeutic modalities for severe asthma still remain as a major unmet need [78]. To overcome these current obstacles, cluster analysis and research for the heterogeneity of severe asthma are actively ongoing. Recent unconventional approach to define the clusters of subjects with severe asthma using TACs seems to be more helpful for the development of precision medicine for severe asthma compared to conventional clinical feature-based clusters, although more future supporting researches are needed. In addition, the heterogeneity of severe asthma is going to be more complex as the cluster analytic tools are advanced.

Recently, accumulating findings suggest that the regulation of ER stress and the restoration of mitochondrial dysfunction are prospective molecular therapeutic approaches for various pulmonary disorders including bronchial asthma. More encouragingly, the inhibition of ER stress overcomes the failure of steroid in attenuating the severe asthmatic features of mice including non-Th2 neutrophilic type (similar to TAC2) as well as the eosinophilic type (similar to TAC3). Furthermore, as we described earlier, therapeutic approach to control ER stress is able to regulate multiple integrated signaling networks concomitantly known as the famous pathogenic mechanisms for steroid-resistant inflammatory responses. In addition, the link between ER stress and mitochondrial ROS generation is very interesting in severe asthma.

Interestingly, in non-Th2 neutrophilic severe asthma, NLRP3 inflammasome assembly is activated and consequently induces IL-1β production and release. In addition, mitochondrial

ROS generation and the mitochondrial DNA damage are closely associated with NLRP3 inflammasome activation in this animal model of severe asthma. Meanwhile, in non-Th2 eosinophilic steroid-resistant asthma induced by fungal extract, mitochondrial dysfunction on their dynamics or morphology as well as ROS generation is observed, which resulted in steroid-resistant airway inflammation and hyperresponsiveness in mice. Therefore, the restoration and inhibition of mitochondrial dysfunction can be a novel promising target for the therapeutics of severe asthma. Considering the link among ER, mitochondria, and inflammasome, their interconnection can be suggested as a more powerful tool for the control of severe asthma (**Figure 1**).

Despite success in mice, to date, there is the shortage of information on molecular mechanisms, explaining these effects of the control for ER stress and mitochondria, and there are also no clinical trials that evaluate the therapeutic effects of the pharmacologic agents targeting subcellular organelles in humans. In addition, since the subcellular organelles play essential roles in the body, the adverse effects of the pharmacologic intervention targeting ER or mitochondria must be considered. However, as for the adverse effects, since this therapeutic approaching concept is aimed to restore the stressful or dysfunctional condition into the physiologic levels, not to block the function or to null, it seems to be superior to other new therapeutics pursuing the single specific target blockade.

In conclusion, the restoration of subcellular organelles in a disease state is a potentially exciting target for developing agents to achieve better management of severe asthma in which steroids and other current agents are less effective.

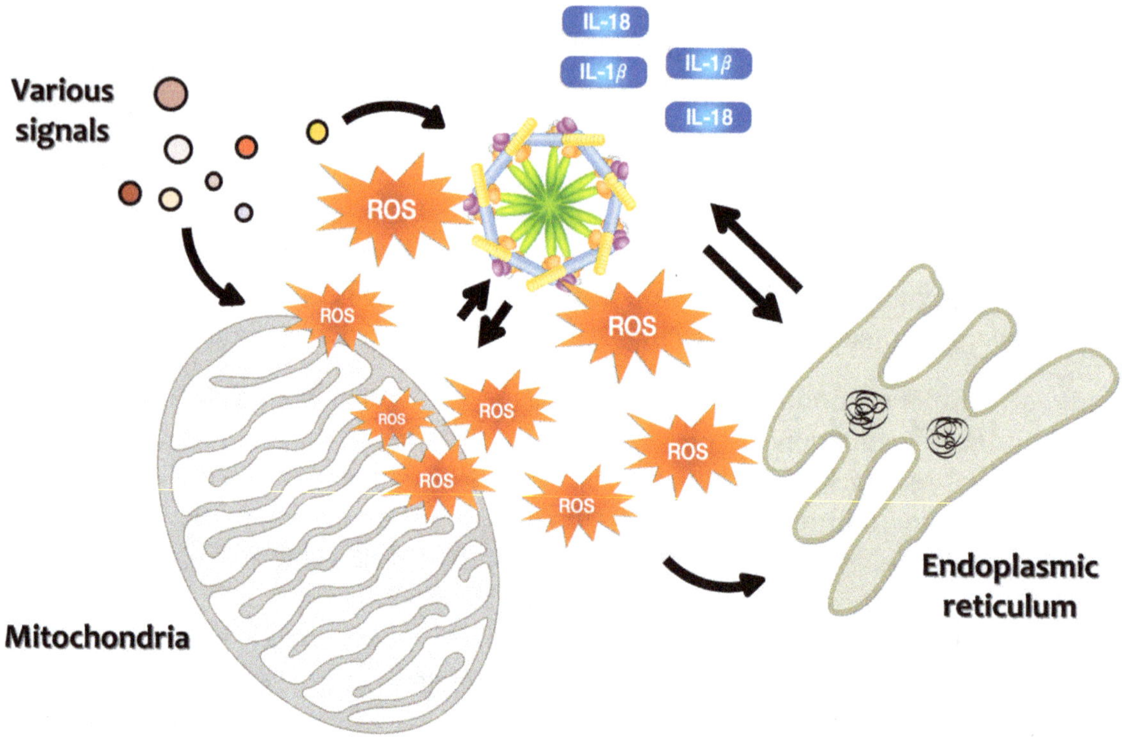

Figure 1. Schematic diagram of the possible interconnection among endoplasmic reticulum, mitochondria, and inflammasome in the pathogenesis of steroid-resistant asthma.

Acknowledgements

This work was supported by the Korea Healthcare Technology R&D Project, Ministry for Health and Welfare, Republic of Korea; Grant HI12C1786, Grant HI16C0062, and by Basic Science Research Program through the National Research Foundation of Korea (NRF) funded by the Ministry of Science, ICT, and future Planning (NRF-2014R1A2A1A01002823).

Author details

Yong Chul Lee and So Ri Kim*

*Address all correspondence to: sori@jbnu.ac.kr

Division of Respiratory Medicine and Allergy, Department of Internal Medicine, Chonbuk National University Medical School, Jeonju, South Korea

References

[1] Kerfeld CA, Sawaya MR, Tanaka S, Nguyen CV, Phillips M, Beeby M, et al. Protein structures forming the shell of primitive bacterial organelles. Science. 2005;**309**(5736):936-938

[2] Reid DW, Nicchitta CV. Diversity and selectivity in mRNA translation on the endoplasmic reticulum. Nature Reviews. Molecular Cell Biology. 2015;**16**(4):221-231

[3] Rapoport TA. Protein translocation across the eukaryotic endoplasmic reticulum and bacterial plasma membranes. Nature. 2007;**450**(7170):663-669

[4] Braakman I, Hebert DN. Protein folding in the endoplasmic reticulum. Cold Spring Harbor Perspectives in Biology. 2013;**5**(5):a013201

[5] Clapham DE. Calcium signaling. Cell. 2007;**131**(6):1047-1058

[6] Westrate LM, Lee JE, Prinz WA, Voeltz GK. Form follows function: The importance of endoplasmic reticulum shape. Annual Review of Biochemistry. 2015;**84**:791-811

[7] Ron D, Walter P. Signal integration in the endoplasmic reticulum unfolded protein response. Nature Reviews. Molecular Cell Biology. 2007;**8**(7):519-529

[8] Kim I, Xu W, Reed JC. Cell death and endoplasmic reticulum stress: Disease relevance and therapeutic opportunities. Nature Reviews. Drug Discovery. 2008;**7**(12):1013-1030

[9] Kim SR, Kim DI, Kang MR, Lee KS, Park SY, Jeong JS, et al. Endoplasmic reticulum stress influences bronchial asthma pathogenesis by modulating nuclear factor kappaB activation. The Journal of Allergy and Clinical Immunology. 2013;**132**(6):1397-1408

[10] Toth A, Nickson P, Mandl A, Bannister ML, Toth K, Erhardt P. Endoplasmic reticulum stress as a novel therapeutic target in heart diseases. Cardiovascular & Hematological Disorders Drug Targets. 2007;**7**(3):205-218

[11] Kelsen SG, Duan X, Ji R, Perez O, Liu C, Merali S. Cigarette smoke induces an unfolded protein response in the human lung: A proteomic approach. American Journal of Respiratory Cell and Molecular Biology. 2008;**38**(5):541-550

[12] Poppek D, Grune T. Proteasomal defense of oxidative protein modifications. Antioxidants & Redox Signaling. 2006;**8**(1-2):173-184

[13] Kim SR, Lee YC. Endoplasmic reticulum stress and the related signaling networks in severe asthma. Allergy, Asthma & Immunology Research. 2015;**7**(2):106-117

[14] Schwarz DS, Blower MD. The endoplasmic reticulum: Structure, function and response to cellular signaling. Cellular and Molecular Life Sciences. 2016;**73**(1):79-94

[15] Emelyanov VV. Mitochondrial connection to the origin of the eukaryotic cell. European Journal of Biochemistry. 2003;**270**(8):1599-1618

[16] Cloonan SM, Choi AM. Mitochondria: Commanders of innate immunity and disease? Current Opinion in Immunology. 2012;**24**(1):32-40

[17] Akundi RS, Huang Z, Eason J, Pandya JD, Zhi L, Cass WA, et al. Increased mitochondrial calcium sensitivity and abnormal expression of innate immunity genes precede dopaminergic defects in Pink1-deficient mice. PLoS One. 2011;**6**(1):e16038

[18] d'Avila JC, Santiago AP, Amancio RT, Galina A, Oliveira MF, Bozza FA. Sepsis induces brain mitochondrial dysfunction. Critical Care Medicine. 2008;**36**(6):1925-1932

[19] Hopps E, Noto D, Caimi G, Averna MR. A novel component of the metabolic syndrome: The oxidative stress. Nutrition, Metabolism, and Cardiovascular Diseases. 2010;**20**(1):72-77

[20] Kim SR, Kim DI, Kim SH, Lee H, Lee KS, Cho SH, et al. NLRP3 inflammasome activation by mitochondrial ROS in bronchial epithelial cells is required for allergic inflammation. Cell Death & Disease. 2014;**5**:e1498

[21] Birsa N, Norkett R, Higgs N, Lopez-Domenech G, Kittler JT. Mitochondrial trafficking in neurons and the role of the Miro family of GTPase proteins. Biochemical Society Transactions. 2013;**41**(6):1525-1531

[22] Westermann B. Mitochondrial fusion and fission in cell life and death. Nature Reviews. Molecular Cell Biology. 2010;**11**(12):872-884

[23] Archer SL. Mitochondrial dynamics—Mitochondrial fission and fusion in human diseases. The New England Journal of Medicine. 2013;**369**(23):2236-2251

[24] Aravamudan B, Thompson MA, Pabelick CM, Prakash YS. Mitochondria in lung diseases. Expert Review of Respiratory Medicine. 2013;**7**(6):631-646

[25] Barnes PJ. New therapies for asthma: Is there any progress? Trends in Pharmacological Sciences. 2010;**31**(7):335-343

[26] Chung KF, Wenzel SE, Brozek JL, Bush A, Castro M, Sterk PJ, et al. International ERS/ATS guidelines on definition, evaluation and treatment of severe asthma. The European Respiratory Journal. 2014;**43**(2):343-373

[27] Chung KF, Godard P, Adelroth E, Ayres J, Barnes N, Barnes P, et al. Difficult/therapy-resistant asthma: The need for an integrated approach to define clinical phenotypes, evaluate risk factors, understand pathophysiology and find novel therapies. ERS Task Force on Difficult/Therapy-Resistant Asthma. European Respiratory Society. The European Respiratory Journal. 1999;**13**(5):1198-1208

[28] Proceedings of the ATS workshop on refractory asthma: Current understanding, recommendations, and unanswered questions. American Thoracic Society. American Journal of Respiratory and Critical Care Medicine. 2000;**162**(6):2341-2351

[29] Bousquet J, Mantzouranis E, Cruz AA, Ait-Khaled N, Baena-Cagnani CE, Bleecker ER, et al. Uniform definition of asthma severity, control, and exacerbations: Document presented for the World Health Organization Consultation on Severe Asthma. The Journal of Allergy and Clinical Immunology. 2010;**126**(5):926-938

[30] The 2016 BTS/SIGN British guideline on the management of asthma. https://www.brit-thoracic.org.uk

[31] Barnes PJ. Severe asthma: Advances in current management and future therapy. The Journal of Allergy and Clinical Immunology. 2012;**129**(1):48-59

[32] Wu W, Bleecker E, Moore W, Busse WW, Castro M, Chung KF, et al. Unsupervised phenotyping of Severe Asthma Research Program participants using expanded lung data. The Journal of Allergy and Clinical Immunology. 2014;**133**(5):1280-1288

[33] Moore WC, Meyers DA, Wenzel SE, Teague WG, Li H, Li X, et al. Identification of asthma phenotypes using cluster analysis in the Severe Asthma Research Program. American Journal of Respiratory and Critical Care Medicine. 2010;**181**(4):315-323

[34] Moore WC, Fitzpatrick AM, Li X, Hastie AT, Li H, Meyers DA, et al. Clinical heterogeneity in the severe asthma research program. Annals of the. American Thoracic Society. 2013;**10**(Suppl):S118-S124

[35] Hastie AT, Moore WC, Meyers DA, Vestal PL, Li H, Peters SP, et al. Analyses of asthma severity phenotypes and inflammatory proteins in subjects stratified by sputum granulocytes. Journal of Allergy and Clinical Immunology. 2010;**125**(5):1028-1036 e13

[36] Kupczyk M, Wenzel S. U.S. and European severe asthma cohorts: What can they teach us about severe asthma? Journal of Internal Medicine. 2012;**272**(2):121-132

[37] Kuo CS, Pavlidis S, Loza M, Baribaud F, Rowe A, Pandis I, et al. T-helper cell type 2 (Th2) and non-Th2 molecular phenotypes of asthma using sputum transcriptomics in U-BIOPRED. The European Respiratory Journal. 2017;**49**(2). DOI: 10.1183/13993003.02135-2016

[38] Chung KF. Defining phenotypes in asthma: A step towards personalized medicine. Drugs. 2014;**74**(7):719-728

[39] Vannuvel K, Renard P, Raes M, Arnould T. Functional and morphological impact of ER stress on mitochondria. Journal of Cellular Physiology. 2013;**228**(9):1802-1818

[40] Jeong JS, Kim SR, Cho SH, Lee YC. Endoplasmic reticulum stress and allergic diseases. Current Allergy and Asthma Reports. 2017;**17**(12):82

[41] Hetz C. The unfolded protein response: Controlling cell fate decisions under ER stress and beyond. Nature Reviews. Molecular Cell Biology. 2012;**13**(2):89-102

[42] Bertolotti A, Zhang Y, Hendershot LM, Harding HP, Ron D. Dynamic interaction of BiP and ER stress transducers in the unfolded-protein response. Nature Cell Biology. 2000;**2**(6):326-332

[43] Shen J, Chen X, Hendershot L, Prywes R. ER stress regulation of ATF6 localization by dissociation of BiP/GRP78 binding and unmasking of Golgi localization signals. Developmental Cell. 2002;**3**(1):99-111

[44] Hotamisligil GS. Endoplasmic reticulum stress and the inflammatory basis of metabolic disease. Cell. 2010;**140**(6):900-917

[45] Grootjans J, Kaser A, Kaufman RJ, Blumberg RS. The unfolded protein response in immunity and inflammation. Nature Reviews. Immunology. 2016;**16**(8):469-484

[46] Arensdorf AM, Diedrichs D, Rutkowski DT. Regulation of the transcriptome by ER stress: Non-canonical mechanisms and physiological consequences. Frontiers in Genetics. 2013;**4**:256

[47] Cao Y, Knochel S, Oswald F, Donow C, Zhao H, Knochel W. XBP1 forms a regulatory loop with BMP-4 and suppresses mesodermal and neural differentiation in Xenopus embryos. Mechanisms of Development. 2006;**123**(1):84-96

[48] Brar GA, Yassour M, Friedman N, Regev A, Ingolia NT, Weissman JS. High-resolution view of the yeast meiotic program revealed by ribosome profiling. Science. 2012;**335**(6068):552-557

[49] Malhotra D, Thimmulappa R, Vij N, Navas-Acien A, Sussan T, Merali S, et al. Heightened endoplasmic reticulum stress in the lungs of patients with chronic obstructive pulmonary disease: The role of Nrf2-regulated proteasomal activity. American Journal of Respiratory and Critical Care Medicine. 2009;**180**(12):1196-1207

[50] Korfei M, Ruppert C, Mahavadi P, Henneke I, Markart P, Koch M, et al. Epithelial endoplasmic reticulum stress and apoptosis in sporadic idiopathic pulmonary fibrosis. American Journal of Respiratory and Critical Care Medicine. 2008;**178**(8):838-846

[51] Kim HJ, Jeong JS, Kim SR, Park SY, Chae HJ, Lee YC. Inhibition of endoplasmic reticulum stress alleviates lipopolysaccharide-induced lung inflammation through modulation of NF-kappaB/HIF-1alpha signaling pathway. Scientific Reports. 2013;**3**:1142-1151

[52] Marciniak SJ. Endoplasmic reticulum stress in lung disease. European Respiratory Review. 2017;**26**(144)

[53] Kim RY, Pinkerton JW, Essilfie AT, Robertson AAB, Baines KJ, Brown AC, et al. Role for NLRP3 inflammasome-mediated, IL-1beta-dependent responses in severe, steroid-resistant asthma. American Journal of Respiratory and Critical Care Medicine. 2017;**196**(3):283-297

[54] Guo Q, Li H, Liu J, Xu L, Yang L, Sun Z, et al. Tunicamycin aggravates endoplasmic reticulum stress and airway inflammation via PERK-ATF4-CHOP signaling in a murine model of neutrophilic asthma. The Journal of Asthma. 2017;**54**(2):125-133

[55] Cabanski M, Steinmuller M, Marsh LM, Surdziel E, Seeger W, Lohmeyer J. PKR regulates TLR2/TLR4-dependent signaling in murine alveolar macrophages. American Journal of Respiratory Cell and Molecular Biology. 2008;**38**(1):26-31

[56] Kim SR, Lee YC, Kim DI, Park HJ. Effects of PKR inhibitor on poly (I:C)-induced exacerbation of severe asthma. The European Respiratory Journal. 2016;**48**:PA1099

[57] Lee KS, Jeong JS, Kim SR, Cho SH, Kolliputi N, Ko YH, et al. Phosphoinositide 3-kinase-δ regulates fungus-induced allergic lung inflammation through endoplasmic reticulum stress. Thorax. 2016;**71**(1):52-63

[58] Ciencewicki J, Trivedi S, Kleeberger SR. Oxidants and the pathogenesis of lung diseases. The Journal of Allergy and Clinical Immunology. 2008;**122**(3):456-468 quiz 69-70

[59] Reddy PH. Mitochondrial dysfunction and oxidative stress in asthma: Implications for mitochondria-targeted antioxidant therapeutics. Pharmaceuticals (Basel). 2011;**4**(3): 429-456

[60] Cheresh P, Kim SJ, Tulasiram S, Kamp DW. Oxidative stress and pulmonary fibrosis. Biochimica et Biophysica Acta. 2013;**1832**(7):1028-1040

[61] Ernster L, Schatz G. Mitochondria: A historical review. The Journal of Cell Biology. 1981;**91**(3 Pt 2):227s-255s

[62] Rizzuto R, Bernardi P, Pozzan T. Mitochondria as all-round players of the calcium game. The Journal of Physiology. 2000;**529**(Pt 1):37-47

[63] Green DR, Kroemer G. The pathophysiology of mitochondrial cell death. Science. 2004;**305**(5684):626-629

[64] Okamoto K, Shaw JM. Mitochondrial morphology and dynamics in yeast and multicellular eukaryotes. Annual Review of Genetics. 2005;**39**:503-536

[65] Song Z, Ghochani M, McCaffery JM, Frey TG, Chan DC. Mitofusins and OPA1 mediate sequential steps in mitochondrial membrane fusion. Molecular Biology of the Cell. 2009;**20**(15):3525-3532

[66] Otera H, Wang C, Cleland MM, Setoguchi K, Yokota S, Youle RJ, et al. Mff is an essential factor for mitochondrial recruitment of Drp1 during mitochondrial fission in mammalian cells. The Journal of Cell Biology. 2010;**191**(6):1141-1158

[67] Kubli DA, Gustafsson AB. Mitochondria and mitophagy: The yin and yang of cell death control. Circulation Research. 2012;**111**(9):1208-1221

[68] Aravamudan B, Kiel A, Freeman M, Delmotte P, Thompson M, Vassallo R, et al. Cigarette smoke-induced mitochondrial fragmentation and dysfunction in human airway smooth muscle. American Journal of Physiology. Lung Cellular and Molecular Physiology. 2014;**306**(9):L840-L854

[69] Rehman J, Zhang HJ, Toth PT, Zhang Y, Marsboom G, Hong Z, et al. Inhibition of mitochondrial fission prevents cell cycle progression in lung cancer. The FASEB Journal. 2012;**26**(5):2175-2186

[70] Loukides S, Bouros D, Papatheodorou G, Panagou P, Siafakas NM. The relationships among hydrogen peroxide in expired breath condensate, airway inflammation, and asthma severity. Chest. 2002;**121**(2):338-346

[71] Chung HK, Kim YK, Park JH, Ryu MJ, Chang JY, Hwang JH, et al. The indole derivative NecroX-7 improves nonalcoholic steatohepatitis in ob/ob mice through suppression of mitochondrial ROS/RNS and inflammation. Liver International. 2015;**35**(4):1341-1353

[72] Park J, Park E, Ahn BH, Kim HJ, Park JH, Koo SY, et al. NecroX-7 prevents oxidative stress-induced cardiomyopathy by inhibition of NADPH oxidase activity in rats. Toxicology and Applied Pharmacology. 2012;**263**(1):1-6

[73] Jin SA, Kim SK, Seo HJ, Jeong JY, Ahn KT, Kim JH, et al. Beneficial effects of necrosis modulator, indole derivative NecroX-7, on renal ischemia-reperfusion injury in rats. Transplantation Proceedings. 2016;**48**(1):199-204

[74] Im KI, Kim N, Lim JY, Nam YS, Lee ES, Kim EJ, et al. The free radical scavenger NecroX-7 attenuates acute graft-versus-host disease via reciprocal regulation of Th1/regulatory T cells and inhibition of HMGB1 release. Journal of Immunology. 2015;**194**(11):5223-5232

[75] Park JH, Seo KS, Tadi S, Ahn BH, Lee JU, Heo JY, et al. An indole derivative protects against acetaminophen-induced liver injury by directly binding to N-acetyl-p-benzoquinone imine in mice. Antioxidants & Redox Signaling. 2013;**18**(14):1713-1722

[76] Davis BK, Wen H, Ting JP. The inflammasome NLRs in immunity, inflammation, and associated diseases. Annual Review of Immunology. 2011;**29**:707-735

[77] Zhou R, Yazdi AS, Menu P, Tschopp J. A role for mitochondria in NLRP3 inflammasome activation. Nature. 2011;**469**(7329):221-225

[78] Lee YC, Kim SR, Severe Asthma CSH. Toward Personalized Patient Management. Singapore: Springer; 2017

10

Severe Asthma: Updated Therapy Approach Based on Phenotype and Biomarker

Marcia Regina Piuvezam,
Laércia Karla Diega Paiva Ferreira,
Talissa Mozzini Monteiro,
Giciane Carvalho Vieira and
Claudio Roberto Bezerra-Santos

Abstract

Asthma is responsible for considerable global morbidity and health-care costs affecting over 300 million people worldwide. This illness is a heterogeneous condition characterized by chronic airway inflammation and pulmonary tissue remodeling resulting in a variety of clinical manifestations and treatment responses. Recent studies have shown an increasing appreciation of heterogeneity in asthma based on molecular phenotyping, biomarkers, and differential responses to therapies. In terms of asthma classification, perhaps the most important distinction to make is whether the patient has evidence of an eosinophilic inflammatory process characterized by type 2 immune response (Th2) or not. Therefore, personalized therapies to asthmatic patients just will be a reality by identifying and characterizing biomarkers. This review approaches the advances in diagnoses and management of asthma and severe asthma and highlights those with difficult-to-treat asthma based on each phenotype and biomarkers, to assist in the optimization of conventional therapy and to guide the use of targeted therapies.

Keywords: severe asthma, phenotypes, endotypes, biomarkers, therapy

1. Introduction: severe asthma definition

Asthma is a heterogeneous disease featured by the airway chronic inflammatory process associated with airway hyper-relativity due to direct and/or indirect stimuli such as exercise, exposure to allergens or irritants, weather change, and respiratory infections. Asthma is characterized by wheezing, shortness of breath, coughing, chest tightness, and variable expiratory airflow limitation. These symptoms may vary over time and intensity and the symptom resolution and airflow limitation can occur spontaneously or in response to pharmacotherapy [1, 2]. The clinical classification of asthma is recent onset asthma, mild and severe forms, or even asymptomatic asthma [1].

The severe asthma (SA) concept is preconized by the European Respiratory Society–American Thoracic Society, which classifies severe asthmatic patients who require treatment with high-dose inhaled (or systemic) corticosteroids (ICS) in combination with a second long-term medication (long-acting β2 agonists—LABA). This definition includes patients who either maintain or are not in control of the disease [3, 4].

The first step to identify SA is to confirm if the patient presents the basic criteria for asthma itself, that is, reversible airway obstruction and bronchial hyper-reactivity and classic clinical symptoms such as wheezing, shortness of breath, cough, and chest tightness. However, many patients with SA do not meet these criteria as those ones with associated obstructive pulmonary disease and vocal cord dysfunction. After confirming the asthmatic condition, the second step is to determine the therapeutic control of the disease, which means adding ICS/LABA combination. However, some asthmatic patients remain poorly controlled independent of therapy leading to exacerbation of clinical symptoms and airway obstruction and might indicate severe and/or frequent asthma [5].

2. Severe asthma epidemiology

Asthma spreads all over the world, affecting more than 300 million people [2, 6]. This milestone makes it one of the most common chronic inflammatory diseases worldwide [5]. Based on standard methods for assessing the asthma symptoms, its global prevalence ranges from 1 to 16% of the population in different countries, while the asthma fatality rate is about 346,000 people around the world [2]. According to epidemiological data, asthma prevalence is higher in developed countries; however, it is also presented in countries with lower economic and social indicators, that is, developing countries [7], with a prevalence of 1%. Another aspect of this disease is the higher prevalence in urban areas in comparison with rural places [2]. Indeed, asthma prevalence has increased in the world over the past decades and is in a constant increasing rate [8, 9].

Asthma development is directly related to immunological factors, immediate hypersensitivity process, age, gender, and obesity. In an overview, around 50% of children under 3 years old and 80% over 6 years old who are diagnosed with asthma are atopic individuals [2, 10]. In most cases, asthma is an inconstant disease throughout the patients' lives, along which they may have periods of remission and asthma attacks [11, 12].

SA accounts for about 5–10% of all confirmed asthma cases in developed countries. Regarding the cost associated with the management of SA, it is about six times higher than the cost of patients with mild-to-moderate asthma [1]. In addition, SA can come up concomitantly with other chronic diseases, such as rhinosinusitis and chronic obstructive pulmonary disease (COPD) [2]. Despite the high asthma prevalence worldwide, its pathophysiology, phenotypes, endotypes, biomarkers, and treatment still need to be elucidated, therefore, being of great interest of study for the scientific community [13].

3. Pathophysiology of severe asthma

The main pathophysiological feature of asthma is the bronchial inflammation resulting from interactions between airway structural cells and the innate/adaptive immune system. Structural cells of the lung, among them, epithelial cells, endothelial cells, and fibroblasts, release inflammatory mediators, mainly chemokines, and actively participate in the inflammatory process by attracting blood cells to the inflamed site. Thus, the development of the inflammatory response initially orchestrated by the lung structural cells in asthma also depends on innate immunity cells such as eosinophils, neutrophils, macrophages, mast cells, NKT cells, γδ-Tcells, inactive lymphoid cells (ILCs) and dendritic cells, and also on adaptive immunity cells represented by T and B cells. Interactions among these cells and the release of various inflammatory proteins, including cytokines, chemokines, adhesion molecules, eicosanoids, histamine, and nitric oxide (NO), promote the bronchial inflammatory process [14–16]. This inflammatory process is a common feature to all atopic asthmatic patients including those with the severe phenotype.

Histological addresses indicate that bronchial biopsies of asthmatic individuals reveal tissue structural changes, such as collagen deposition under the epithelium, which is described as the thickening of the basement membrane and of the smooth muscle layer of the airways due to the hyperplasia and the hypertrophy of the smooth muscle, which is most commonly observed in patients with severe asthma [17].

Further, there is an increase if the number of blood vessels (angiogenesis) in response to increased secretion of the vessel-endothelial growth factor (VEGF) [18] as well as an increase in mucus secretion commonly observed in biopsies of asthmatic patients, due to an increase in the number of secreting-mucus goblet cell in the epithelium and in the size of submucosal glands [19].

Once asthma presents a complex inflammatory process regulated by immune cells and structural bronchial cells collaborating for the initiation, exacerbation, and maintenance of the inflammatory process, all of these events might lead to irreversible bronchial structural changes and the airway remodeling which strongly contribute to severe development of asthma [15].

3.1. Airway remodeling

Airway remodeling can be defined as a set of changes in the composition, content and organization of the cellular and molecular constituents of the airway wall. The airway remodeling includes epithelial damage, cilial dysfunction, increased thickness of sub-epithelial basement membrane, angiogenesis, and neuronal proliferation. Also, it increases airway smooth muscle mass and goblet cell hyperplasia with mucus production which causes stress and injury to epithelial cells [20, 21].

Epithelial damage is characterized by the thickening of the sub-epithelial basement membrane with deposition of collagens type I, III, V and VI, periostin, tenascin, osteopontin and fibronectin. Periostin is expressed in epithelial and matrix cells, upregulated by type 2 cytokines, and is implicated in the basement membrane fibrosis [22]. In addition, the epithelium is a source of members of the epidermal growth factor family (neurotrophins, angiogenic factors, and TGF-β) that promotes the neuronal and microvascular proliferation present in the airway remodeling. This process leads to mucosal fibrosis, muscle hyperplasia, and the reduction in distance between airway smooth muscle cells and the epithelium [20].

4. Phenotypes, endotypes and biomarkers

Traditionally, two clinical forms of asthma have been defined: allergic asthma and non-allergic asthma. About 80% of children and 50% of adults have allergic asthma characterized by an allergic sensitization defined by the presence of serum immunoglobulin E (IgE) and/or a positive allergy skin test for common proteins of inhaled allergens such as house dust mites, animal dander, fungal spores, plant pollen, or ingested allergens as peanuts. In 80% of the cases, patients with allergic asthma have concomitant allergic rhinitis. The "united airway disease" hypothesis proposes that allergic rhinitis and asthma are manifestations of the same underlying disease process and that each influences the severity of the other. Non-allergic asthma usually develops later in life with no IgE reactivity to allergens or any obvious involvement of the adaptive immune system such as Th2 cells. This form of disease is more common in women and it is often associated with chronic rhinosinusitis, nasal polyps, obesity, and is difficult to treat, often requiring long-term treatment with systemic steroids [15].

Currently, the division of asthma into only two clinical forms is oversimplified due to the discovery of diverse asthma phenotypes, each one with a distinct pathophysiology as better described further in this chapter. The asthma phenotypes differ in terms of genetic susceptibility, environmental risk factors, onset age, clinical presentation, prognosis, and response to therapies [23]; therefore, asthma is seen as a syndrome rather than a single disease [20]. It is also described as a considerable clinical overlap with COPD among smokers with asthma [2]. On the other hand, endotypes represent molecular mechanisms' underlying observable characteristics of phenotypes and characterization of mediators (biomarkers) as the pharmacological target for each phenotype is desirable to personalize each asthma syndrome [24, 25].

According to the spectrum of asthma, SA affects a group of patients with high medical needs, whose pathophysiology and clinical characteristics vary widely [7, 23]. Therefore, the clinical aspects of SA vary from those based purely on airway obstruction [13, 26] to those related to corticosteroid resistance [1, 3, 27] and to those based on life-threatening (or life-ending) diseases. Therefore it becomes sine qua non to classify SA by specific phenotype(s), endotype(s), and their biomarkers [28, 29].

4.1. Phenotypes of severe asthma

Phenotypes of SA involve a complex interaction of many genetic and environmental factors in association with observable characteristics, such as specific IgE responsiveness (biomarker) to particular allergens and lung functions [7, 23, 30] (**Figure 1**). Therefore, characterization of these phenotypes has involved biased and unbiased approaches to grouping clinical, physiologic, and hereditary characteristics [7, 31–33]. Nowadays, SA phenotypes are mainly composed of the following classification: type 2 asthma and non-type 2 asthma (**Figure 1**).

4.1.1. Type 2 asthma

Allergic asthma, which has been described as Th2 immune response (type 2), is a hallmark with an increase of $CD4^+$ T cells that produce IL-4, IL-5, and IL-13 detected on the bronchoalveolar fluid as well as on mucosal biopsies and correlated with blood and airway eosinophilia and

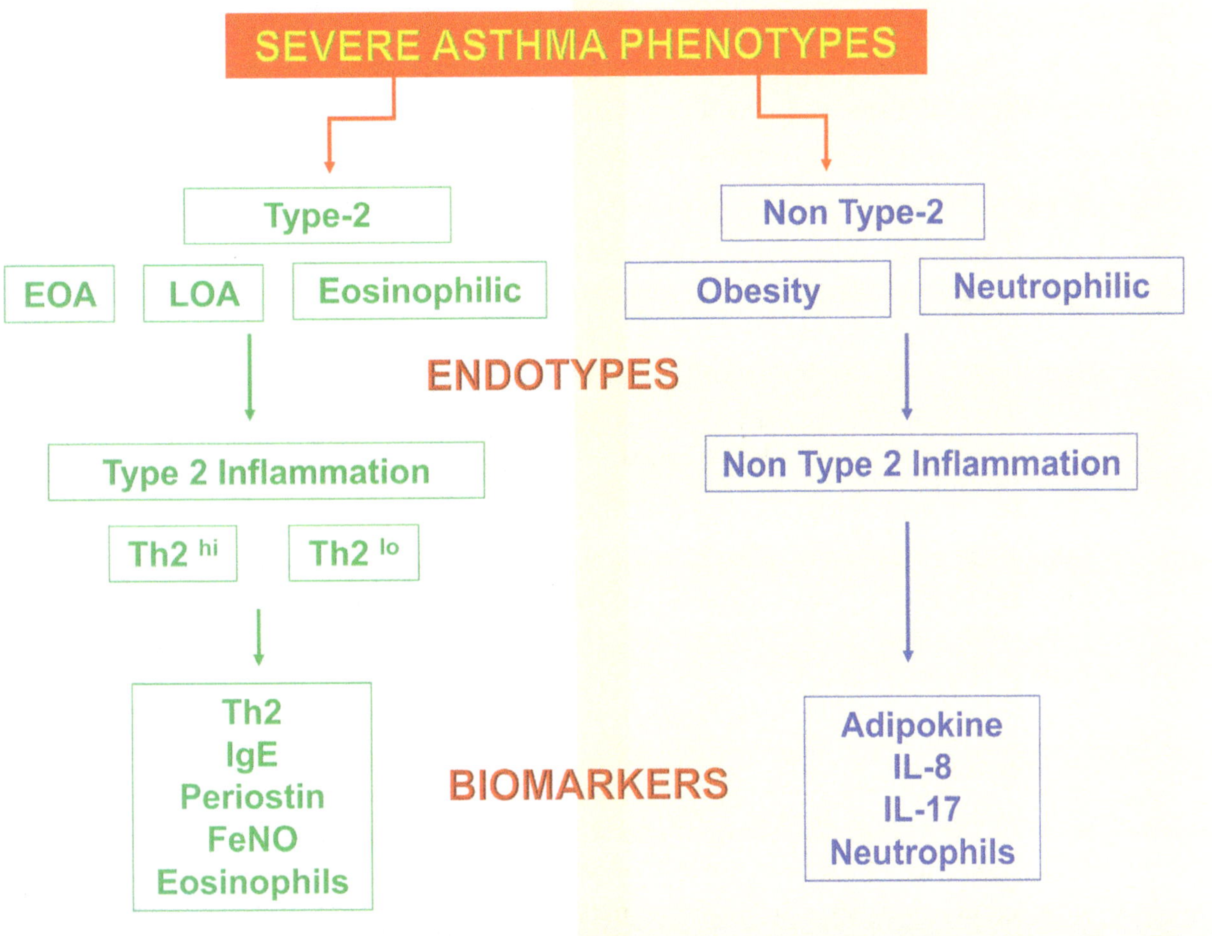

Figure 1. Phenotypes, endotypes, and biomarkers in severe asthma. Asthma is divided into phenotypes: type 2 inflammation and non-type 2 inflammation. Type 2 phenotype: early onset asthma (EOA), late onset asthma (LOA), and eosinophilic asthma; biomarkers: Th2 cytokines, IgE, Periostin, FeNO (fraction of nitric oxide expired), and eosinophilia. Non-type 2 phenotypes: asthma associated with obesity and neutrophilic asthma; biomarkers: adipokine, IL-8 or IL-17, and neutrophilia.

high-serum titer of allergen-specific IgE as biomarkers [34]. The presence or absence of these cytokines, allergen-specific IgE and eosinophilia, is a feature of $Th2^{hi}$ and $Th2^{lo}$ endotype clusters, respectively [35, 36]. The type 2 asthma phenotype is divided into early-onset asthma (EOA), late-onset asthma, and eosinophilic asthma [37].

4.1.1.1. *Early-onset asthma (EOA)*

EOA phenotype originates in early childhood, is characterized by an allergic component, and might be observed on the most asthmatic patients. However, the lack of responsiveness to corticosteroids and the lower concentrations of IgE in some children with asthma suggest that not all EOA is type 2-associated phenotype, and this may be important in the development of SA [38].

Recent researches have shown the importance of age at the onset to the SA phenotype [7, 13, 39]. Early onset better identifies "allergic asthma" than clinically available tests of atopy/allergy. Classification of adult asthma into EOA is widely used in the literature. A recent review included 12 studies comparing early- and late-onset current asthma in adults. The most common age used to delineate the 2 age-of-onset phenotypes was 12 years [40, 41]. EOA can be present with mild-to-severe disease, but it is unclear whether mild allergic asthma progresses to a severe disease or whether severe allergic asthma arises in childhood and remains severe [32].

The Severe Asthma Research Program (SARP) cluster analysis showed that people with the most severe EOA had greater numbers of skin-test reactions and poorer lung functions than individuals with mild asthma and that they were more likely to be of African descent. It also linked SA to a longer duration of disease and a history of pneumonia [42]. These data suggest that both genetic and environmental factors are important in asthma pathogenesis [13]. It is likely that as the severity of allergic early-onset type 2 asthma increases, non-Th2 immune pathways including those related to Th17 and Th1 are also engaged, as is innate immunity [43, 44].

The prognosis for children with initial severe atopic phenotypes is worse than for other phenotypes and this poor prognosis of allergic asthma with early onset has also been described in numerous prospective birth cohorts [23, 40]. In adults, mold sensitization in allergic asthma is associated with severe exacerbations requiring hospitalization and uncontrolled asthma despite high doses of ICS usage [13, 42].

4.1.1.2. *Late-onset asthma*

LOA is prevalent in adults over 65 and is also denominated as adult-onset asthma. The rate of morbidity and mortality of patients directly attributable to LOA is 4–15% higher than young patients with asthma [45, 46]. In addition, these numbers are underestimated due to the presence of comorbid diseases that complicate the diagnosis, as wheezing, breathlessness, and cough can also be caused by cardiovascular diseases [47]. The prevalence of asthma in the elderly is higher than was previously thought and considering the rapid aging of the global population the burden of asthma in the elderly is expected to rise significantly [15, 37]. In addition, older adults are more likely to be diagnosed with COPD without consideration of asthma, especially if they have a history of smoking [30]. Taking together these factors, the differential diagnosis of asthma in adults is potentially more challenging than in children, and asthma costs may be higher among older patients due to increase of hospitalization.

The role of genetic predisposition in LOA is less clear than in atopic childhood-onset asthma. In LOA, a family history of asthma is often lacking and atopy is not more common than in the general population. Occupational asthma has become the most common type of LOA in many industrialized countries [48]. Forward, female sex hormones are associated with non-atopic LOA [49] whereas no sex difference was observed for the incidence of allergic asthma. Alternatively, asthma prevalence decreases with the number of years of oral contraceptive pill use [50]. In addition to that, there is evidence that the incidence of asthma decreases after menopause [51], whereas hormone replacement therapy in post-menopausal females is associated with an increased risk of asthma onset [52, 53].

Adult-onset asthma with highly elevated numbers of eosinophils often is related to sinusitis and nasal polyps. This phenotype indicates an association to type 2 cytokines and inflammatory cells such mast cells and basophils [54]. However, the lack of allergy clinical symptoms in this phenotype suggests that the Th2 process differs from and is probably more complex than the one associated with the early-onset asthma phenotype. As type 2 cytokines are also upregulated in cancer, inflammatory bowel disease, and interstitial fibrosis, a Th2 inflammatory process in the lung without mucosal-allergen-specific IgE and associated clinical allergic reactions is clearly possible [55, 56].

Also, some asthmatics present a mix of sputum neutrophilia and eosinophilia which might imply that there are interactions of additional immune pathways (endotypes) with Th2 immunity, including activation of pathways related to IL-33 and IL-17 by Th17 cells [57–59].

The phenotype named late-onset non-allergic asthma of the elderly [54] occurs in individuals beyond 65 years with a frequency of 8–10%. This phenotype can be grouped into two subphenotypes: (i) the persistent asthma and (ii) the newly diagnosed asthma [13, 20, 60] where atopy and elevated IgE levels are less frequent.

The physiologic and histopathologic findings in the airways of aging subjects are driven by important cellular age-associated changes. The immune system is complex and with increasing age, there are alterations in both the innate and adaptive immune responses, termed "immunosenescence." Research on this subject has focused primarily on cancer and autoimmunity but not in asthma. However, immunosenescence likely has important consequences in elderly asthmatics and increases susceptibility to airway infections, which in turn may exacerbate underlying SA or potentially play a role in the inception of LOA patients [22]. Another important issue in the airway of aging individuals is the increase in the number of sputum neutrophils [22, 26] and neutrophil mediators including MMP-9, neutrophil elastase, and IL-8, biomarkers for this phenotype, resembling changes seen in a phenotype of SA noted in some younger adults [1].

4.1.1.3. Eosinophilic severe asthma

Eosinophils are granulocytic effector cells that produce and store biologically active molecules, including cytotoxic proteins, that is, major basic protein (MBP), eosinophil peroxidase (EPX), eosinophil cationic protein (ECP), eosinophil-derived neurotoxin (EDN), lipid mediators, chemotactic peptides, as well as cytokines [61] against pathogens. However, the eosinophil-derived granule proteins are not only toxic to pathogens but also to other cells within immune responses, causing tissue damage and consequently organ dysfunction. In addition, eosinophils can contribute to inflammatory pathways through their capacity to synthesize and secrete a remarkable number of pro-inflammatory cytokines and chemokines [61–63].

Indeed, eosinophils produce type-2 cytokines (IL-4, IL-5, IL-13, and IL-25) and chemokines (CCL5/RANTES, CCL11/eotaxin, and CCL3) and are able to recruit leukocytes to the inflamed site [64, 44]. Alternately, following the allergen challenge, airway eosinophils have been shown to express GM-CSF and CXCL8/IL-8 [65, 66], thereby inducing neutrophil recruitment.

Therefore, eosinophils may contribute to airway remodeling in SA through release of transforming growth factor (TGFβ-1) [64]. It has also been reported that interferon-gamma (IFN-γ) might also potently activate eosinophils [67] and is elevated in the serum of some acute severe asthmatic patients [68], underscoring the importance of these pathways in SA.

Recently, a multiple-biomarker approach has been described to predict eosinophilic SA. These ones are represented by high-exhaled nitric oxide (FeNO) and elevated serum levels of periostin which correlate with increased eosinophil numbers in sputum, poor asthma control, and severe disease phenotype [69, 70]. FeNO is secreted by epithelial cells, macrophages, and other inflammatory cells in response to different stimuli into the asthmatic lung; however, the mechanisms involved in FeNO enhances still remain poorly unknown. On the other hand, periostin is mainly secreted by airway fibroblasts and epithelial cells in response to type 2 cytokines IL-4/IL-13 and TGF-β. Elevated levels of this biomarker have also been reported to correlate with eosinophil adhesion, recruitment and activation, airway remodeling, as well as chronic eosinophilic rhinosinusitis [70].

4.1.2. Non-type 2 asthma

Absence of type 2 profile in asthmatics represents half of all asthmatic patients and the lack of described biomarkers makes difficult phenotype-based therapy [71–73]. Some patients might lack type 2 inflammation profiles simply because corticosteroids have substantially reduced that pathway. Non-type 2 patients generally have LOA often in association with obesity, post-infectious, neutrophilia, smoking-related factors and are less likely to be atopic or allergic [7, 74].

4.1.2.1. Obesity-related asthma

Obesity and asthma are important public health problems [75], and the symptoms of asthma in obese individuals are more severe once these patients present development of steroid resistance, destabilization or lack of asthma control, and the worst quality of life [76]. Obese asthmatics are characterized in two phenotypes based in the Th2 profile: (i) an early-onset atopic asthma (EOA)—this phenotype presents $Th2^{hi}$ profile, where allergic asthma is complicated by the presence of obesity and (ii) late-onset non-atopic asthma (LOA)—this phenotype presents the $Th2^{lo}$ profile, occurring preferably in women and where the development of asthma is a consequence of obesity [77].

In the EOA phenotype, obese asthmatics have a history of atopy, increased airway obstruction, greater bronchial hyper-reactivity, higher IgE serum level, and a greater likelihood of allergic sensitization and reactions compared with late-onset obese asthmatics [78]. In contrast, late-onset obese asthmatics had less atopy, less bronchial hyper-reactivity, less airway obstruction, and fewer exacerbations [77]. There is a clear association between obesity and asthma and probably childhood obesity precedes the onset of asthma. However, more studies that clarify the characteristics of the two described phenotypes are needed [78].

Adiponectin is an important adipokine secreted by the adipocytes and its levels have been reported to be lower in obese patients [78]. In the asthma context, it appears that adiponectin does not protect against the development of inflammation and may in fact exacerbate the

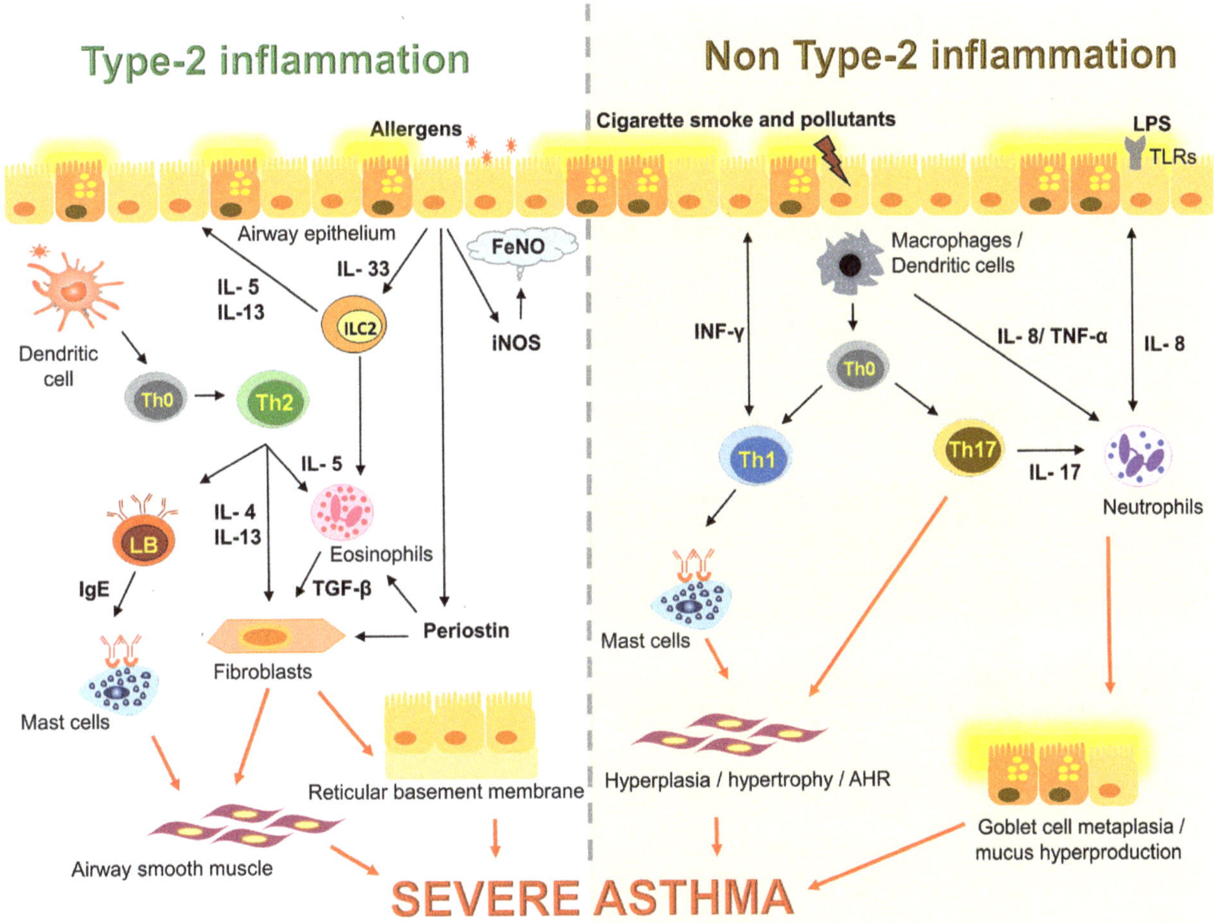

Figure 2. Type 2 inflammation and non-type 2 inflammation and its relation to structural changes in severe asthma. In type 2 inflammation, self-maintenance of the inflammatory process occurs through the following mechanism: Type 2 cytokines are generated by Th2. Lymphocytes and ILC2 cells, which activate several cells downstream, inducing remodeling of the airways through the thickening of the MBR, metaplasia/hyperplasia of goblet cells, mucus overproduction, and airway smooth muscle hyperplasia/hypertrophy. Factors involved in the development of non-type 2 inflammation in asthma include pollutants, cigarette smoke and microorganisms. These factors can activate innate immunity as well as Th1 and Th17 inflammatory processes. *Abbreviations*: AHR, hyper reactivity of the airways; FeNO, fraction of nitric oxide expired; IL, interleukin; ILC2, innate lymphoid cell; iNOS, nitric inducible oxide synthase; RBM, reticular basilar membrane; TGF-β, transforming growth factor-β; LPS, lipopolysaccharide; TLRs, toll-like receptors; TNF-α, tumor necrosis factor-α; IFN-γ, interferon-γ.

disease via anti-Th1 inflammatory effects, allowing type 2 differentiation and a more severe allergic response [75]. Another pro-inflammatory adipokine is resistin [29] whose levels of resistin: adiponectin ratio have been found to be higher in asthmatic uncontrolled subjects than in control subjects [78].

4.1.2.2. Neutrophilic asthma

Neutrophilia has been inconsistently associated with SA for several years although it is generally seen in corticosteroid-treated patients [79–81]. In affected individuals, lung neutrophilia has been associated with lower lung function, more trapping of air, thicker airway walls, and greater expression of matrix metalloproteinases compared to people with non-neutrophilic asthma; however, neutrophilia has not been associated with airway hyper reactivity [82, 83].

In SA, the number of neutrophils, in bronchi, is elevated compared to healthy subjects [58]. These cells were characterized by a high expression of the high affinity receptor for IgE (FcεRI) and released IL-8 (CXCL8) [84]. The expression of FcεRI on neutrophils seems to depend on the presence of type 2 cytokines [85]. The number of neutrophils in the airways of asthmatic individuals depends on IL-8 and TNF-α concentrations, both being chemotactic cytokines released from macrophages, epithelial cells, and neutrophils [86, 87].

Transcripts for IL17A were found to be elevated in the sputum of patients with asthma and were correlated with IL-8 transcripts and sputum neutrophils as well as with asthma severity [88]. Although, type 2 cells are predominant in the course of atopic diseases, the recruitment of neutrophils in the course of non-atopic asthma is driven by Th17—a subset of T helper cells releasing IL-17 [89, 90]. Neutrophilia can also coexist with eosinophilia, and this characteristic identifies people with disease severity and emphasizes the complexity of the immunobiology of SA in respect of the multiple different innate and adaptive immune pathways and cell functions involved in asthma phenotypes and endotypes [57, 91] (**Figure 2**).

5. Severe asthma management: classical and biological therapies

Several endotypes are targeted to control SA symptoms by reducing future asthma attacks. The most classical strategy to approach such outcomes in asthma pharmacological therapy is linked to regulation of the smooth muscle cell contraction/relaxation machinery. These targets are represented by an array of cell receptors reported as β2 adrenergic, muscarinic, and glucocorticoid receptors, phosphodiesterases enzymes, leukotrienes receptors, and leukotriene synthase enzyme [20]. These receptor functions are largely regulated by the classical pharmacological therapies used to treat asthma and they have been mentioned to cause a satisfactory disease control when administrated as monotherapy or in combination in different dosages for children, adolescents, adults, or special population which are the ones with comorbidities, that is, obesity, food allergy, anxiety, and depression and others [3].

Medications used for SA control and risk reduction so far represent the main strategy to attenuate the illness symptoms. In case of SA the combination of higher dose ICS and LABA is recommended. These medications are pharmacologically classified as gold-standard steroid/bronchodilator drugs. Their effects occur by linking on nuclear cell receptors leading to strong inhibition of several inflammatory asthma parameters such as type-2 cytokine production, eosinophil activation, and mucus-secreting goblet cells, which are key components to asthma symptoms initiation, maintenance, and exacerbation [92, 93]. Also, the long-acting muscarinic agonist—LAMA named tiotropium—has been used as an add-on pharmacotherapy for SA control [94]. See below the main SA management medication/procedures in **Table 1**.

Adapted from [3].

However, classical pharmacological therapy causes side-effects and adverse drug events affecting for instance adrenal, growth suppression, and other organ malfunction [95]. Additionally, it has been reported that ≥40% of asthmatic patients are not well controlled which may require escalated treatment [96]. Therefore, new asthma targets/biomarkers have been searched in the perspective of improving asthma therapy considering the different disease endotype such as type 2, non-type 2, and bronchial epithelium-derived factors [28].

5.1. Endotypes/biomarkers-based asthma therapy

Anti-IgE therapy was previously described to treat SA patients that do not respond to classical therapy. High allergen-specific-IgE serum level has been reported as the type 2 asthma biomarker. Its secretion is crucial to eosinophil and basophil sensitization that is defined as a previous step to mast cell degranulation, and posterior pro-inflammatory and spasmogenic molecules stimulate smooth muscle cells, blood vessels, sensory nerves, and mucus-secreting goblet cells which are altogether pivotal to induce hyper-reactivity and lung inflammation [97]. Therefore, inhibiting IgE response is an important approach to control SA symptoms and in this perspective the anti-IgE medication omalizumab has provided good outcomes [98].

Treatment and strategies	Medication/procedure	Dosage
Higher-dose ICS/LABA combination	Prednisolone, formoterol	ICS: Max 2000 mcg/day LABA: Max. 72 mcg/day
Oral corticosteroids	Prednisone or prednisolone	Adults: 1 mg/kg/day Children: 1–2 mg/kg/day
Add-on therapy without phenotyping	Tiotropium (LAMA)	5 μg, 2.5 μg or 1.25 μg once daily during 4-week period
Add-on therapy with phenotyping	Omalizumab (anti-IgE), mepolizumab and reslizumab (anti-IL-5)	Omalizumab: 150–1200 mg once every 2 or 4 weeks Mepolizumab: 750 mg once every 4 weeks Reslizumab: 3 mg/kg every 4 weeks up to 24 months
Non-pharmacological therapy	Bronchial thermoplasty, high-altitude treatment and psychological interventions	

Table 1. Severe asthma management.

Therapy based on anti-IL-5 administration, mepolizumab, has been shown effective to reduce severe eosinophilic asthma symptoms by inhibiting IL-5 actions highly on eosinophils but also in basophil cells [61]. It is well documented that IL-5 is a key cytokine implicated in maturation, activation, proliferation, and survival of eosinophils. Then, part of difficult-to-treat eosinophilic asthma patients does not respond to both ICS and systemic glucocorticoids, which points to IL-5 as an important biomarker to be targeted in SA therapy. Also, a placebo-controlled trial in patients with eosinophilic severe asthma has revealed the safety and efficacy of the anti-IL-5 therapy named reslizumab which reduces asthma exacerbation and improves lung function as asthma control [99].

Another endotype-based therapy for SA has emerged and the use of anti-IL-4 and anti-IL-13 therapies indicates satisfactory outcomes [41]. Both cytokines present a crucial role in IgE synthesis, eosinophil activation, mucus secretion, and airway remodeling indicating that neutralizing these biomarkers might collaborate to SA control. Additionally, prostaglandin D (PGD) 2 receptor expressed by type 2 cells named CRTH2 has been implicated in SA symptoms which might be controlled by the use of a CRTH2 antagonist. PGD2 is an arachidonic acid derivative mainly secreted by mast cells and activates several cells. In response to activation, these cells secrete an array of pro-inflammatory cytokines present into the asthmatic lung [100].

Besides classical pharmacological and/or biological asthma therapy, other therapies (i.e., allergen immunotherapy, vaccinations, bronchial thermoplasty, and vitamin D), non-pharmacological treatments (i.e., avoidance of allergens, air pollutants, some foods and medicines, healthy diet, physical activity, weight reduction, dealing with emotional stress, and others), and complementary and alternative medicine have been reported in the literature. However, the last one has been not recommended for use by severe adult asthmatic patients due its limited evidence of effectiveness [101].

Individualized management protocol should be taken into account for asthmatic special population, for instance, exercise-induced bronchoconstriction in adolescents, elderly, pregnant, and aspirin-exacerbated respiratory disease; however, the management of SA is importantly challenging and the endotype-based therapies might be the better strategy to approach the illness control.

6. Conclusion

Human severe asthma is a heterogeneous disease and an emerging health public issue affecting hundreds of million people worldwide and such a complex inflammatory condition which has led this to be classified as a syndrome. Recent cluster analyses on severe asthma based on phenotypes, endotypes, and biomarkers have hardly classified this illness to better improving its management. Updated asthma phenotypes known as type 2, non-type 2, eosinophilic, or neutrophilic raise the necessity of new biomarker identification, mainly a single one, for diagnosis and therapy purposes. In this chapter, we reviewed the advances on severe asthma phenotypes/endotypes, diagnoses, and management based on classical medication composed of high doses of inhaled corticosteroids and long-acting β2 agonist combination as well as those add-on therapies represented by long-acting muscarinic agonists, biological/monoclonal antibodies, and non-pharmacological approaches routinely used to control difficult-to-treat asthma. Finally, taking all these new concepts and management strategies on severe asthma, it has been agreed by international consensus on the urgent need for the development of a new phenotype/endotype-based therapy to treat severe asthma.

Author details

Marcia Regina Piuvezam[1*], Laércia Karla Diega Paiva Ferreira[2], Talissa Mozzini Monteiro[2], Giciane Carvalho Vieira[3] and Claudio Roberto Bezerra-Santos[1]

*Address all correspondence to: mrpiuvezam@ltf.ufpb.br

1 Department of Physiology and Pathology, Federal University of Paraíba, João Pessoa, Paraiba, Brazil

2 Federal University of Paraíba, João Pessoa, Paraiba, Brazil

3 Department of Morphology, Center of Health Science, Federal University of Paraíba, João Pessoa, Paraiba, Brazil

References

[1] Trejo Bittar HE, Yousem SA, Wenzel SE. Pathobiology of severe asthma. Annual Review of Pathology: Mechanisms of Disease. 2015;**10**:511-545. DOI: 10.1146/annurev-pathol-012414-040343

[2] GINA. Global Strategy for Asthma Management and Prevention, Glob. Initiat. Asthma. 2017. http://ginasthma.org/2017-gina-report-global-strat. DOI: 10.1183/09031936.00138707

[3] GINA. Pocket guide for asthma management and prevention, Glob. Initiat. Asthma. 2017. pp. 1-29. http://ginasthma.org/2017-pocket-guide-for-asthma-management-and-prevention/

[4] Tan WC, Vollmer WM, Lamprecht B, Mannino DM, Jithoo A, Nizankowska-Mogilnicka E, Mejza F, Gislason T, Burney PGJ, Buist AS. BOLD collaborative research group, worldwide patterns of bronchodilator responsiveness: Results from the burden of obstructive lung disease study. Thorax. 2012;**67**:718-726. DOI: 10.1136/thoraxjnl-2011-201445

[5] Chung KF, Wenzel SE, Brozek JL, Bush A, Castro M, Sterk PJ, Adcock IM, Bateman ED, Bel EH, Bleecker ER, Boulet L-P, Brightling C, Chanez P, Dahlen S-E, Djukanovic R, Frey U, Gaga M, Gibson P, Hamid Q, Jajour NN, Mauad T, Sorkness RL, Teague WG. International ERS/ATS guidelines on definition, evaluation and treatment of severe asthma. The European Respiratory Journal. 2014;**43**:343-373. DOI: 10.1183/09031936.00202013

[6] Boulet L-P, FitzGerald JM, Reddel HK. The revised 2014 GINA strategy report. Current Opinion in Pulmonary Medicine. 2015;**21**:1-7. DOI: 10.1097/MCP.0000000000000125

[7] Wu W, Bleecker E, Moore W, Busse WW, Castro M, Chung KF, Calhoun WJ, Erzurum S, Gaston B, Israel E, Curran-Everett D, Wenzel SE. Unsupervised phenotyping of severe asthma research program participants using expanded lung data. The Journal of Allergy and Clinical Immunology. 2014;**133**:1280-1288. DOI: 10.1016/j.jaci.2013.11.042

[8] Moffatt MF, Gut IG, Demenais F, Strachan DP, Bouzigon E, Heath S, von Mutius E, Farrall M, Lathrop M, Cookson WOCM, GABRIEL Consortium. A large-scale, consortium-based genomewide association study of asthma. The New England Journal of Medicine. 2010; **363**:1211-1221. DOI: 10.1056/NEJMoa0906312

[9] Reddel HK, Taylor DR, Bateman ED, Boulet L-P, Boushey HA, Busse WW, Casale TB, Chanez P, Enright PL, Gibson PG, de Jongste JC, Kerstjens HAM, Lazarus SC, Levy ML, O'Byrne PM, Partridge MR, Pavord ID, Sears MR, Sterk PJ, Stoloff SW, Sullivan SD, Szefler SJ, Thomas MD, Wenzel SE. American Thoracic Society/European Respiratory Society Task Force on Asthma Control and Exacerbations, An Official American Thoracic Society/European Respiratory Society Statement: Asthma Control and Exacerbations. American Journal of Respiratory and Critical Care Medicine. 2009;**180**:59-99. DOI: 10.1164/rccm.200801-060ST

[10] Siroux V, Gonzalez JR, Bouzigon E, Curjuric I, Boudier A, Imboden M, Anto JM, Gut I, Jarvis D, Lathrop M, Omenaas ER, Pin I, Wjst M, Demenais F, Probst-Hensch N, Kogevinas M, Kauffmann F. Genetic heterogeneity of asthma phenotypes identified by a clustering approach. The European Respiratory Journal. 2014;**43**:439-452. DOI: 10.1183/09031936.00032713

[11] Spruit MA, Singh SJ, Garvey C, ZuWallack R, Nici L, Rochester C, Hill K, Holland AE, Lareau SC, Man WD-C, Pitta F, Sewell L, Raskin J, Bourbeau J, Crouch R, Franssen FME, Casaburi R, Vercoulen JH, Vogiatzis I, Gosselink R, Clini EM, Effing TW, Maltais F, van der Palen J, Troosters T, Janssen DJA, Collins E, Garcia-Aymerich J, Brooks D, Fahy BF, Puhan MA, Hoogendoorn M, Garrod R, Schols AMWJ, Carlin B, Benzo R, Meek P, Morgan M, Rutten-van Mölken MPMH, Ries AL, Make B, Goldstein RS, Dowson CA, Brozek JL, Donner CF, Wouters EFM. ATS/ERS Task Force on Pulmonary Rehabilitation, An Official American Thoracic Society/European Respiratory Society Statement: Key concepts and advances in pulmonary rehabilitation. American Journal of Respiratory and Critical Care Medicine. 2013;**188**:e13-e64. DOI: 10.1164/rccm.201309-1634ST

[12] Kurland G, Deterding RR, Hagood JS, Young LR, Brody AS, Castile RG, Dell S, Fan LL, Hamvas A, Hilman BC, Langston C, Nogee LM, Redding GJ. American Thoracic Society Committee on Childhood Interstitial Lung Disease (chILD) and the chILD Research Network, An Official American Thoracic Society Clinical Practice Guideline: Classification, evaluation, and management of childhood interstitial lung disease in infancy. American Journal of Respiratory and Critical Care Medicine. 2013;**188**:376-394. DOI: 10.1164/rccm.201305-0923ST

[13] Moore WC, Meyers DA, Wenzel SE, Teague WG, Li H, Li X, D'Agostino R, Castro M, Curran-Everett D, Fitzpatrick AM, Gaston B, Jarjour NN, Sorkness R, Calhoun WJ, Chung KF, Comhair SAA, Dweik RA, Israel E, Peters SP, Busse WW, Erzurum SC, Bleecker ER, National Heart, Lung, and Blood Institute's Severe Asthma Research Program. Identification of asthma phenotypes using cluster analysis in the severe asthma research program. American Journal of Respiratory and Critical Care Medicine. 2010; **181**:315-323. DOI: 10.1164/rccm.200906-0896OC

[14] Lambrecht BN, Hammad H. The airway epithelium in asthma. Nature Medicine. 2012; **18**:684-692. DOI: 10.1038/nm.2737

[15] Lambrecht BN, Hammad H. The immunology of asthma. Nature Immunology. 2015;**16**: 45-56. DOI: 10.1038/ni.3049

[16] Barnes PJ. Cellular and molecular mechanisms of asthma and COPD. Clinical Science. 2017;**131**:1541-1558. DOI: 10.1042/CS20160487

[17] Benayoun L, Druilhe A, Dombret M-C, Aubier M, Pretolani M. Airway structural alterations selectively associated with severe asthma. American Journal of Respiratory and Critical Care Medicine. 2003;**167**:1360-1368. DOI: 10.1164/rccm.200209-1030OC

[18] Siddiqui S, Sutcliffe A, Shikotra A, Woodman L, Doe C, McKenna S, Wardlaw A, Bradding P, Pavord I, Brightling C. Vascular remodeling is a feature of asthma and nonasthmatic eosinophilic bronchitis. The Journal of Allergy and Clinical Immunology. 2007;**120**:813-819. DOI: 10.1016/j.jaci.2007.05.028

[19] Ordoñez CL, Khashayar R, Wong HH, Ferrando R, Wu R, Hyde DM, Hotchkiss JA, Zhang Y, Novikov A, Dolganov G, Fahy JV. Mild and moderate asthma is associated with airway goblet cell hyperplasia and abnormalities in Mucin gene expression. American Journal of Respiratory and Critical Care Medicine. 2001;**163**:517-523. DOI: 10.1164/ajrccm.163.2.2004039

[20] Holgate ST, Wenzel S, Postma DS, Weiss ST, Renz H, Sly PD. Asthma. Nature Reviews Disease Primers. 2015;**1**:15025. DOI: 10.1038/nrdp.2015.25

[21] Al-Muhsen S, Johnson JR, Hamid Q. Remodeling in asthma. The Journal of Allergy and Clinical Immunology. 2011;**128**:451-462. DOI: 10.1016/j.jaci.2011.04.047

[22] Boulet L-P. Airway remodeling in asthma. Current Opinion in Pulmonary Medicine. 2018;**24**:56-62. DOI: 10.1097/MCP.0000000000000441

[23] Wenzel SE. Asthma phenotypes: The evolution from clinical to molecular approaches. Nature Medicine. 2012;**18**:716-725. DOI: 10.1038/nm.2678

[24] Lötvall J, Akdis CA, Bacharier LB, Bjermer L, Casale TB, Custovic A, Lemanske RF Jr, Wardlaw AJ, Wenzel SE, Greenberger PA. Asthma endotypes: A new approach to classification of disease entities within the asthma syndrome. The Journal of Allergy and Clinical Immunology. 2011;**127**:355-360. DOI: 10.1016/j.jaci.2010.11.037

[25] Agache I, Akdis C, Jutel M, Virchow JC. Untangling asthma phenotypes and endotypes. Allergy. 2012;**67**:835-846. DOI: 10.1111/j.1398-9995.2012.02832.x

[26] Chakir J, Shannon J, Molet S, Fukakusa M, Elias J, Laviolette M, Boulet L-P, Hamid Q. Airway remodeling-associated mediators in moderate to severe asthma: Effect of steroids on TGF-beta, IL-11, IL-17, and type I and type III collagen expression. The Journal of Allergy and Clinical Immunology. 2003;**111**:1293-1298 http://www.ncbi.nlm.nih.gov/pubmed/12789232 [Accessed: January 12, 2018

[27] Adcock IM, Lane SJ. Corticosteroid-insensitive asthma: Molecular mechanisms. The Journal of Endocrinology. 2003;**178**:347-355 http://www.ncbi.nlm.nih.gov/pubmed/12967328 [Accessed: January 12, 2018

[28] Agache I, Akdis CA. Endotypes of allergic diseases and asthma: An important step in building blocks for the future of precision medicine. Allergology International. 2016;**65**: 243-252. DOI: 10.1016/j.alit.2016.04.011

[29] Akdis CA, Ballas ZK. Precision medicine and precision health: Building blocks to foster a revolutionary health care model. The Journal of Allergy and Clinical Immunology. 2016;**137**:1359-1361. DOI: 10.1016/j.jaci.2016.03.020

[30] Wenzel SE. Asthma: Defining of the persistent adult phenotypes. Lancet. 2006;**368**: 804-813. DOI: 10.1016/S0140-6736(06)69290-8

[31] Wenzel SE. Complex phenotypes in asthma: Current definitions. Pulmonary Pharmacology & Therapeutics. 2013;**26**:710-715. DOI: 10.1016/j.pupt.2013.07.003

[32] Fitzpatrick AM, Teague WG, Meyers DA, Peters SP, Li X, Li H, Wenzel SE, Aujla S, Castro M, Bacharier LB, Gaston BM, Bleecker ER, Moore WC, National Institutes of Health/National Heart, Lung, and Blood Institute Severe Asthma Research Program. Heterogeneity of severe asthma in childhood: Confirmation by cluster analysis of children in the National Institutes of Health/National Heart, Lung, and Blood Institute Severe Asthma Research Program. Journal of Allergy and Clinical Immunology. 2011; **127**:382-389.e13. DOI: 10.1016/j.jaci.2010.11.015

[33] Just J, Gouvis-Echraghi R, Couderc R, Guillemot-Lambert N, Saint-Pierre P. Novel severe wheezy young children phenotypes: Boys atopic multiple-trigger and girls nonatopic uncontrolled wheeze. Journal of Allergy and Clinical Immunology. 2012;**130**: 103-110.e8. DOI: 10.1016/j.jaci.2012.02.041

[34] Robinson DS, Hamid Q, Ying S, Tsicopoulos A, Barkans J, Bentley AM, Corrigan C, Durham SR, Kay AB. Predominant Th2-like Bronchoalveolar T-lymphocyte population in atopic asthma. Clinical and Experimental Allergy. 1992;**326**:298-304. DOI: 10.1056/NEJM199201303260504

[35] Woodruff PG, Boushey HA, Dolganov GM, Barker CS, Yang YH, Donnelly S, Ellwanger A, Sidhu SS, Dao-Pick TP, Pantoja C, Erle DJ, Yamamoto KR, Fahy JV. Genome-wide profiling identifies epithelial cell genes associated with asthma and with treatment response to

corticosteroids. Proceedings of the National Academy of Sciences. 2007;**104**:15858-15863. DOI: 10.1073/pnas.0707413104

[36] Spellberg B, Edwards JE. Type 1/type 2 immunity in infectious diseases. Clinical Infectious Diseases. 2001;**32**:76-102. DOI: 10.1086/317537

[37] Ray A, Raundhal M, Oriss TB, Ray P, Wenzel SE. Current concepts of severe asthma. The Journal of Clinical Investigation. 2016;**126**:2394-2403. DOI: 10.1172/JCI84144

[38] Masoli M, Fabian D, Holt S, Beasley R. The global burden of asthma: Executive summary of the GINA dissemination committee report. Allergy. 2004;**59**:469-478. DOI: 10.1111/j.1398-9995.2004.00526.x

[39] Haldar P, Pavord ID, Shaw DE, Berry MA, Thomas M, Brightling CE, Wardlaw AJ, Green RH. Cluster analysis and clinical asthma phenotypes. American Journal of Respiratory and Critical Care Medicine. 2008;**178**:218-224. DOI: 10.1164/rccm.200711-1754OC

[40] Just J, Bourgoin-Heck M, Amat F. Clinical phenotypes in asthma during childhood. Clinical and Experimental Allergy. 2017;**47**:848-855. DOI: 10.1111/cea.12939

[41] Bagnasco D, Ferrando M, Varricchi G, Passalacqua G, Canonica GW. A critical evaluation of anti-IL-13 and anti-IL-4 strategies in severe asthma. International Archives of Allergy and Immunology. 2016;**170**:122-131. DOI: 10.1159/000447692

[42] Fitzpatrick AM, Baena-Cagnani CE, Bacharier LB. Severe asthma in childhood: Recent advances in phenotyping and pathogenesis. Current Opinion in Allergy and Clinical Immunology. 2012;**12**:193-201. DOI: 10.1097/ACI.0b013e32835090ac

[43] Zhao J, Lloyd CM, Noble A. Th17 responses in chronic allergic airway inflammation abrogate regulatory T-cell-mediated tolerance and contribute to airway remodeling. Mucosal Immunology. 2013;**6**:335-346. DOI: 10.1038/mi.2012.76

[44] Loutsios C, Farahi N, Porter L, Lok LS, Peters AM, Condliffe AM, Chilvers ER. Biomarkers of eosinophilic inflammation in asthma. Expert Review of Respiratory Medicine. 2014;**8**:143-150. DOI: 10.1586/17476348.2014.880052

[45] Moorman JE, Akinbami LJ, Bailey CM, Zahran HS, King ME, Johnson CA, Liu X. National surveillance of asthma: United States, 2001–2010. Vital & Health Statistics. Series 3, Analytical and Epidemiological Studies. 2012:1-58 http://www.ncbi.nlm.nih.gov/pubmed/24252609 [Accessed: January 12, 2018

[46] Tsai C-L, Lee W-Y, Hanania NA, Camargo CA. Age-related differences in clinical outcomes for acute asthma in the United States, 2006–2008. Journal of Allergy and Clinical Immunology. 2012;**129**:1252-1258.e1. DOI: 10.1016/j.jaci.2012.01.061

[47] Gonzalez-Garcia M, Caballero A, Jaramillo C, Maldonado D, Torres-Duque CA. Prevalence, risk factors and underdiagnosis of asthma and wheezing in adults 40 years and older: A population-based study. The Journal of Asthma. 2015;**52**:823-830. DOI: 10.3109/02770903.2015.1010733

[48] Dykewicz MS. Occupational asthma: Current concepts in pathogenesis, diagnosis, and management. The Journal of Allergy and Clinical Immunology. 2009;**123**:519-528. DOI: 10.1016/j.jaci.2009.01.061

[49] Melgert BN, Ray A, Hylkema MN, Timens W, Postma DS. Are there reasons why adult asthma is more common in females? Current Allergy and Asthma Reports. 2007;**7**:143-150 http://www.ncbi.nlm.nih.gov/pubmed/17437685 [Accessed: January 12, 2018

[50] Jenkins MA, Dharmage SC, Flander LB, Douglass JA, Ugoni AM, Carlin JB, Sawyer SM, Giles GG, Hopper JL. Parity and decreased use of oral contraceptives as predictors of asthma in young women. Clinical and Experimental Allergy. 2006;**36**:609-613. DOI: 10.1111/j.1365-2222.2006.02475.x

[51] Troisi RJ, Speizer FE, Willett WC, Trichopoulos D, Rosner B. Menopause, postmenopausal estrogen preparations, and the risk of adult-onset asthma. A prospective cohort study. American Journal of Respiratory and Critical Care Medicine. 1995;**152**:1183-1188. DOI: 10.1164/ajrccm.152.4.7551368

[52] Romieu I, Fabre A, Fournier A, Kauffmann F, Varraso R, Mesrine S, Leynaert B, Clavel-Chapelon F. Postmenopausal hormone therapy and asthma onset in the E3N cohort. Thorax. 2010;**65**:292-297. DOI: 10.1136/thx.2009.116079

[53] van den Berge M, Heijink HI, van Oosterhout AJM, Postma DS. The role of female sex hormones in the development and severity of allergic and non-allergic asthma. Clinical and Experimental Allergy. 2009;**39**:1477-1481. DOI: 10.1111/j.1365-2222.2009.03354.x

[54] Koczulla AR, Vogelmeier CF, Garn H, Renz H. New concepts in asthma: Clinical phenotypes and pathophysiological mechanisms. Drug Discovery Today. 2017;**22**:388-396. DOI: 10.1016/j.drudis.2016.11.008

[55] Heller F, Florian P, Bojarski C, Richter J, Christ M, Hillenbrand B, Mankertz J, Gitter A, Burgel N, Fromm M, Zeitz M, Fuss I, Strober W, Schulzke JD. Interleukin-13 is the key effector Th2 cytokine in ulcerative colitis that affects epithelial tight junctions, apoptosis, and cell restitution. Gastroenterology. 2005;**129**:550-564. DOI: 10.1016/j.gastro.2005.05.002

[56] Hoshino T, Kato S, Oka N, Imaoka H, Kinoshita T, Takei S, Kitasato Y, Kawayama T, Imaizumi T, Yamada K, Young HA, Aizawa H. Pulmonary inflammation and emphysema. American Journal of Respiratory and Critical Care Medicine. 2007;**176**:49-62. DOI: 10.1164/rccm.200603-316OC

[57] Hastie AT, Moore WC, Meyers DA, Vestal PL, Li H, Peters SP, Bleecker ER, National Heart, Lung, and Blood Institute Severe Asthma Research Program. Analyses of asthma severity phenotypes and inflammatory proteins in subjects stratified by sputum granulocytes. Journal of Allergy and Clinical Immunology. 2010;**125**:1028-1036.e13. DOI: 10.1016/j.jaci.2010.02.008

[58] Ciepiela O, Ostafin M, Demkow U. Neutrophils in asthma—A review. Respiratory Physiology & Neurobiology. 2015;**209**:13-16. DOI: 10.1016/J.RESP.2014.12.004

[59] Fahy JV. Type 2 inflammation in asthma—Present in most, absent in many. Nature Reviews Immunology. 2015;**15**:57-65. DOI: 10.1038/nri3786

[60] Manni ML, Trudeau JB, Scheller EV, Mandalapu S, Elloso MM, Kolls JK, Wenzel SE, Alcorn JF. The complex relationship between inflammation and lung function in severe asthma. Mucosal Immunology. 2014;**7**:1186-1198. DOI: 10.1038/mi.2014.8

[61] Pelaia C, Vatrella A, Busceti MT, Gallelli L, Terracciano R, Savino R, Pelaia G. Severe eosinophilic asthma: From the pathogenic role of interleukin-5 to the therapeutic action of mepolizumab. Drug Design, Development and Therapy. 2017;**11**:3137-3144. DOI: 10.2147/DDDT.S150656

[62] Brusselle GG, Maes T, Bracke KR. Eosinophils in the spotlight: Eosinophilic airway inflammation in nonallergic asthma. Nature Medicine. 2013;**19**:977-979. DOI: 10.1038/nm.3300

[63] Yousefi S, Simon D, Simon H-U. Eosinophil extracellular DNA traps: Molecular mechanisms and potential roles in disease. Current Opinion in Immunology. 2012;**24**:736-739. DOI: 10.1016/j.coi.2012.08.010

[64] Possa SS, Leick EA, Prado CM, Martins MA, Tibério IFLC. Eosinophilic inflammation in allergic asthma. Frontiers in Pharmacology. 2013;**4**:46. DOI: 10.3389/fphar.2013.00046

[65] Louis R, Lau LCK, Bron AO, Roldaan AC, Radermecker M, Djulanovic R. The relationship between airways inflammation and asthma severity. American Journal of Respiratory and Critical Care Medicine. 2000;**161**:9-16. DOI: 10.1164/ajrccm.161.1.9802048

[66] Fahy JV. Eosinophilic and neutrophilic inflammation in asthma: Insights from clinical studies. Proceedings of the American Thoracic Society. 2009;**6**:256-259. DOI: 10.1513/pats.200808-087RM

[67] George L, Brightling CE. Eosinophilic airway inflammation: Role in asthma and chronic obstructive pulmonary disease. Therapeutic Advances in Chronic Disease. 2016;**7**:34-51. DOI: 10.1177/2040622315609251

[68] Pelaia G, Vatrella A, Busceti MT, Gallelli L, Calabrese C, Terracciano R, Maselli R. Cellular mechanisms underlying eosinophilic and neutrophilic airway inflammation in asthma. Mediators of Inflammation. 2015;**2015**:879783. DOI: 10.1155/2015/879783

[69] Shimoda T, Obase Y, Nagasaka Y, Asai S. Phenotype classification using the combination of lung sound analysis and fractional exhaled nitric oxide for evaluating asthma treatment. Allergology International. 2017:1-6. DOI: 10.1016/j.alit.2017.09.004

[70] Nagasaki T, Matsumoto H, Izuhara K, Kanemitsu Y, Tohda Y, Horiguchi T, Kita H, Tomii K, Fujimura M, Yokoyama A, Nakano Y, Hozawa S, Ito I, Oguma T, Izuhara Y, Tajiri T, Iwata T, Yokoyama T, Niimi A, Mishima M. Utility of serum periostin in combination with exhaled nitric oxide in the management of asthma. Allergology International. 2017;**66**:404-410. DOI: 10.1016/j.alit.2017.02.003

[71] Dweik RA, Sorkness RL, Wenzel S, Hammel J, Curran-Everett D, Comhair SAA, Bleecker E, Busse W, Calhoun WJ, Castro M, Chung KF, Israel E, Jarjour N, Moore W, Peters S, Teague G, Gaston B, Erzurum SC, National Heart, Lung, and Blood Institute Severe Asthma Research Program. Use of exhaled nitric oxide measurement to identify a reactive, at-risk phenotype among patients with asthma. American Journal of Respiratory and Critical Care Medicine. 2010;**181**:1033-1041. DOI: 10.1164/rccm.200905-0695OC

[72] McGrath KW, Icitovic N, Boushey HA, Lazarus SC, Sutherland ER, Chinchilli VM, Fahy JV, Asthma Clinical Research Network of the National Heart, Lung, and Blood Institute. A large subgroup of mild-to-moderate asthma is persistently noneosinophilic. American Journal of Respiratory and Critical Care Medicine. 2012;**185**:612-619. DOI: 10.1164/rccm.201109-1640OC

[73] Fajt ML, Wenzel SE. Asthma phenotypes and the use of biologic medications in asthma and allergic disease: The next steps toward personalized care. The Journal of Allergy and Clinical Immunology. 2015;**135**:299-310. DOI: 10.1016/j.jaci.2014.12.1871

[74] Dixon AE, Pratley RE, Forgione PM, Kaminsky DA, Whittaker-Leclair LA, Griffes LA, Garudathri J, Raymond D, Poynter ME, Bunn JY, Irvin CG. Effects of obesity and bariatric surgery on airway hyperresponsiveness, asthma control, and inflammation. Journal of Allergy and Clinical Immunology. 2011;**128**:508-515.e2. DOI: 10.1016/j.jaci.2011.06.009

[75] Rasmussen F, Hancox RJ. Mechanisms of obesity in asthma. Current Opinion in Allergy and Clinical Immunology. 2014;**14**:35-43. DOI: 10.1097/ACI.0000000000000024

[76] Sutherland ER, Goleva E, King TS, Lehman E, Stevens AD, Jackson LP, Stream AR, Fahy JV, Leung DYM. Asthma clinical research network, cluster analysis of obesity and asthma phenotypes. PLoS One. 2012;**7**:e36631. DOI: 10.1371/journal.pone.0036631

[77] Holguin F, Bleecker ER, Busse WW, Calhoun WJ, Castro M, Erzurum SC, Fitzpatrick AM, Gaston B, Israel E, Jarjour NN, Moore WC, Peters SP, Yonas M, Teague WG, Wenzel SE. Obesity and asthma: An association modified by age of asthma onset. Journal of Allergy and Clinical Immunology. 2011;**127**:1486-1493.e2. DOI: 10.1016/j.jaci.2011.03.036

[78] Gomez-Llorente M, Romero R, Chueca N, Martinez-Cañavate A, Gomez-Llorente C. Obesity and asthma: A missing link. International Journal of Molecular Sciences. 2017; **18**:1490. DOI: 10.3390/ijms18071490

[79] Wenzel SE, Szefler SJ, Leung DYM, Sloan SI, Rex MD, Martin RJ. Bronchoscopic evaluation of severe asthma. American Journal of Respiratory and Critical Care Medicine. 1997;**156**:737-743. DOI: 10.1164/ajrccm.156.3.9610046

[80] Jatakanon A, Uasuf C, Maziak W, Lim S, Chung KF, Barnes PJ. Neutrophilic inflammation in severe persistent asthma. American Journal of Respiratory and Critical Care Medicine. 1999;**160**:1532-1539. DOI: 10.1164/ajrccm.160.5.9806170

[81] Kato T, Takeda Y, Nakada T, Sendo F. Inhibition by dexamethasone of human neutrophil apoptosis in vitro. Natural Immunity. 1995;**14**:198-208. http://www.ncbi.nlm.nih.gov/pubmed/8696009 [Accessed: January 12, 2018

[82] Busacker A, Newell JD, Keefe T, Hoffman EA, Granroth JC, Castro M, Fain S, Wenzel S. A multivariate analysis of risk factors for the air-trapping asthmatic phenotype as measured by quantitative CT analysis. Chest. 2009;**135**:48-56. DOI: 10.1378/chest.08-0049

[83] Gupta S, Siddiqui S, Haldar P, Raj JV, Entwisle JJ, Wardlaw AJ, Bradding P, Pavord ID, Green RH, Brightling CE. Qualitative analysis of high-resolution CT scans in severe asthma. Chest. 2009;**136**:1521-1528. DOI: 10.1378/chest.09-0174

[84] Gounni AS, Lamkhioued B, Koussih L, Ra C, Renzi PM, Hamid Q. Human neutrophils express the high-affinity receptor for immunoglobulin E (Fc epsilon RI): Role in asthma. The FASEB Journal. 2001;**15**:940-949. http://www.ncbi.nlm.nih.gov/pubmed/11292654 [Accessed: January 12, 2018]

[85] Alphonse MP, Saffar AS, Shan L, HayGlass KT, Simons FER, Gounni AS. Regulation of the high affinity IgE receptor (Fc epsilonRI) in human neutrophils: Role of seasonal allergen exposure and Th-2 cytokines. PLoS One. 2008;**3**:e1921. DOI: 10.1371/journal.pone.0001921

[86] Lavinskiene S, Bajoriuniene I, Malakauskas K, Jeroch J, Sakalauskas R. Sputum neutrophil count after bronchial allergen challenge is related to peripheral blood neutrophil chemotaxis in asthma patients. Inflammation Research. 2014;**63**:951-959. DOI: 10.1007/s00011-014-0770-0

[87] Macdowell AL, Peters SP. Neutrophils in asthma. Current Allergy and Asthma Reports. 2007;**7**:464-468. http://www.ncbi.nlm.nih.gov/pubmed/17986378 [Accessed: January 12, 2018]

[88] Bullens DM, Truyen E, Coteur L, Dilissen E, Hellings PW, Dupont LJ, Ceuppens JL. IL-17 mRNA in sputum of asthmatic patients: Linking T cell driven inflammation and granulocytic influx? Respiratory Research. 2006;**7**:135. DOI: 10.1186/1465-9921-7-135

[89] Cosmi L, Annunziato F, MIG G, RME M, Nagata K, Romagnani S. CRTH2 is the most reliable marker for the detection of circulating human type 2 Th and type 2 T cytotoxic cells in health and disease. European Journal of Immunology. 2000;**30**:2972-2979. DOI: 10.1002/1521-4141(200010)30:10<2972::AID-IMMU2972>3.0.CO;2-#

[90] Monteseirín J, Camacho MJ, Bonilla I, De la Calle A, Guardia P, Conde J, Sobrino F. Respiratory burst in neutrophils from asthmatic patients. The Journal of Asthma. 2002;**39**:619-624. http://www.ncbi.nlm.nih.gov/pubmed/12442951 [Accessed: January 12, 2018]

[91] Bourgeois EA, Levescot A, Diem S, Chauvineau A, Bergès H, Milpied P, Lehuen A, Damotte D, Gombert J-M, Schneider E, Girard J-P, Gourdy P, Herbelin A. A natural protective function of invariant NKT cells in a mouse model of innate-cell-driven lung inflammation. European Journal of Immunology. 2011;**41**:299-305. DOI: 10.1002/eji.201040647

[92] Rodrigo GJ, Price D, Anzueto A, Singh D, Altman P, Bader G, Patalano F, Fogel R, Kostikas K. LABA/LAMA combinations versus LAMA monotherapy or LABA/ICS in COPD: A systematic review and meta-analysis. International Journal of Chronic Obstructive Pulmonary Disease. 2017;**12**:907-922. DOI: 10.2147/COPD.S130482

[93] Wynn TA. Type 2 cytokines: Mechanisms and therapeutic strategies. Nature Reviews. Immunology. 2015;**15**:271-282. DOI: 10.1038/nri3831

[94] Beeh K-M, Moroni-Zentgraf P, Ablinger O, Hollaenderova Z, Unseld A, Engel M, Korn S. Tiotropium Respimat® in asthma: A double-blind, randomised, dose-ranging study in adult patients with moderate asthma. Respiratory Research. 2014;**15**:61. DOI: 10.1186/1465-9921-15-61

[95] Leung JS, Johnson DW, Sperou AJ, Crotts J, Saude E, Hartling L, Stang A. A systematic review of adverse drug events associated with administration of common asthma medications in children. PLoS One. 2017;**12**:e0182738. DOI: 10.1371/journal.pone.0182738

[96] Bengtson LGS, Yu Y, Wang W, Cao F, Hulbert EM, Wolbeck R, Elliott CA, Buikema AR. Inhaled corticosteroid-containing treatment escalation and outcomes for patients with asthma in a U.S. Health Care Organization. Journal of Managed Care & Specialty Pharmacy. 2017;**23**:1149-1159. DOI: 10.18553/jmcp.2017.23.11.1149

[97] Navinés-Ferrer A, Serrano-Candelas E, Molina-Molina G-J, Martín M. IgE-related chronic diseases and anti-IgE-based treatments. Journal of Immunology Research. 2016; **2016**:1-12. DOI: 10.1155/2016/8163803

[98] Chipps BE, Lanier B, Milgrom H, Deschildre A, Hedlin G, Szefler SJ, Kattan M, Kianifard F, Ortiz B, Haselkorn T, Iqbal A, Rosén K, Trzaskoma B, Busse WW. Omalizumab in children with uncontrolled allergic asthma: Review of clinical trial and real-world experience. The Journal of Allergy and Clinical Immunology. 2017;**139**:1431-1444. DOI: 10.1016/j.jaci.2017.03.002

[99] Murphy K, Jacobs J, Bjermer L, Fahrenholz JM, Shalit Y, Garin M, Zangrilli J, Castro M. Long-term safety and efficacy of reslizumab in patients with eosinophilic asthma. Journal of Allergy and Clinical Immunology: In Practice. 2017;**5**:1572-1581.e3. DOI: 10.1016/j.jaip.2017.08.024

[100] Fahy JV. Type 2 inflammation in asthma—Present in most, absent in many. Nat. Rev. Immunol. 2015;**15**:57-65. DOI: 10.1038/nri3786

[101] Kohn CM, Paudyal P. A systematic review and meta-analysis of complementary and alternative medicine in asthma. European Respiratory Review. 2017;**26**:160092. DOI: 10.1183/16000617.0092-2016

11

Monoclonal Antibodies for Asthma Management

Dolly V. Rojas, Diana L. Silva and Carlos D. Serrano

Abstract

Asthma is a multifactorial and complex disease, with different degrees of risks and severity, as well as the response to treatment. Medications currently available are most effective in severe asthma; nonetheless, there is a percentage of patients that have no response to the treatment that guidelines suggest in their recommendations. In the last years, there have been new insights in inflammatory molecules that contribute to asthma physiopathology and a lot of them have been considered to be possible targets in the management of severe asthma. As a consequence of this, a few monoclonal antibodies have been developed evidencing their effectiveness in the treatment of the disease. The study of these new therapies has allowed the identification of specific inflammatory pathways. This chapter intends to offer a critical perspective of the current guidelines for the management of severe asthma, as well as to discuss current treatments and the future on new molecules. Through an adequate characterization, different phenotypes will be recognized and associated with a determinate biomarker and should be used to select the treatment that can offer the highest efficiency in these patients. In this way, the treatment will be directed to a personalized medicine.

Keywords: severe asthma, inflammation, phenotype, treatment, monoclonal antibodies

1. Introduction

Asthma is a heterogeneous disease characterized by chronic airway inflammation. The GINA guidelines indicate that inflammation control is a key for management goals and as such is considered a treatment priority. Severe asthma represents a good part of the health spending, with significant impact on patients' quality of life. Hence, the identification and correct treatment of severe asthma may help to control exacerbations and the inflammatory process, thus improving the personal, social, and economic impact of the disease [1]. In the pathophysiology of asthma, there are multiple processes mediated by various cytokines and cells that cause inflammation. Management goals have been directed toward these molecules and cell targets through the use of corticosteroids, which have meant a dramatic change in the control of the disease. However, these drugs act in a nonspecific way. Furthermore, the development of new monoclonal antibodies could represent a significant milestone for treatment of asthma, reinforcing the essential idea of personalized medicine. In 1984, researchers Jerne, Köhler, and Milstein received the Nobel Prize in Medicine for their work on plasma cell and multiple myeloma cell fusion, which allowed the generation of specific antibodies with the appropriate genetic information, but at high speed. In subsequent years, immunoglobulins synthesized from this new technology, with specific target molecules, such as the endotoxin of Gram-negative bacteria in sepsis, demonstrated an initial benefit. Subsequently, the concept of personalized medicine began to take shape, and in recent years, biomedical research has focused on deepening the molecular mechanisms underlying various pathologies, parallel to the production of new drugs that act at crucial points of specific immunological cascades. Therefore, monoclonal antibodies are an effective and safe therapeutic alternative in many chronic diseases such as rheumatoid arthritis, cancer, and asthma and are seen as a hopeful option in many other diseases. The challenge now is not to get lost in the wide variety of clinical studies that can be found in the literature, as well as in connecting a particular patient with the appropriate management based on the evidence.

2. Critical view of current guidelines and treatment

Large studies on severe asthma have expanded our knowledge about the characteristics of the disease. Severity is defined as the requirement for systemic corticosteroids more than twice a year, the need for at least one hospitalization, previous admission to an intensive care unit, the need for mechanical ventilation in the previous year, impaired pulmonary function determined by a forced expiratory volume in the first second (FEV1) less than 80% of the predicted in the presence of forced vital capacity (FVC) below normal limits after the administration of bronchodilator, or the use of high doses of corticosteroids inhaled and long-acting beta-2-agonists without achieving control of symptoms [2]. In fact, it is estimated that 50% of patients are not well-controlled despite receiving optimal treatment, and that 5–10% do not respond to treatment. Also, receiving high doses of inhaled or systemic corticosteroids increases the risk for adverse effects, which implies an affectation of the additional quality of life due to the sum of other secondary diseases [3]. The GINA guidelines include evidence-based diagnostic and therapeutic recommendation derived from studies that meet all criteria of scientific validity. However, it is possible that in selected patients, guidelines do not accurately reflect what a clinician is trying to address.

The guidelines suggest management according to severity and control, symptom dynamics and pulmonary function, but these are directed to the total population of patients with asthma [1]. In this sense, there will always be a percentage of patients who either receive a suboptimal treatment or who remain unresponsive despite being in the most serious step. Finally, the guidelines are not based on the characteristics of the specific inflammation related to the different phenotypes, which are the ones that could define with greater precision what would be the ideal treatment to stop a specific pathophysiological mechanism [4]. It is not sufficient then to establish a management based only on severity, since there are several aspects that arise from the very concept that asthma is a heterogeneous disease and with different molecular and genetic bases, so if a patient should be typecast within a general parameter, reduce their therapeutic options [5]. On the other hand, the control of severe asthma represents a challenge for specialists in allergology and pneumology due to the high impact of this disease on the quality of life of patients. The GINA guidelines establish levels of disease control according to the response to treatment as follows: well-controlled, partially controlled, and uncontrolled. However, it can differ as patients cataloged in one of the degrees, in reality corresponding to another, taking into account that probably a partially controlled asthma is actually an uncontrolled asthma and that this has therapeutic implications. In daily practice, middle terms cannot be established to define management. Some patients persist without control despite established therapeutic recommendations, which allows us to infer that as with severity, there are other aspects that should be evaluated from the pathophysiology of the disease and not only based on the degree of control of the disease. Additionally, the classification based on control is very strict and poorly documented.

2.1. Approach by phenotypes

It is clear that some characteristics can be identified in some asthmatic patients and not in others; from this arises the concept of "phenotype," which is defined as the presence of different characteristics that are the product of the interaction of genes with the environment. There may be overlap between them and that the same patient can migrate transiently or definitively from one phenotype to another. The challenge, therefore, is to determine in each patient the individual characteristics.

Several years ago, Chung and Adcock [6] published a review about phenotyping of asthma. The first systematic study of severe asthma carried out in Europe by the group ENFUMOSA (European Network for Understanding Mechanisms of Severe Asthma) [7] consolidated the concept that asthma has a heterogeneous expression, and thus, severe asthma should be considered a different form of the disease, more than simply an increase in the symptoms of it. Subsequent studies included in the Severe Asthma Research Program (SARP) of the United States, together with the results of the ENFUMOSA group, and subsequently of the BIOAIR (Longitudinal Assessment of Clinical Course and BIOmarkers in severe chronic AIRway Disease) [8], have extended the knowledge of clinical expressions and generated new hypotheses about the pathophysiology of severe asthma. In this way, five phenotypes have been established:

1. Early onset atopic asthma with airway dysfunction, eosinophilic inflammation, and high number of hospitalizations.
2. Asthma with noneosinophilic inflammation, obesity, and present in the female sex.
3. Early onset asthma, with few symptoms and minimal eosinophilic inflammation.
4. Asthma with eosinophilic inflammation, with few symptoms and delayed onset.
5. Asthma with neutrophilic inflammation.

2.1.1. Severe asthma early onset

It comprises 40% of all severe asthmatics. Patients develop the disease in childhood and have a history of atopy, increased bronchial hyperresponsiveness, higher levels of total immunoglobulin E (IgE), and a higher eosinophil count both peripherally and in sputum, as well as a tendency to subendothelial fibrosis and overexpression of the mucin gene. In general terms, they respond to management with inhaled corticosteroids. Family history suggests a genetic component; in fact, multiple studies have reported associations between genes related to the expression of the Th2 phenotype and multiple polymorphisms related to greater severity. The Th2 pattern of cytokines, including interleukins (IL) 2, 4, 5, 9, and 13, is expressed in the bronchial submucosa of these patients. These cytokines contribute to the allergic inflammation of the airway, generating the activation and the recruitment of B lymphocytes producing specific IgE, mast cells, basophils, and eosinophils. IL-13 also acts as an inducer of the genes of regulator 1 of the chlorine channels, periostin, and the inhibitor of serpin peptidase.

Recently, the role of thymic stromal lymphopoietin (TSLP) has been described as an inducer of IL-4, -5, and -13 production in the initiation of cellular response mediated by Th2 pattern cells, as well as IL-25 and -33, which are produced in response to exposure to allergens, contaminants, and viruses. IL-33, which is a member of the cytokine family of IL-1, possesses potent induction and chemotactic activity of Th2 lymphocytes. Elevated levels of IL-33 and TSLP have been observed in patients with asthma, especially in severe cases [9].

2.1.2. Phenotypes with and without eosinophilia

An increased presence of eosinophils in induced sputum and in peripheral blood can identify the eosinophilic subgroup. The cutoff points are at least 3% of eosinophils in the sputum and peripheral eosinophilia greater than 350 (absolute number). The noneosinophilic phenotype has been defined as asthma with eosinophils in induced sputum less than 3% and increased neutrophilic infiltration. The mechanisms that explain neutrophilia in the airway are not very clear. It has been suggested that this phenotype reflects a "non-Th2" pattern with all its molecular implications. In addition, it is associated with a poor response to treatment with inhaled corticosteroids (even inducing even more neutrophilia), suggesting a Th1 pattern orchestrated by the tumor necrosis factor alpha (TNFα), which is assumed to have an important role. Both Th17 cells and bacterial colonization of the airway secondary to defects in phagocytosis have been implicated as causes of neutrophilia [10].

The identification of phenotypes results in a large number of treatments with specific objectives, which have been developed for some years. The challenge is to unify the physiopathology with clinical phenotypes and use that knowledge to discover other phenotypes that have not yet been recognized. None of the clinical phenotypes established to date has a detailed identification of their pathophysiology, biomarkers, genetic elements, stability over time, or the response to a specific treatment. Probably, all the factors that influence a phenotype will need to be incorporated into an endotype, which is nothing else than the subtype defined by the functional or pathophysiological mechanism of the disease for a particular individual.

The support of the evidence regarding the conformation of phenotypes and endotypes continues to be limited by the lack of large-scale longitudinal studies that may intertwine the pathophysiology with the clinical findings. However, there are already phenotypes that seem to be clearly defined in terms of their clinical and molecular bases, and in which the pharmacological intervention with monoclonal antibodies constitutes an important starting point in the management of severe asthma [2].

3. Monoclonal antibodies

Monoclonal antibodies are specialized glycoproteins produced by B cells from a stem cell, forming identical clones of it. They can recognize specific molecules, such as cytokines or receptors.

3.1. Chimeric monoclonal antibodies

They are artificial molecules in which the constant portions of the heavy and light chains come from a human immunoglobulin and the variable regions VL and VH (variable region of the light and heavy chain, respectively) are obtained from an antibody of murine origin. The goal with the construction of a chimeric antibody is to reduce immunogenicity without affecting the selectivity of the antibody for the antigen. These molecules have 66% of human component and 33% of murine origin; they are less immunogenic than the first-generation monoclonal antibodies, but they can still induce an immune response against them. Antibodies of this type end with the prefix ximab (e.g. infliximab, rituximab).

3.2. Humanized antibodies

These molecules have 90% of human origin, so when it is injected into the patients, there is no response from the immune system. Only the antigen binding site (paratope) is of murine origin and is formed from the spatial combination of the hypervariable loops. The rest of the variable region (called M) only works as a scaffold whose function is to serve as structural support to the paratope. In this way, the epitopes associated with the murine M regions, which are present in the chimeric antibodies, are not found in the humanized antibodies. This type of antibody ends with the prefix zumab (e.g., omalizumab, trastuzumab).

3.3. Human antibodies

Almost 100% of its structure is human. However, while the production of mouse monoclonal antibodies is routinely carried out by hybridoma technology, the production of human monoclonal antibodies by this technology has been difficult, because the human hybridomas and cell lines derived from multiple myeloma have been difficult to develop and immunization in vivo is not feasible for many antigens. However, several techniques make it possible to generate human monoclonal antibodies, such as the expression of immunoglobulin fragments, the single-chain variable fractions, and the single strands of the variable fraction. Currently, the development of recombinant monoclonal antibodies by phage library technology with genes that encode the immunoglobulin variable regions has proven useful in basic and clinical research. This type of antibody ends with the prefix mumab or numab (e.g. adalimumab, secukinumab) [11–13].

The traditional production process of monoclonal antibodies is outlined in Figure 1

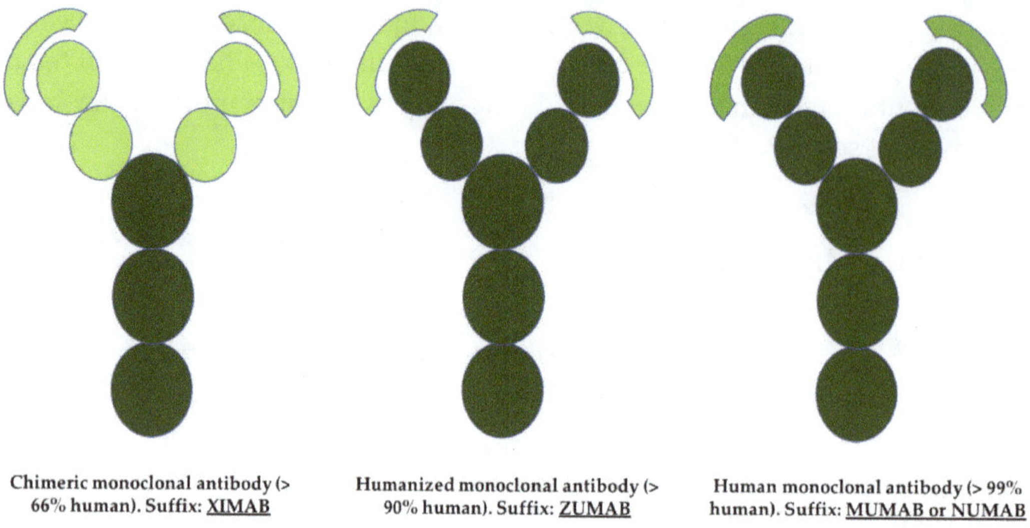

Figure 1. Types of monoclonal antibodies according to their humanization.

3.4. Development and production

The production of monoclonal antibodies is based on the method of fusion of B lymphocytes from an immunized animal (usually a mouse), with an immortal myeloma cell line and the culture of the cells in a medium in which the nonfused normal and tumoral cells cannot survive. The resulting fused cells that are obtained are called hybridomas and each hybridoma produces only one immunoglobulin, derived from a B lymphocyte of the immunized animal [11]. The method as such consists of the fusion of spleen cells from a mouse immunized to an antigen or mixture of known antigens, with a myeloma cell line, with the subsequent formation of hybrid cells that preserve many chromosomes of the fused pairs. These cells are then placed in a selection medium that allows the survival only of immortalized hybrids, which in turn are cultured as cell clones that secrete the antibody of interest. This method of selection includes hypotaxine,

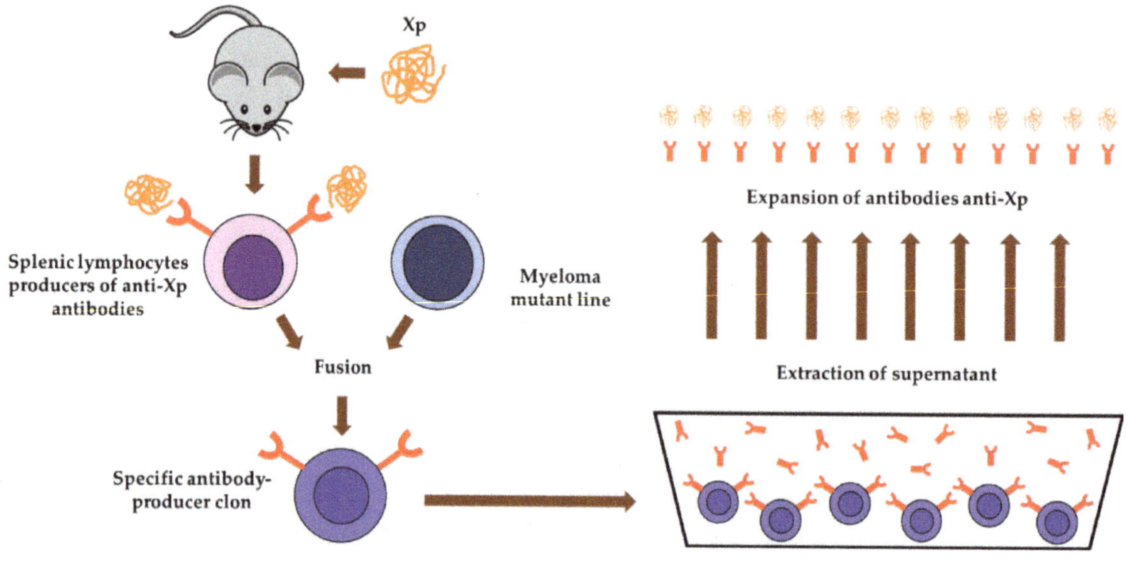

Figure 2. Schematic process for the production of monoclonal antibodies. Xp: "X" protein.

aminopterin, and thymidine, and is therefore called HAT [14]. Antibody-producing hybridomas are expanded in larger capacity culture vessels, and the cells are harvested by centrifugation, suspended in culture medium supplemented with fetal calf serum and dimethyl sulfoxide (DMSO) to freeze, first at −70°C and then in liquid nitrogen. The production of the monoclonal antibody is made from the supernatant of bulk cultures or after intraperitoneal inoculation of the hybridoma in histocompatible animals. In the latter case, an antibody-producing tumor is produced that generates an ascitic fluid rich in these. In both cases, the monoclonal antibodies are separated and purified by conventional methods [15] (**Figure 2**).

4. Current and future targets in the management of asthma

4.1. Current targets

4.1.1. Nonspecific blockade of inflammation (corticosteroids and leukotriene antagonists)

At present, asthma control focuses on the use of inhaled corticosteroids, either alone or in association with leukotriene antagonists, and/or long-acting beta-2 agonists. Numerous studies have documented the efficacy of corticosteroids in reducing inflammation, both in children and adults and at any degree of severity. Currently, they are considered the most effective drugs to achieve control in most cases. Its action requires binding to a cytoplasmic receptor (alpha GR), which is associated with heat shock proteins (Hsp90-Hsp60). The binding of the corticoid to its receptor induces the dissociation of these proteins and the translocation of the complex toward the nucleus where several events occur that lead to the activation of the transcription of anti-inflammatory genes and the blocking of those pro-inflammatory. Additionally, corticosteroids interact directly with transcription factors, such as the nuclear factor kB, further blocking the expansion of the inflammatory process.

The use of these drugs has made it possible to reduce both the symptoms and the frequency and severity of the exacerbations, improving quality of life, lung function, and reducing bronchial hyperreactivity. However, their lack of specificity makes them susceptible to generating adverse effects in different organs. In addition, there is a percentage of patients resistant to corticosteroids, a phenomenon explained, among other causes, by the presence of a receptor isoform unable to bind to the glucocorticoid [16].

It is difficult to know if in the medium or long term, corticosteroids will continue to be the standard asthma therapy. Likewise, it is uncertain whether the advent of monoclonal antibodies will allow the reduction of the dose of corticosteroids and/or their total clearance in patients with severe asthma. The cysteinyl leukotrienes comprise C4, D4, and E4 leukotrienes. They are mediators that play an important role in inflammation, mucus secretion, bronchospasm, and remodeling. The antagonists of the type 1 receptors of cysteinyl leukotrienes (montelukast) are potent and selective and block their action in a competitive manner, generating an interruption of the pro-inflammatory intracellular cascade with a subsequent reduction of its effects. Clinical studies show that antagonism of these receptors is beneficial to some degree and percentage of the population. However, it is never superior to the effects achieved with corticosteroids used as monotherapy or in combination with long-acting beta-2 agonists. The precise indications for use in asthma have not been completely defined. It seems that its administration in transient early wheeze triggered by virus and without atopy works to a certain extent [17].

4.1.2. Long-acting β-agonists (LABA) combined

The agonist stimulation of the beta 2 adrenergic receptors generates smooth muscle relaxation of the central and peripheral airways, reversing the bronchial obstruction in asthmatics. The effect is given by the activation of adenylate cyclase (it catalyzes the conversion of adenosine triphosphate—ATP—into cyclic adenosine monophosphate—AMPc), generating the decrease in intracellular calcium, and thus causing muscle relaxation. This treatment always associated with a corticoid is a choice when control is not achieved with the inhaled corticosteroid alone [18].

4.1.3. Anti-IgE therapy

IgE is a clear therapeutic goal in allergic diseases. It is released by the plasmocyte, binds to its receptor of high affinity in the mast cell, and later, upon exposure to the allergen involved, induces several effector responses including the release of mediators responsible of allergic reaction. Omalizumab, a recombinant humanized monoclonal antibody, binds specifically to free serum IgE in its CH3 domain, near the high-affinity receptor binding site, thereby blocking its interaction with mast cells, basophils, antigen-presenting cells, and other inflammatory cells that express the receptor. That binding results in the decrease of free IgE, generating a negative feedback of the receptor of high affinity, and therefore, an interruption of the inflammatory cascade evident by the reduction of the levels of tissue eosinophils and peripheral blood, as well as of the GM-CSF, and IL-2, -4, and -13. They also decrease the presentation of allergens to T cells and the production of cytokines that stimulate differentiation toward the Th2 phenotype [19] (**Figure 3**).

The efficacy and safety of omalizumab treatment in severe asthma has been demonstrated in several controlled studies, showing a significant reduction in exacerbations, a steroid-sparing effect, and improvement in quality of life. The greatest benefit has been observed in patients with allergic asthma, particularly those of greater severity, who failed to respond to conventional treatment [20]. Since 2003, this continues to be its main indication, when it was approved by the Food and Drug Administration (FDA). In 2005, it was approved by the European Medicines Agency (EMA) as an additional therapy in adult patients and in children older than 6 years with persistent severe uncontrolled allergic asthma, with decreased lung function (FEV1 less than 80% of predicted), despite the chronic management with high doses of inhaled corticosteroids plus long-acting beta 2-agonists and with evidence of sensitization to at least one aeroallergen in the skin test or by determination of specific IgE in blood [21]. In Colombia, Invima has approved it since 2005 with the same indication.

4.1.4. Interleukins 4 and 13

IL-4 and -13 are considered the most important cytokines in allergic inflammation in the respiratory tract for a long time; they are essential for the differentiation of CD4+ lymphocytes toward the Th2 phenotype. In addition, they are the promoters of the Ig class switch toward the production

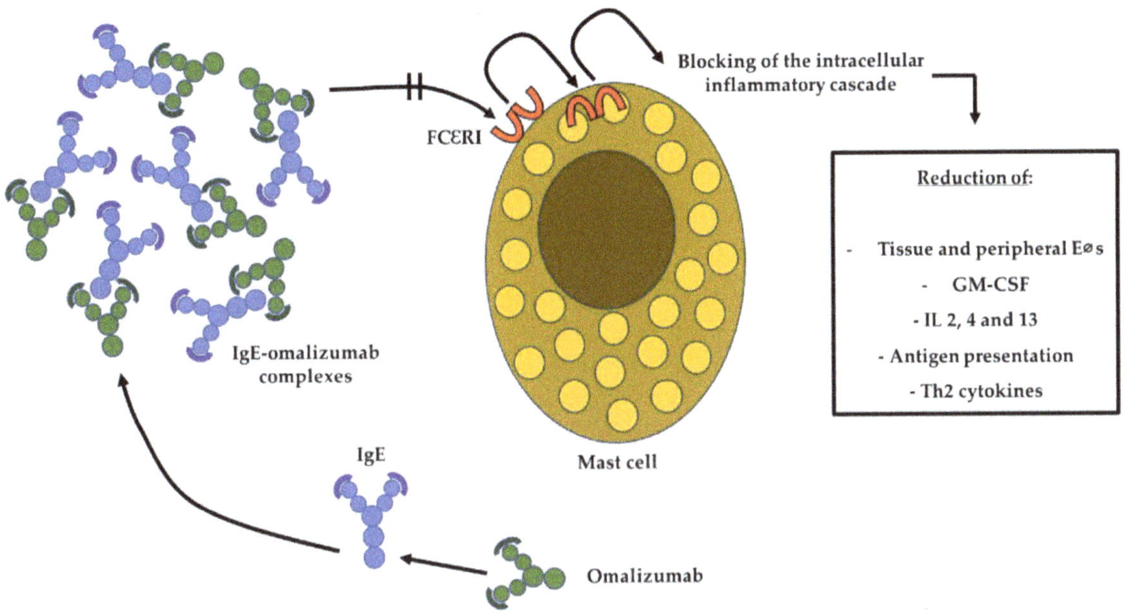

Figure 3. Molecular effects of omalizumab. This antibody binds to soluble immunoglobulin E (IgE), preventing its binding to the high-affinity receptor on the mast cell membrane. This generates a negative feedback that induces the internalization of this receptor and the blockade of the entire intracellular inflammatory cascade with the subsequent anti-inflammatory effects. FCεRI: high-affinity receptor for IgE; Eøs: eosinophils; GM-CSF: colony-stimulating factor of granulocytes and monocytes.

of IgE, of the differentiation of the B cells in plasma producing specific Ig E, and of the recruitment of eosinophils to the airway through the receptors for them that are expressed in them. They also stimulate mast cells and other pro-inflammatory cells. IL-13 favors the development of airway fibrosis and mucus hypersecretion, and in conjunction with IL-4, induces inflammation, remodeling, and the proliferation of bronchial fibroblasts and smooth muscle cells [22].

4.1.5. Interleukin 5

It is produced mostly by Th2 cells, mast cells, basophils, and eosinophils. This cytosine mainly conditions the population of eosinophils, from their medullary differentiation to their maturation, survival, and activation. It is a potent inhibitor of eosinophilic apoptosis [23].

4.2. Future targets

4.2.1. Interleukin 9

It is produced by Th2, Th9, basophil, eosinophil, and mast cells, and is thought to be also by neutrophils. This cytokine acts by binding to its IL-9R alpha receptor, generating an increase in the proliferation and attraction of mast cells. It plays a very important role in the differentiation and activation of Th2 cells. Together with interleukins 4 and 13, it acts on the smooth muscle and the airway epithelium, contributing to bronchial hyperreactivity [23].

4.2.2. Granulocyte macrophage colony-stimulating factor

It is a growth factor involved in the differentiation and survival of eosinophils [23].

4.2.3. *Thymic stromal lymphopoietin*

It is an epithelial cytokine similar to IL-7, produced in response to a pro-inflammatory stimulus. It acts by inducing the release of cytokines from the Th2 pattern. Patients with asthma have elevated levels of this cytokine in their airway, showing a correlation between the degree of elevation and the severity of the disease. In fact, several studies have shown that some polymorphisms in the locus for the TSLP gene have a protective effect for the development of asthma and bronchial hyperreactivity [24].

4.2.4. *Prostaglandin D2 receptor (PTGDR)*

It is a receptor located in Th2 cells, innate lymphoid type 2 cells (ILC2), and in eosinophils. Prostaglandin D2 is its natural ligand. PTGDR activation stimulates the synthesis of Th2 cytokines.

4.2.5. *Interleukin 25*

It is produced by epithelial cells in response to different stimuli. Through the induction of GATA 3, it favors the differentiation toward Th2 and ILC2 cells. It has an essential role in inflammation of the airway and in the remodeling process [25].

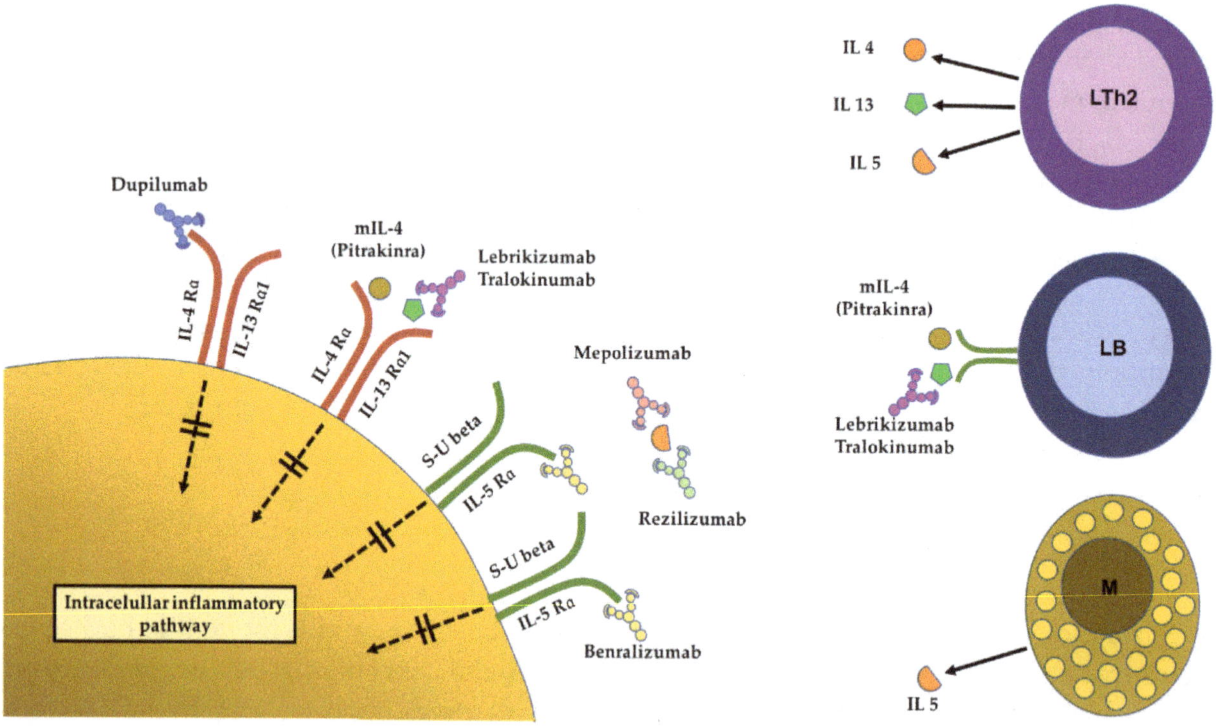

Figure 4. Different monoclonal antibodies with their respective therapeutic targets within the inflammatory cascade of asthma. The neutralization of the different receptors and mediators blocks the intracellular cascade of kinases that amplify the inflammatory process. IL-4Rα: alpha receptor for interleukin 4; IL-13 Rα1: alpha 1 chain of the interleukin 13 receptor; rIL-4: inactive recombinant interleukin 4; S-U: subunit.

Antibody (references)	Type	Target	Study phase	Clinic outcomes	Inflammatory outcomes	Dose/route/interval
Benralizumab [27–31]	Humanized	IL-5Rα	II–III	- Reduction of exacerbations, and hospitalization - Improvement of FEV1 - Improvement of the quality of life	- ↓ eosinophilia - ↓ sputum eosinophils - ↓ECP	20–100 mg SC/4–8 weeks
Mepolizumab [32–35]	Humanized	IL-5S	II–III	- Reduction of exacerbations - Reduction of dose of oral corticosteroids - Improvement of the ACT - Improvement of FEV1	- ↓ eosinophilia - ↓ sputum eosinophils	75 mg IV/month 100 mg SC/month
Reslizumab [36, 37]	Humanized	IL-5S	III	- Improvement of FEV1 - Improvement of the ACT - Improvement of symptoms - Reduction of exacerbations	- ↓ sputum eosinophils	3 mg/kg IV/month
Dupilumab [38, 39]	Human	IL-4Rα	II–III	- Reduction of exacerbations - Improvement of FEV1 -Improvement of the quality of life	- ↓ FeNO - ↓ total IgE - ↓ eotaxin 1	200 mg SC/2 weeks
Pitrakinra [40, 41]	rIL-4	IL-4Rα	II	- Reduction of exacerbations* - Reduction of night awakenings* - Reduction of activities limitation by asthma* - Reduction of exacerbations in patients with eosinophilia - Reduction of need for beta-2's rescue -FEV1 improvement	- ↓ FeNO	3–10 mg inhaled/12 h

Antibody (references)	Type	Target	Study phase	Clinic outcomes	Inflammatory outcomes	Dose/route/interval
Lebrikizumab [42, 43]	Humanized	IL-13	II–III	- Reduction of exacerbations - Improvement of FEV1	- ↓ periostin	125–250 mg SC/month
Tralokinumab [44, 45]	Human	IL-13	II–III	- Reduction of bronchial hyperreactivity - Reduction of need for beta-2's rescue - Improvement of FEV1	- ↓ eosinophilia	300 mg SC/2–4 weeks

*Defects associated with specific polymorphisms. Other monoclonal antibodies that have been studied: anti-TSLP [46]; enokisumab (anti IL-9) [47]; anti-GM-CSF [48]; anti IL-25 [49]; anti IL-33 [50].

rIL-4: inactive recombinant interleukin 4; IL-5Rα: alpha receptor for interleukin 5; IL-5S: soluble interleukin 5; IL-4Rα: alpha receptor for interleukin 4; IL-13: interleukin 13; FEV1: forced expiratory volume in the first second; NS: not significant difference; ACT: asthma control test; ECP: eosinophilic cationic protein; FeNO: expired fraction of nitric oxide; IgE: immunoglobulin E; SC: subcutaneous route; IV: intravenous route.

Table 1. Main monoclonal antibodies that have been studied for the treatment of asthma [27–45].

4.2.6. Interleukin 33

IL-33 origin and actions are very similar to IL-25. Its effect is even greater and more potent on innate lymphoid cells compared to IL-25. In addition, it activates mast cells and basophils and is a survival factor for eosinophils [26].

4.2.7. Tumoral necrosis factor (TNF-a)

It is produced by epithelial cells, Th1 and Th17 cells. TNF-a promotes the recruitment of eosinophils and neutrophils to the airway by dysregulation of adhesion molecules. It activates macrophages for the production of growth factors and GM-CSF [25].

4.2.8. Intervention in the Th2 pathway with monoclonal antibodies

The possible therapeutic interventions with monoclonal antibodies for the treatment of asthma are outlined in **Figure 4**. The characteristics of the main molecules and the current evidence available for each of them are detailed in **Table 1** [27–45]. Other monoclonal antibodies have fewer studies and possibly have a residual role in the treatment of asthma [46–50].

5. Conclusion(s)

A significant percentage of patients with severe asthma do not achieve control of the disease despite receiving adequate treatment. Current guidelines are outdated and will be even more if biomarkers and specific molecular susceptible of an intervention are not included in future guideline versions.

For now, omalizumab, the only biological treatment available for the management of severe asthma, continues influencing future studies aiming to evaluate new molecules and possible newer targets in selected patients. Linking the characteristics of each patient's disease, with the effects of a specific monoclonal antibody, will surely imply a much more effective and timely control of the disease.

The detailed approach of the phenotypic characteristics and their molecular basis should lead to a personalized treatment of great precision and effectiveness. A very promising new era in the treatment of asthma is approaching.

Author details

Dolly V. Rojas*, Diana L. Silva and Carlos D. Serrano

*Address all correspondence to: dollyvanessa@gmail.com

Allergy Unit, Fundación Valle del Lili, Faculty of Health Sciences, ICESI University, Cali, Colombia

References

[1] Bagnasco D, Ferrando M, Bernardi S, Passalacqua G, Canonica GW. The path to personalized medicine in asthma. Expert Review of Respiratory Medicine. 2016;**10**:957-965. DOI: 10.1080/17476348.2016.1205490

[2] Wensel S. Severe asthma: From characteristics to phenotypes to endotypes. Clinical and Experimental Allergy. 2012;**42**:650-658. DOI: 10.1111/j.1365-2222.2011.03929.x

[3] Dahlen SE. Asthma phenotyping: Noninvasive biomarkers suitable for bedside science are the next step to implement precision medicine. Journal of Internal Medicine. 2016;**279**:205-207. DOI: 10.1111/joim.12466

[4] Boluyt N, Rottier BL, de Jongste JC, Riemsma R, Vrijlandt EJ, Brand PL. Assessment of controversial pediatric asthma management options using GRADE. Pediatrics. 2012;**130**: 658-668. DOI: 10.1542/peds.2011-3559

[5] Bel EH. Clinical phenotypes of asthma. Current Opinion in Pulmonary Medicine. 2004; **10**:44-50. PMID: 14749605

[6] Chung F, Adcock I. Asthma: Application of cell and molecular biology techniques to unravel causes and pathophysiological mechanisms. Methods in Molecular Medicine. 2000;**44**:1-29. DOI: 10.1385/1-59259-072-1:1

[7] Abraham B, Anto JME, Barreiro E, Bel EHD, Bonsignore G, Bousquet J, et al. The ENFUMOSA cross-sectional European multicentre study of the clinical phenotype of chronic severe asthma. The European Respiratory Journal. 2003;**22**:470-477. PMID: 14516137

[8] Kupczyk M, Dahlén B, Sterk PJ, Nizankowska-Mogilnicka E, Papi A, Bel EH, et al. Stability of phenotypes defined by physiological variables and biomarkers in adults with asthma. Allergy. 2014;**69**:1198-1204. DOI: 10.1111/all.12445

[9] Woodruff PG, Modrek B, Choy DF, Jia G, Abbas AR, Ellwanger A, et al. T helper type 2-driven inflammation defines major subphenotypes of asthma. American Journal of Respiratory and Critical Care Medicine. 2009;**180**:388-395. DOI: 10.1164/rccm.200903-0392OC

[10] Zhang Q, Illing R, Hui CK, Downey K, Carr D, Stearn M, et al. Bacteria in sputum of stable severe asthma and increased airway wall thickness. Respiratory Research. 2012;**18**: 13-45. DOI: 10.1186/1465-9921-13-35

[11] Almagro JC, Fransson J. Humanization of antibodies. Frontiers in Bioscience. 2008;**13**: 1619-1633. PMID: 17981654

[12] Ballow M. -ximab this and -zumab that! Has the magic bullet arrived in the new millennium of medicine and science? The Journal of Allergy and Clinical Immunology. 2005;**116**:738-743. DOI: 10.1016/j.jaci.2005.07.020

[13] Reichert JM, Rosensweig CJ, Faden LB, Dewitz MC. Monoclonal antibody successes in the clinic. Nature Biotechnology. 2005;**23**:1073-1078. DOI: 10.1038/nbt0905-1073

[14] Abbas A, Lichtman A. Cellular and Molecular Immunology. 8th ed. Elsevier; 2015. pp. 94-98

[15] Yamada T. Therapeutic monoclonal antibodies. The Keio Journal of Medicine. 2011;**60**:37-46. PMID: 21720199

[16] Torrego A, Pujols L, Picado C. Response to glucocorticoid treatment in asthma. The role of alpha and beta isoforms of the glucocorticoid receptor. Archivos de Bronconeumología. 2002;**38**:436-440. PMID: 12237016

[17] Peters-Golden M, Henderson WR. Leukotrienes. The New England Journal of Medicine. 2007;**357**:1841-1854. DOI: 10.1056/NEJMra071371

[18] Barnes PJ. Scientific rationale for inhaled combination therapy with long-acting beta2-agonist and corticosteroids. The European Respiratory Journal. 2002;**19**:182-191. PMID: 11843317

[19] Normansell R, Walker S, Milan SJ, Walters EH, Nair P. Omalizumab for asthma in adults and children. Cochrane Database of Systematic Reviews. 2014;**139**:28-35. DOI: 10.1002/14651858.CD003559.pub4

[20] Kopp MV. Omalizumab: Anti-IgE therapy in allergy. Current Allergy and Asthma Reports. 2011;**11**:101-106. DOI: 10.1007/s11882-010-0173-4

[21] Humbert M, Beasley R, Ayres J, Slavin R, Hebert J, Bousquet J, et al. Benefits of omalizumab as add-on therapy in patients with severe persistent asthma who are inadequately controlled despite best available therapy (GINA 2002 step 4 treatment): INNOVATE. Allergy. 2005;**60**:309-316. DOI: 10.1111/j.1398-9995.2004.00772.x

[22] Wills-Karp M. Interleukin 13 in asthma pathogenesis. Immunological Reviews. 2004; **202**:175-190. DOI: 10.1111/j.0105-2896.2004.00215.x

[23] Sokol CL, Barton GM, Farr AG, Medzhitov R. A mechanism for the initiation of allergen-induced T helper type 2 responses. Nature Immunology. 2008;**9**:310-318. DOI: 10.1038/ni1558

[24] Brusselle GG, Maes T, Bracke KR. Eosinophils in the spotlight: Eosinophilic airway inflammation in nonallergic asthma. Nature Medicine. 2013;**19**:977-979. DOI: 10.1038/nm.3300

[25] Boyman O, Kaegi C, Akdis M, Bavbek S, Bossios A, Chatzipetrou A, et al. EAACI IG Biologicals task force paper on the use of biologic agents in allergic disorders. Allergy. 2015;**70**:727-754

[26] Oboki K, Nakae S, Matsumoto K, Saito H. IL-33 and airway inflammation. Allergy, Asthma & Immunology Research. 2011;**3**(2):81-88

[27] Laviolette M, Gossage DL, Katial R, Leigh R, Olivenstein R, Katial R, et al. Effects of benralizumab on airway eosinophils in asthmatic patients with sputum eosinophilia. The Journal of Allergy and Clinical Immunology. 2013;**132**:1086-1096. DOI: 10.1016/j.jaci.2013.05.020

[28] Busse WW, Katial R, Gossage D, Sari S, Wang B, Kolbeck R, et al. Safety profile, pharmacokinetics, and biologic activity of MEDI-563, an anti-IL-5 receptor alpha antibody, in a phase I study of subjects with mild asthma. The Journal of Allergy and Clinical Immunology. 2010;**125**:1237-1244. DOI: 10.1016/j.jaci.2010.04.005

[29] Bleecker ER, FitzGerald JM, Chanez P, Papi A, Weinstein SF, Barker P, et al. Efficacy and safety of benralizumab for patients with severe asthma uncontrolled with high-dosage inhaled corticosteroids and long-acting β2-agonists (SIROCCO): A randomised, multicentre, placebo-controlled phase 3 trial. Lancet. 2016;**388**:2115-2127. DOI: 10.1016/S0140-6736(16)31324-1

[30] FitzGerald JM, Bleecker ER, Nair P, Korn S, Ohta K, Lommatzsch M, et al. Benralizumab, an anti-interleukin-5 receptor α monoclonal antibody, as add-on treatment for patients with severe, uncontrolled, eosinophilic asthma (CALIMA): A randomised, double-blind, placebo-controlled phase 3 trial. Lancet. 2016;**388**:2128-2141. DOI: 10.1016/S0140-6736(16)31322-8

[31] Wang FP, Liu T, Lan Z, Li SY, Mao H. Efficacy and safety of anti-interleukin-5 therapy in patients with asthma: A systematic review and meta-analysis. PLoS One. 2016; **11**:e0166833.32. DOI: 10.1371/journal.pone.0166833

[32] Nair P, Pizzichini MM, Kjarsgaard M, Inman MD, Efthimiadis A, Pizzichini E, et al. Mepolizumab for prednisone dependent asthma with sputum eosinophilia. The New England Journal of Medicine. 2009;**360**:985-993. DOI: 10.1056/NEJMoa0805435

[33] Flood-Page P, Swenson C, Faiferman I, Matthews J, Williams M, Brannick L, et al. A study to evaluate safety and efficacy of mepolizumab in patients with moderate persistent asthma. American Journal of Respiratory and Critical Care Medicine. 2007;**176**:1062-1071. DOI: 10.1164/rccm.200701-085OC

[34] Haldar P, Brightling CE, Hargadon B, Gupta S, Monteiro W, Sousa A, et al. Mepolizumab and exacerbations of refractory eosinophilic asthma. The New England Journal of Medicine. 2009;**360**:973-984. DOI: 10.1056/NEJMoa0808991

[35] Ortega HG, Liu MC, Pavord ID, Brusselle GG, FitzGerald JM, Chetta A, et al. Mepolizumab treatment in patients with severe eosinophilic asthma. The New England Journal of Medicine. 2014;**371**:1198-1207. DOI: 10.1056/NEJMoa1403290

[36] Brusselle G, Germinaro M, Weiss S, Zangrilli J. Reslizumab in patients with inadequately controlled late-onset asthma and elevated blood eosinophils. Pulmonary Pharmacology & Therapeutics. 2017;**43**:39-45. DOI: 10.1016/j.pupt.2017.01.011

[37] Li J, Lin C, Du J, Xiao B, Du C, Sun J, et al. The efficacy and safety of reslizumab for inadequately controlled asthma with elevated blood eosinophil counts: A systematic review and meta-analysis. The Journal of Asthma. 2017 Apr;**54**(3):300-307. DOI: 10.1080/02770903.2016.1212371

[38] Wensel S, Ford L, Pearlman D, Spector S, Sher L, Skobieranda F, et al. Dupilumab in persistent asthma with elevated eosinophil levels. The New England Journal of Medicine. 2013;**368**:2455-2466

[39] Wenzel S, Castro M, Corren J, Maspero J, Wang L, Zhang B, et al. Dupilumab efficacy and safety in adults with uncontrolled persistent asthma despite use of medium-to-high-dose inhaled corticosteroids plus a long-acting β2 agonist: A randomized double-blind placebo-controlled pivotal phase 2b dose-ranging trial. Lancet. 2016;**388**:31-44. DOI: 10.1016/S0140-6736(16)30307-5

[40] Wenzel S, Wilbraham D, Fuller R, Getz EB, Longphre M. Effect of an interleukin-4 variant on late phase asthmatic response to allergen challenge in asthmatic patients: Results of two phase 2a studies. Lancet. 2007;**370**:1422-1431. DOI: 10.1016/S0140-6736(07)61600-6

[41] Slager RE, Otulana BA, Hawkins GA, Yen YP, Peters SP, Wenzel SE, et al. IL-4 receptor polymorphisms predict reduction in asthma exacerbations during response to an anti-IL-4 receptor α antagonist. The Journal of Allergy and Clinical Immunology. 2012;**130**:516-522. DOI: 10.1016/j.jaci.2012.03.030

[42] Corren J, Lemanske RF, Hanania NA, Korenblat PE, Parsey MV, Arron JR, et al. Lebrikizumab treatment in adults with asthma. The New England Journal of Medicine. 2011;**365**:1088-1098. DOI: 10.1056/NEJMoa1106469

[43] Hanania NA, Noonan M, Corren J, Korenblat P, Zheng Y, Fischer SK, et al. Lebrikizumab in moderate-to-severe asthma: Pooled data from two randomised placebo-controlled studies. Thorax. 2015;**70**:748-756. DOI: 10.1136/thoraxjnl-2014-206719

[44] Piper E, Brightling C, Niven R, Oh C, Faggioni R, Poon K, et al. A phase II placebo-controlled study of Tralokinumab in moderate-to-severe asthma. The European Respiratory Journal. 2013;**41**:330-338. DOI: 10.1183/09031936.00223411

[45] Brightling CE, Chanez P, Leigh R, O'Byrne PM, Korn S, She D, et al. Efficacy and safety of Tralokinumab in patients with severe uncontrolled asthma: A randomised, double-blind, placebo-controlled, phase 2b trial. The Lancet Respiratory Medicine. 2015;**3**:692-701. DOI: 10.1016/S2213-2600(15)00197-6

[46] Gauvreau GM, O'Byrne PM, Boulet LP, Wang Y, Cockcroft D, Bigler J, et al. Effects of an anti-TSLP antibody on allergen induced asthmatic response. The New England Journal of Medicine. 2014;**370**:2102-2110. DOI: 10.1056/NEJMoa1402895

[47] Parker JM, Oh CK, LaForce C, Miller SD, Pearlman DS, Le C, et al. Safety profile and clinical activity of multiple subcutaneous doses of MEDI-58, a humanized anti-interleukin-9 monoclonal antibody, in two randomized phase 2a studies in subjects with asthma. BMC Pulmonary Medicine. 2011;**11**:14-23. DOI: 10.1186/1471-2466-11-14

[48] Krinner EM, Raum T, Petsch S, Bruckmaier S, Schuster I, Petersen L, et al. A human monoclonal IgG1 potently neutralizing the pro-inflammatory cytokine GM-CSF. Molecular Immunology. 2007;**44**:916-925. DOI: 10.1016/j.molimm.2006.03.020

[49] Ballantyne SJ, Barlow JL, Jolin HE, Nath P, Williams AS, Chung KF, et al. Blocking IL-25 prevents airway hyperresponsiveness in allergic asthma. The Journal of Allergy and Clinical Immunology. 2007;**120**:1324-1331. DOI: 10.1016/j.jaci.2007.07.051

[50] Liu X, Li M, Wu Y, Zhou Y, Zeng L, Huang T, et al. Anti-IL-33 antibody treatment inhibits airway inflammation in a murine model of allergic asthma. Biochemical and Biophysical Research Communications. 2009;**386**:181-185. DOI: 10.1016/j.bbrc.2009.06.008

12

The Asthma Obese Phenotype

Marina Ruxandra Oțelea and Agripina Rașcu

Abstract

Asthma is a very heterogeneous disease, with two major asthma phenotypes, the allergic and the late onset asthma, differentiated by the triggers, the cellular dominance, the Th1/Th2 inflammation pattern and the local and serological markers. As there were many overlapping biological markers between these two phenotypes, different types of tentative classification followed. A clinical one makes a difference between the predominant eosinophilic one (with better response to glucocorticoid) and the predominant neutrophilic one with more severe evolution and low rate of therapeutical improvement. Another approach was based on cluster analysis of asthma characteristics (onset, atopic status, and body mass index (BMI)), sensitivity to methacholine test, peak flow variability, bronchodilatation response, postbronchodilator level of FEV1, sputum eosinophil and neutrophil count, FeNO test, clinical symptom scores, treatment scheme to control symptoms, exacerbations, and severity. Emerging data suggest a distinct late onset obese-asthma phenotype, with a specific pathophysiology, comorbidities, and clinical evolution. This chapter reviews the main characteristics of this phenotype: the specific lung function impairment, the underlying inflammation, the adipokine profile, the comorbidities and the therapeutical approach. The mutual influence between obesity and asthma will be illustrated, whenever scientific data are available.

Keywords: asthma-obese phenotype, metabolic changes in asthma, inflammation in asthma, asthma biomarkers

1. Introduction

Obesity became in recent years a recurrence and one of the major concerns in asthma research. This chapter presents the relation between obesity and asthma, underlining the influences on pathological mechanisms, evolution, and treatment, in order to give an overview of the current knowledge about the asthma-obese phenotype (AOP). Inside the AOP, two distinct forms have been described: an early onset, atopic asthma with no gender differences in incidence and a late onset, non-atopic asthma predominantly in women [1]. We interpret the first as an atopic asthma aggravated by obesity and the second as a form of asthma favored by obesity. They have common characteristics related to the pathological consequences of obesity, the subject of our review.

2. Incidence

Worldwide, 15–20% of the population suffers from asthma [2, 3]. The prevalence have different slopes in different countries, with higher incidence in developing countries [4] and apparently constant rate in recent years or even with a tendency of reduction in current wheezing in countries with previous higher prevalence [2].

The trends of incidence of asthma and obesity are similar: a flat curve of high prevalence in developed countries and an increasing prevalence in less developed countries [2, 5]. However, the recently published analysis from the US national survey, comparing the 8.5% population attributable fraction for overweight/obesity between 1988 and 1994 with the 11.9% one, in 2011–2014, found this increase statistically non-significant [6]. Studies from developing countries, in prospective cohorts, confirmed the parallel increase in incidence of obesity and asthma, [7], particularly in obese women [8].

The AOP could be, in fact, related not to obesity but to the metabolic syndrome. A Norway study confirmed, but another large longitudinal study with 25 years of follow-up contradicted this assumption and found that independent factors to the metabolic syndrome play significant roles in the association of asthma with obesity [9]. Waist circumference was negatively associated with eosinophilia [10] and gave an odds ratio (OR) = 1.46 for asthma in females [11]. The relation between asthma and metabolic syndrome seems to be reciprocal, as asthma increases the risk for metabolic syndrome [12] and for obesity [13].

High BMI is also associated with the severity of asthma, particularly in women [14], with a reduced FEV1 %, a higher readmission rate and longer hospitalization stay [15]. In a large cross-sectional Israeli study, obesity was associated with mild and moderate to severe asthma in male, and to moderate to severe asthma in females [16]. Differences in severity between obese and non-obese were maintained after adjustment for demographics, smoking status, medication or gastroesophageal reflux [17].

Genomic studies also support this association. A twin-based research concluded that 8% of the genetic component of the obesity is shared with asthma [18]. A large case control sample of population with European origin revealed a protection for asthma-obesity co-occurrence with the 16p11.2 inversion [19]. Several gene polymorphisms (TNF-α, -β or leptin receptors) with interrelated physiopathological mechanisms for the AOP seem to be involved in risk and/or the therapeutical response [20–23].

3. Pathogenic pathways

Impressive research data have been accumulated to explain the relationship between obesity and asthma. Among them, two pathogenic processes draw special attention: the lung function impairment and the specific airways inflammation.

3.1. Lung function impairment

3.1.1. Structural changes

In normal obese, forced vital capacity (FVC) is smaller than slow vital capacity (SVC), and this points to the possibility of even underdiagnosis obstruction, when using FEV1/FVC data [24]. Reduced SVC and total lung capacity (TLC), increased inspiratory reserve volume, decreased expiratory reserve volume (ERV) and maximal voluntary ventilation volume (MVV) was found in severe obesity [25]. The reduction in FVC%, FEV1%, MVV% was parallel with the BMI increase [26]. The reduction in the functional residual capacity (FRC) was more pronounced than of the TLC until BMI exceeded 35 kg/m^2, after which the decrease was proportionate [27]. While VC and TLC are markers of restriction, the MVV integrates the endurance and strength of the respiratory muscles with the airway diameter and resistance and is interpreted as an obstructive dysfunction. Another argument against a pure restrictive pattern in obesity is that the FRC reduction is due to the ERV reduction, with normal or even increased RV and reflects a lower airways caliber [28]. The volume of FRC is the expression of the equilibrium between the inward elastic recoil of the lung and outward elastic recoil of the chest wall. Obesity, particularly the abdominal one, reduces the expansion of the diaphragm and of the excursions of the thoracic cage, limiting the elastic recoil of the lung. Ventilation occurs at lower lung volumes, the transpulmonary pressure is lower. These changes affect the retractive forces of the lung parenchyma and the airways caliber and unload the airway smooth muscle (ASM); as consequence, the ASM shortens more in response to external stimuli. Even more, due to the decreased expansion of the airways, actin and myosin attach closer and are more difficult to detach during relaxation. A confirmation of these mechanisms is obtaining no difference in the fall of FEV1 after methacholine test with or without a previous avoidance of deep inspiration in nonasthmatic obese (NAO) persons [29].

3.1.2. Metabolic changes

Obesity increases the respiratory demand, with greater energy expenditure for breathing. Obesity-related inflammatory cytokines (such as TNF-α or leptin) and hormones (insulin) increase the ASM contractility. The insulin growth factor 1 stimulates the proliferation of the ASM. Insulin raises the expression of β1-containing laminins, promoting contractility [30].

Successful weight loss programs reverse the lung function changes and have an important role in asthma management in these patients. Weight loss reduces airway resistance, airways obstruction, improves peak expiratory flow (PEF) variability, and increases FRC and ERV [31].

Weight loss in obese asthmatics (OA) with high IgE and dominant Th2 inflammation improved the resting respiratory system mechanics, assessed by oscillometry, but had no effect on the sensitivity of air closure during the methacholine test, reflected by FVC % reduction. Certain differences in response, according to the underlying inflammation of the AOP subtypes, have been noticed [32] serving as argument that weight loss cumulates the benefit of the structural, the metabolic, and of the inflammatory improvement in OA.

3.2. Influences of the obesity inflammation pattern on asthma

Obesity generates a low-grade inflammation, switches blood monocytes and tissue macrophages to the M1 activation pathway, and impairs the ratio between regulatory T-lymphocytes (Treg) and Th17. Changes from the lean to obese pattern involve the switch of macrophages from M2 to M1 domination, switch from Th2 to Th1 cells, and switch from the Treg cells and NKT to B cells, mast cells and neutrophils. Together with the adipokine profile modification, a pro-inflammatory pattern develops (**Figure 1**).

3.2.1. Polarization of the macrophages

Macrophages are polarized to the M1 state by interferon-γ and by inducers of TNF-α, such as lipopolysaccharides (LPS). M1 macrophages upregulate pro-inflammatory cytokines as TNF-α, interleukin IL-1β, IL-6, IL-12, IL-15, and IL-23 and oxidative stress.

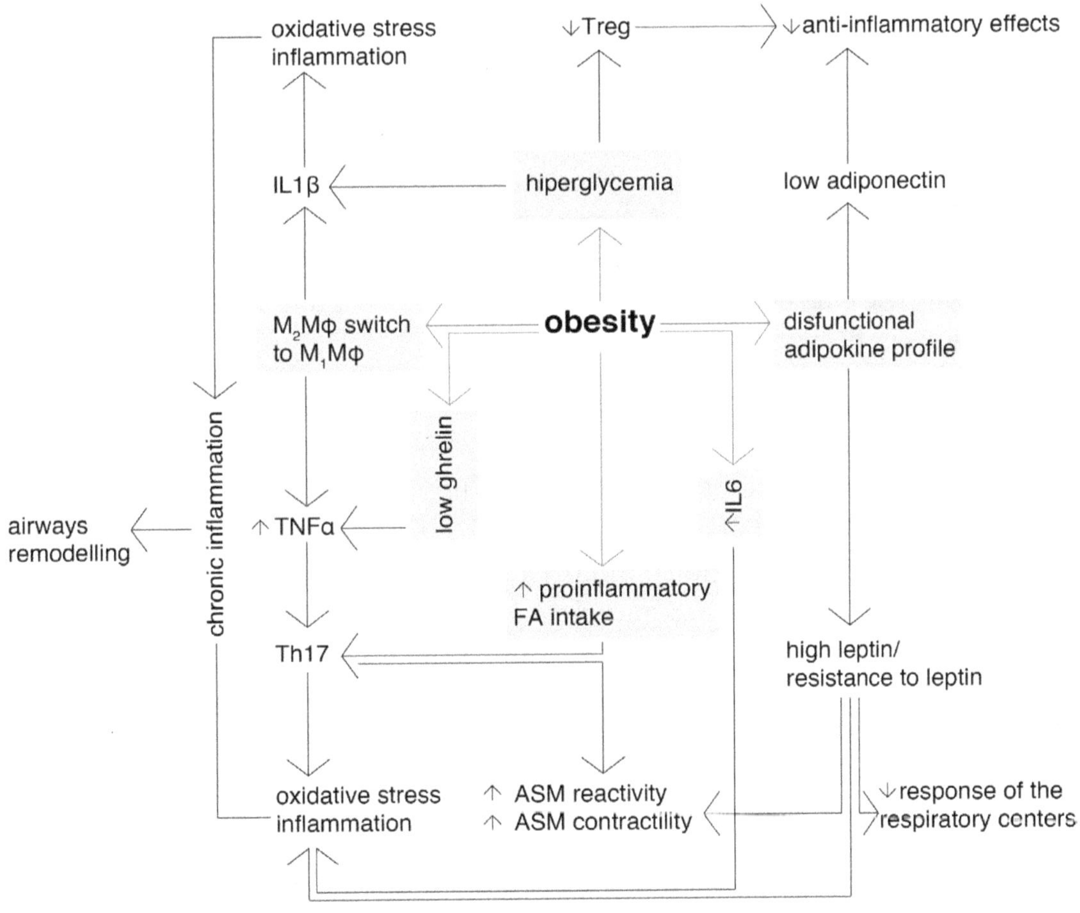

Figure 1. Obesity-related inflammation in asthma. ASM = airway smooth muscle; FA = fatty acids; IL1β = interleukin 1β, IL6 = interleukin 6; M1Mϕ = M1 macrophage; M2Mϕ = M2 macrophage; Th17 = T helper 17 cells; TNFα = tumor necrosis factor α; Treg = regulatory T cells.

Lung macrophages are a heterogeneous population divided into alveolar and interstitial macrophages. In non-allergic asthma, M1 macrophages are increased and pathogenic, while in allergic forms, they seem to be protective. Due to their defense capacity against pathogens, they have a role in preventing the asthma exacerbation. The most extensively investigated negative effects of the M1 polarization specific cytokine signature are TNF-α and IL-1β in asthma. Exogenous administration of recombinant TNF-α shifts to the left the curve of responsiveness to methacholine in normal subjects [33]. In asthma patients, high levels of TNF-α in bronchoalveolar lavage or bronchial biopsies are associated with severity [34]. How TNF-α induces airways hypersensitivity is not completely understood, but experimental research showed that TNF-α increases ASM contractility by intracellular calcium increase. The intimate process involves a variety of G-protein coupled agonists (methacholine, histamine and serotonine). After binding to TNF receptor 2, TNF-α increases the Th17 differentiation and induces vascular modifications through endothelin and neurotrophic tyrosine kinase receptor type 2. Of interest for obesity, a condition associated with low ghrelin levels is that the raise of TNF-α level in the bronchoalveolar lavage after ovalbumin challenge is attenuated by this orexigenic factor [35].

The IL-1β is a pro-inflammatory cytokine with special interest for bronchoconstriction, particularly if primed by IL-5. IL-1β is a result of activation of numerous lung cells, including lymphocytes, macrophages, mastocytes and even ASM. IL-1β could be the link between toll-like receptors (TLR) and nucleotide-binding oligomerization domain-like receptors (NLR), the NLRP3 inflammasome and the activation of the TH17 cells, as both TLR and NLR that sense the external signals promote IL-1β secretion [36]. From macrophages cytoplasm, IL-1 is secreted through lipid pores requiring the presence of gasdermin D (GSDMD), a protein identified from genomic-wide studies as a possible asthma marker [37]. Experimental data showed that GSDMD expression regulates cell growth of ASM and promotes fibrosis with remodeling of airways [38]. Cellular stress-related inflammation, with high extracellular release of adenosine triphosphate (ATP), uric acid crystals, and cholesterol also involve the IL-1β signal [39]. The expression of IL-1β is upregulated by prolonged hyperglycemic state [40], with possible impact on AOP.

3.2.2. The predominant Th1/Th17 activation

The level of Th17 increases in obese, if a certain threshold of the BMI is achieved, in absence of an acute or chronic inflammation [41]. An inhibition effect on adipogenesis in mesenchymal cells and on the adipocyte differentiation raised the hypothesis that IL-17 could be a regulatory cytokine of obesity itself, providing a negative feedback on the adipose tissue expansion [42]. Several mechanisms have been proposed to explain how Th17 increases in obesity. The higher metabolic activity related to nutrients intake raises the ATP level and the release of ATP molecules to the extracellular space; ATP binds to P2X7, a purinergic receptor, capable of driving Th17 responses during inflammation and secretion of pro-inflammatory cytokines [43]. Unhealthy diet, with high pro-inflammatory, long chain, saturated free fatty acid (FFA), and low anti-inflammatory ω3- polyunsaturated fatty acids (PUFAs) and monounsaturated fatty acids (MUFA) activates the TLR in adipocytes and macrophages, and the Th1/Th17 pathways in dendritic cells [44]. Micronutrient deficiencies, such as low levels of vitamin D, are also frequent in obese persons. The enhanced infection susceptibility is due to the decreased levels of cathelicidin in the primary defense cells, aggravating the clinical evolution.

In obesity, the adipocytes have a significant contribution to the circulating IL-6, promoting the differentiation of TH17 and naive CD4 T-cells. Leptin, another cytokine of the IL-6 family, is also increased, with many pathological implications for asthma. Among these, leptin modulates Th17 response by conditioning the signal transducer and activator of transcription 3 (STAT3) expression and phosphorylation in CD4 cells [45]. Th1 and Th17 differentiation require mammalian Target of Rapamycin 1 (mTORC1) signals [46], which are known to be activated by growth factors, amino acids or insulin, all being raised at obesity.

Through IL-17 secretion, Th17 cells recruit and activate neutrophils to produce pro-inflammatory cytokines (IL-6, IL-8) [41], chemokines, and adhesion molecules. IL-17 upregulates IL-8 secretion in airway epithelial cells and initiates airway remodeling, increasing the levels of fibroblast-derived inflammatory mediators, such as the α-chemokines, IL-8, and growth-related oncogene-α [41]. Pathogenic Th17 cells express IL-1R1, a type of IL-1β receptor, with bronchoconstriction effect [47].

Epigenetic markers, such as promoter methylation of transcription factors associated with increased Th1 differentiation, were found in OA preadolescent compared to non obese asthmatic patients (NOA) [48].

3.2.3. Reduction of Treg

Tregs have a significant role in suppression of allergy and asthma, as they are sources of anti-inflammatory cytokines (IL-10, TGFβ1 and IL-35) and have suppressor function on a variety of immune cells (B cells, NK cells, CD4+, CD8+) and dendritic cells. Tregs are even able to kill effector lymphocytes in a perforin-dependent manner. The number of studies related to the Treg number and function in asthma is increasing but are far from being conclusive: in allergic inflammation, Tregs are generally low and less able to control the inflammation process. An increased number of Tregs were found in more severe asthma, an effect that could be also due to the inhaled corticoids [49].

Concerning AOP, a reduction of Treg is present in insulin resistance OA [50]. Particularly with high amount of abdominal fat, Treg is reduced, contributing to the low-grade inflammation and insulin resistance development. Leptin has similar inhibitory effect on Treg [51]. Treg expresses the insulin receptor, and hyperinsulinemia affects their IL-10 production and the suppressor functionality [52]. As insulin levels are frequently elevated in obese subjects, the insulin effect on Treg could be a part of the explanation of the severity of asthma of the AOP.

3.2.4. The adipokine profile

The inflammation pattern in obesity is closely related to the adipokine profile. A meta-analysis of 13 studies with 3642 patients concluded that the high leptin and low adiponectin are associated with the diagnosis of asthma [53].

The leptin receptor is constitutively expressed in epithelial lung cells but also on immune cells. **Leptin** directly stimulates respiratory centers, increases frequency, minute and tidal volume. These positive effects on the respiratory function are lost in obesity, a state of leptin resistance, but high dose of leptin administered to obese mice was able to restore the breathing pattern and the arterial CO_2 [54].

Compared to obese non-asthmatic, leptin levels are increased in OA [55]. The difference is higher in women [56] and in patients with lung neutrophilia [57]. High leptin level upregulates the expression of inflammatory proteins, such as cPLA2-α [58] or phospholipase D1 [59], raises leukotrienes (LT) production [60] and bronchial responsiveness. Again, the effect was manifest particularly in obese women [61]. LT synthesis in neutrophils depends on circulatory arachidonic acid, on nuclear localization of the 5-lipooxigenase [62], and on the level of extracellular signal regulated kinases (ERK) activity, significantly influenced by androgens. This might contribute to the gender differences in AOP.

Attenuation of the constitutive muscarinic activation of the ASM cells via the central nervous system (a normal dilatator effect and leptin) has been proposed as part of leptin resistance [63]. Leptin resistance seems to be selective, as the pro-inflammatory effects are maintained in obesity. Leptin effects on airway remodeling could be related to reduction in α1-antitripsin expression, enhanced intercellular adhesion molecule 1 (ICAM-1) expression and increase in the CCL11, G-CSF, VEGF, and IL-6 production [64].

The circadian secretion of leptin is the highest at midnight; in obese subjects, the basal and the evening increase is higher than in lean subjects [65]. This could be an influencer of the nocturnal asthma attacks and of the overall severity of asthma.

In contrast with leptin increase, plasma adiponectin is decreased in asthma [66], independent of the BMI [67]. The adiponectin is correlated with the FEV1 decline, and with the high serum and sputum IgE [68]. Adiponectin is able to polarize the macrophages to an M2 state [69], switches the balance by inhibition of pro-inflammatory cytokines (TNFα), stimulates the anti-inflammatory ones (IL10), diminishes Nf-Kb activation, and negatively correlates with protein C and IL6. Despite experimental data to confirm these actions, adiponectin's role in predicting asthma severity remains controversial.

Adiponectin circulates as trimer (the low molecular weight form) or hexamers (the high molecular weight form), and the inconsistent findings of these studies could be explained by different serum adiponectin components that were measured, as only high low-molecular-weight isoform was strongly associated with the asthma risk and lung function decrease [70].

4. Clinical and therapeutic particularities of OA

4.1. Biomarkers

The specific physiopathology of the AOP was translated in different attempts to define biomarkers. Particular biomarkers or different cut points for predicting airway inflammation were proposed. Classification and relevant examples of proposed biomarkers are summarized in **Table 1**. Most of these studies were not reproduced on larger scales, and currently there are no guidelines on their clinical utilization.

Category	Biological sample	Type	Comments
Inflammatory biomarkers	Sputum	High MMP1, MMP2, and MMP8	Study design primarily for asthma severity: these MMP not found in other clusters [71]
		IL-5	Comparison between OA and LA inside the group of severe asthma [72]
		14 differentially expressed genes encoding proteins related to the cell cycle and growth factor regulating pathways (MAPK1, E2F1, and SPRY2) and to the interferon signaling pathway (OASL, OAS3 and TRIM14)	Study design for cluster identification; the results selected refer to the comparison between late onset asthma, severe, high proportion of atopic, nonsmokers and obese female asthmatics, high frequency of exacerbations despite near normal lung function, 73.6% atopy. [73]
		Gene expression of calcium signal transmission (*S100P, S100A16*), lymphocyte differentiation (*MAL*), and mucin (*MUC1*) increase	Comparison of diet (high fat meal)-induced metabolism in asthma and healthy controls. No specific analysis related to BMI, but mean BMI was in the obesity range in asthma and in overweight range in controls [74]
	Exhaled breath condensate	Increase in glucose, n-valerate, acetoin, isovalerate, and 1,2-propanediol levels and a decrease in formate, ethanol, methanol, acetone, propionate, acetate, lactate, and saturated fatty acid levels	Relatively small cross-sectional study, well designed to differentiate AOP from obese-non asthma and lean-asthma, strong statistical power of correlation [75]
	Bronchial submucosa	Increased eosinophil count	In a severe asthma population, eosinophil number in submucosa correlated with BMI [72]
	Bronchial submucosa	No increase in eosinophil count	In mild to moderate OA, eosinophil number in submucosa not different from obese without asthma [76]
	Blood	Low periostin l	Study design primarily for asthma severity: low levels found also in other clusters, no difference between OAP and other cluster presented [71]
	Blood	CCL17, IL-4, IL-13	Cross-sectional study. Comparison of lean asthma and obese asthma [77]
	Expired air	FeNO test	Large cross-sectional study; low FeNO associated with adiposity indicators; in high FeNO group, adiposity indicators associated with worse asthma severity or control [78]
Adipokine profile	Blood	Leptin	Cross-sectional study, comparison to lean asthma AO, leptin mediates asthma control [77]

Category	Biological sample	Type	Comments
	Blood	Adiponectin	Review of the controversial epidemiological results in human studies mainly to heterogeneity of the design of these studies [79]
	Blood	Resistin	Post-weight management intervention Δ resistin negatively associated to Δ FRC and Δ RV [80]
Functional test (bronchial reactivity)		Challenge test with ozone	Comparison between obese and non-obese; post-exposure decrease of FVC in obese, similar bronchial reactivity and IL-6 increase [81]
		Challenge test with mannitol	Airway hyper-responsiveness to mannitol in obese non-asthmatic without asthma comparative to non-obese subjects [82]

Table 1. Asthma-obese phenotype biomarkers.

4.2. Comorbidities

The clinical manifestations and the treatment response appear to be influenced by comorbidities. They can be summarized as allergic (rhinitis, eczema), smoking-related, psychogenic (hyperventilation, depression, and anxiety disorders), metabolic syndrome, gastroesophageal reflux disease and obstructive sleep apnea [83]. Comorbidities become significant when there is reciprocal impact. As a disease is the expression of a certain number of dysregulated functional mechanisms, comorbidities, by cumulating more abnormalities, will always have a potential negative impact. Comorbidities might share co-determination factors or potentiate mechanisms for the related comorbidity. The asthma-obesity relation suits very well in these last categories.

In terms of co-determination factors, the chronic asthma inflammation is influenced by the metabolic inflammation, as previously described. Certain comorbidities, such as the gastroesophageal reflux disease (GERD) and obstructive sleep apnea (OSA) have an independent high prevalence in asthma and in obesity but aggravate each other when they coexist.

4.2.1. Gastroesophageal reflux disease

To evaluate prevalence, different definitions of Gastroesophageal reflux disease (GERD) are used in the epidemiological studies: the presence of the reflux symptoms, the pH measurement, the endoscopic findings of the gastroesophageal mucosal disease or presence of the hiatal hernia. Despite the variation in methodology, the incidence was significantly higher than in the non-asthmatic population no matter what criteria were used. On the obesity side, a meta-analysis showed that the risk for GERD progressively increases with the increase in BMI

[84]. The asthma-GERD relation is bilateral. GERD is the cause for the abnormal acid reflux that leads to microaspiration into the airways, initiating reflex cough and bronchoconstriction via vago-vagal reflexes. Asthma bronchoconstriction triggers acid reflux, as happens in some patients during the methacholine test. Theophylline increases gastric acid secretion and lowers low esophagus sphincter tone [85]. Both obesity and asthma increase the transdiaphragmatic and intragastric pressures and favor hiatal hernia.

Despite common agreement that GERD was associated with more severe asthma symptoms, apparently, no association between GERD and the severity of asthma was found in a subpopulation of OA [86]. This emphasizes the need for dedicated studies to this particular phenotype.

Indirect arguments that asthma control might have positive influence on GERD are the presence of the silent reflux in asthma patients and the relative risk of development of GERD [87], but there are no published data to confirm this hypothesis.

GERD influences also obesity, by changing type and frequency of meals. Reduction in weight has favorable effects on GERD-related symptoms.

Due to the presence of the increased cholinergic tone in both asthma and GERD, the use of anticholinergic medication might be of interest.

4.2.2. *Obstructive sleep apnea*

Obstructive sleep apnea (OSA) has a higher prevalence in men, while OA is more prevalent in women. Due to the high association rate between OSA and asthma [86] and the worse asthma control in the presence of OSA, an overlap asthma-OSA syndrome was proposed [88]. As with the GERD, asthma increases the risk of the new-onset OSA [89]. Obesity is the major risk factor for OSA, but OSA also leads to obesity: impaired sleep architecture changes leptin signal with a reduction in satiety along with craving for high energy foods [90], modifies transcriptional networks in visceral fat, and reduces secretion of growth hormone. The excessive daytime sleepiness reduces physical activity, increases the proportion of the fat mass compared to the free fat mass and makes weight loss programs more difficult to succeed.

OSA has negative impact on asthma. During apnea episodes, the upper way vibration and suction collapse, activate vagal tone, and induce reflex bronchoconstriction. The more negative intrathoracic pressure developed during apnea increases the pulmonary capillary volume. These pathological processes trigger asthma attacks. Repeated mechanical trauma is associated with upper and lower airway inflammation [91]. OSA aggravates nocturnal asthma, lowers the quality of life, and leads to more frequent exacerbations.

Asthma has negative effects on OSA. In asthma patients, OSA is more severe, with lower apnea-hypopnea index (AHI). Sleep efficiency and arousal index were higher in severe asthma compared to moderate asthma, but apparently no correlation have been found between OSA severity and measures of the asthma severity evaluated by FEV1 or with the asthma quality of life score [92]. High dose, long-term corticosteroid treatment, particularly in poorly controlled asthma could be a contributing factor to obesity and OSA [93].

Nocturnal GERD links asthma, GERD, and OSA under a common aggravating factor. The increase of the respiratory effort exacerbates asthma and OSA symptoms and is associated with higher AHI and inflammation in the exhaled breath condensate [94].

4.2.3. Metabolic syndrome-related comorbidities

Increased incidence of type 2 diabetes and cardiovascular events (hypertension, ischemic heart disease, cerebrovascular disease) is also expected to happen, as directly influenced by obesity. In a very large adult study, elevated waist circumference and triglyceride (TG) and low high-density lipoprotein (HDL) were significantly associated with wheezing [95]. In this respect, statins represent a potential treatment modality in severe asthma; their anti-inflammatory effects and the enhancement of the corticosteroid sensitivity make them good candidates for AO treatment, particularly in cases with metabolic syndrome [96].

4.3. Therapeutical challenges

Current guidelines do not differentiate pharmacotherapy between OA and NOA, but studies have confirmed that AO is more severe and more difficult to control, with the regular medication [83, 97].

AOP benefits from **lifestyle** changes: weight reduction is a priority goal, but all other general asthma interventions should be addressed: smoking cessation, allergen exposure avoidance, occupational risk assessment, and so on. Diet and/or bariatric surgery is correlated with reduction of exacerbations and improvements in the lung function, clinical manifestations, and quality of life [98, 99]. Successful interventions increase in efficacy of the inhaled corticosteroids (ICS) after smoking cessation [100] and after losing weight [98].

Treatment of **comorbidities** related to overweight directly impacting asthma. Positive effects on asthma control have been reported from continuous positive airway pressure (CPAP) therapy of OSA [92]. There is also a benefit on the pulmonary function in OA with diabetes treated with dipeptydil-peptidase4 inhibitors related to the correction of the oxidative/antioxidative imbalances [101].

Proton pomp inhibitors and histamine H2 receptor improve GERD-related symptoms and quality of life but does not influence asthma control [102]. However, improvement of symptoms in severe, selected cases was obtained from different surgical procedures [103, 104]. However, the common high cholinergic tone in GERD and asthma raised the hypothesis that anticholinergic therapy could be a common solution [104]. A Cochrane systematic review provided some evidence that long-acting muscarinic antagonists added to ICS show some benefits on FEV1 [105], but prospective studies should confirm if there is also benefit in the AOP, and if this effect is higher in asthma-GERD association. The anti-inflammatory effect of statins in asthma is not consistent across studies [106]. Whether their effect on asthma evolution is increased in those OA with dyslipidemia remains to be demonstrated.

If standard step-increase asthma medication is not efficient, specific endotype treatment (precision medicine approach) would be desirable.

OA is associated with some specific inflammatory pathways activation, one of which is 5-lipoxygenase pathway inflammation; leukotriene antagonists have similar efficacy with ICS in the presence of obesity [107]. Some biological therapies for severe forms of asthma were proven beneficial also in OA. For example, in OA patients with raised eosinophils and high airways reversibility, Mepolizumab was more efficient in the reduction of exacerbations [108]. Nevertheless, the ones that targeted commonly upregulated pathways were not successful. For example, a 12 weeks treatment with Brodalumab (a human anti-IL-17 receptor) had no clinically meaningful effects [109]. Golimumab, an anti-THF-α humanized antibody, provided some improvements, but limited use due to the risks associated with this therapy: infections, congestive heart failure, malignancies, and demyelinating disorders [110]. However, in a small selected group of overweight and obese severe asthma patients this treatment reduced the oral steroid dose and hospitalizations [111].

5. Conclusions

To conclude, the AOP is supported by epidemiological, pathophysiological, and clinical data. There are still many uncertainties about the OAP and even more about the two subtypes, described until now only from the epidemiological perspective; further research is needed to elucidate common and specific mechanisms and to improve our knowledge about the specific biomarkers and the therapeutical approaches for the subtypes of AOP.

Author details

Marina Ruxandra Oțelea[1*] and Agripina Rașcu[1,2]

*Address all correspondence to: marina.otelea@umfcd.ro

1 University of Medicine and Pharmacy "Carol Davila", Bucharest, Romania

2 Colentina Clinical Hospital, Occupational Medicine Department, Bucharest, Romania

References

[1] Ather JL, Poynter ME, Dixon AE. Immunological characteristics and management considerations in obese patients with asthma. Expert Review of Clinical Immunology. 2015;**11**:793-803

[2] Asher MI, Montefort S, Björkstén B, et al. Worldwide time trends in the prevalence of symptoms of asthma, allergic rhinoconjunctivitis, and eczema in childhood: ISAAC phases one and three repeat multicountry cross-sectional surveys. Lancet. 2006;**368**(9537):733-743

[3] Gershon AS, Wang C, Guan J, To T. Burden of comorbidity in individuals with asthma. Thorax. 2010;**65**:612-618

[4] Huang C, Liu W, Hu Y, et al. Updated prevalences of asthma, allergy, and airway symptoms, and a systematic review of trends over time for childhood asthma in shanghai, China. PLoS One. 2015;**10**:e0121577

[5] Abarca-Gómez L et al. Worldwide trends in body-mass index, underweight, overweight, and obesity from 1975 to 2016: A pooled analysis of 2416 population-based measurement studies in 128·9 million children, adolescents, and adults. The Lancet. 2017, pii: S0140-6736;(17):32129-32123

[6] Akinbami LJ, Rossen LM, Fakhouri THI, Fryar CD. Asthma prevalence trends by weight status among US children aged 2-19 years. Pediatric Obesity. 2017:1988-2014

[7] Forno E, Acosta-Pérez E, Brehm JM, et al. Obesity and adiposity indicators, asthma, and atopy in Puerto Rican children. The Journal of Allergy and Clinical Immunology. 2014;**133**:1308-1314

[8] Mishra V. Effect of obesity and asthma among adult Indian women. International Journal of Obesity and Related Metabolic Disorders. 2004;**28**:1048-1058

[9] Assad N, Qualls C, Smith LJ, et al. Body mass index is a stronger predictor than the metabolic syndrome for future asthma in women. The longitudinal CARDIA study. American Journal of Respiratory and Critical Care Medicine. 2013;**188**:319-326

[10] Lessard A, Turkotte H, Cornier Y, Boulet LP. Obesity and asthma. A specific phenotype? Chest. 2008;**134**:317-323

[11] Brumpton B, Langhammer A, Romundstad P, et al. General and abdominal obesity and incident asthma in adults: The HUNT study. The European Respiratory Journal. 2013;**41**:323-329

[12] Del-Rio-Navarro BE, Castro-Rodriguez JA, Garibay Nieto N, et al. Higher metabolic syndrome in obese asthmatic compared to obese nonasthmatic adolescent males. The Journal of Asthma. 2010;**47**:501-506

[13] Renosto LC, Acatauassu C, Andrade I, et al. Growth velocity and weight gain in prepubertal asthmatic children. Revista da Associação Médica Brasileira. 2017;**63**:236-241

[14] The ENFUMOSA Study Group. The ENFUMOSA cross-sectional European multicentre study of the clinical phenotype of chronic severe asthma. The European Respiratory Journal. 2003;**22**:470-477

[15] Okubo Y, Michihata N, Yoshida K, et al. Impact of pediatric obesity on acute asthma exacerbation in Japan. Pediatric Allergy and Immunology. 2017;**00**:1-5

[16] Machluf Y, Farkash R, Fink D, Chaiter Y. Asthma severity and heterogeneity: Insights from prevalence trends and associated demographic variables and anthropometric indices among Israeli adolescents. The Journal of Asthma. 2017;**5**:1-11

[17] Schatz DM, Magid DJ, Camargo CA. The relationship between obesity and asthma severity and control in adults. The Journal of Allergy and Clinical Immunology. 2008;**122**:507-511

[18] Hallstrand TS, Fischer ME, Wurfel MM, Afari N, Buchwald D, Goldberg J. Genetic pleiotropy between asthma and obesity in a community-based sample of twins. The Journal of Allergy and Clinical Immunology. 2005;**116**:1235-1241

[19] González JR, Cáceres A, Esko T, et al. A common 16p11.2 inversion underlies the joint susceptibility to asthma and obesity. American Journal of Human Genetics. 2014;**94**:361-372

[20] Yang Y-H, Liu Y-Q, Zhang L, et al. Genetic polymorphisms of the TNF-α-308G/a are associated with metabolic syndrome in asthmatic patients from Hebei province, China. International Journal of Clinical and Experimental Pathology. 2015;**8**:13739-13746

[21] Rosmond R. Association studies of genetic polymorphisms in central obesity: A critical review. International Journal of Obesity. 2003;**27**:1141-1151

[22] Kaya Z, Caglayan S, Akkiprik M, et al. Impact of glucocorticoid receptor gene (NR3C1) polymorphisms in Turkish patients with metabolic syndrome. Journal of Endocrinological Investigation. 2016;**39**:557-566

[23] Ishiyama-Shigemoto S, Yamada K, Yuan X, et al. Association of polymorphisms in the beta2-adrenergic receptor gene with obesity, hypertriglyceridaemia, and diabetes mellitus. Diabetologia. 1999;**42**:98e101

[24] Fortis S, Corazalla E, Wang Q, Kim HJ. The difference between slow and forced vital capacity increases with increasing body mass index: A paradoxical difference in low and normal body mass indices. Respiratory Care. 2015;**60**:113-118

[25] Costa D, Barbalho MC, Miguel GPS, Forti EMP, Azevedo JLMC. The impact of obesity on pulmonary function in adult women. Clinics. 2008;**63**:719-724

[26] Ladosky W, Botelho MA, Albuquerque JP Jr. Chest mechanics in morbidly obese non-hypoventilated patients. Respiratory Medicine. 2001;**95**:281-286

[27] Jones RL, Nzekwu MMU. The effects of body mass index on lung volumes. Chest. 2006;**130**:827-833

[28] King GG, Brown NJ, Diba C, et al. The effects of body weight on airway caliber. The European Respiratory Journal. 2005;**25**:896-901

[29] Boulet LP, Turcotte H, Boulet G, Simard B, Robichaud P. Deep inspiration avoidance and airway response to methacholine: Influence of body mass index. Canadian Respiratory Journal. 2005;**12**:371-376

[30] Dekkers BGJ, Schaafsma D, Tran T, Zaagsma J, Meurs H. Insulin- induced laminin expression promotes a hypercontractile airway smooth muscle phenotype. American Journal of Respiratory Cell and Molecular Biology. 2009;**41**:494-504

[31] Hakala K, Stenius-Aarniala B, Sovijarvi A. Effects of weight loss on peak flow variability, airways obstruction, and lung volumes in obese patients with asthma. Chest. 2000;**118**:1315-1321

[32] Chapman DG, Irvin CG, Kaminsky DA, et al. Influence of distinct asthma phenotypes on lung function following weight loss in the obese. Respirology. 2014;**19**:1170-1177

[33] Thomas PS, Yates DH, Barnes PJ. Tumor necrosis factor-alpha increases airway responsiveness and sputum neutrophilia in normal human subjects. American Journal of Respiratory and Critical Care Medicine. 1995;**152**:76-80

[34] Yang T, Li Y, Lyu Z, et al. Characteristics of proinflammatory cytokines and chemokines in airways of asthmatics: Relationships with disease severity and infiltration of inflammatory cells. Chinese Medical Journal. 2017;**130**:2033-2204

[35] Fu T, Wang L, Zeng Q, Zhang Y, Sheng B, Han L. Ghrelin ameliorates asthma by inhibiting endoplasmic reticulum stress. The American Journal of the Medical Sciences. 2017;**354**:617-625

[36] Besnard AG, Togbe D, Couillin I, et al. Inflammasome–IL-1–Th17 response in allergic lung inflammation. Journal of Molecular Cell Biology. 2012;**4**:3-10

[37] Moffatt MF, Gut IG, Demenais F, et al. A large-scale, consortium-based genomewide association study of asthma. The New England Journal of Medicine. 2010;**363**:1211-1221

[38] Das S, Miller M, Beppu AK, et al. GSDMB induces an asthma phenotype characterized by increased airway responsiveness and remodeling without lung inflammation. Proceedings of the National Academy of Sciences of the United States of America. 2016;**113**:13132-13137

[39] Gasse P, Riteau N, Charron S, et al. Uric acid is a danger signal activating NALP3 inflammasome in lung injury inflammation and fibrosis. American Journal of Respiratory and Critical Care Medicine. 2009;**179**:903-913

[40] Schroder K, Zhou R, Tschopp J. The NLRP3 inflammasome: A sensor for metabolic danger? Science. 2010:296-300

[41] Schindler TI, Wagner J-J, Goedicke-Fritz S, et al. TH17 cell frequency in peripheral blood is elevated in overweight children without chronic inflammatory diseases. Frontiers in Immunology. 2017;**8**:1543

[42] Ahmed M, Gaffen SL. IL-17 in obesity and adipogenesis. Cytokine & Growth Factor Reviews. 2010;**21**(6):449-453

[43] Pandolfi JB, Ferraro AA, Sananez I, et al. ATP-induced inflammation drives tissue-resident Th17 cells in metabolically unhealthy obesity. Journal of Immunology. 2016;**196**: 3287-3296

[44] Stelzner K, Herbert D, Popkova Y, et al. Free fatty acids sensitize dendritic cells to amplify TH1/TH17-immune responses. European Journal of Immunology. 2016;**46**:2043-2053

[45] Reis BS, Lee K, Fanok MH, et al. Leptin receptor signaling in T cells is required for Th17 differentiation. Journal of Immunology. 2015;**194**:5253-5260

[46] Delgoffe GM, Pollizzi KN, Waickman AT, et al. The mammalian target of Rapamycin (mTOR) regulates T helper cell differentiation through the selective activation of mTORC1 and mTORC2 signaling. Nature Immunology. 2011;**12**:295-303

[47] Chehimi M, Vidal H, Eljaafari A. Pathogenic role of IL-17-producing immune cells in obesity, and related inflammatory diseases. Journal of Clinical Medicine. 2017;**6**:68

[48] Rastogi D, Siuzuki M, Greally JM. Differential epigenome-wide DNA methylation patterns in childhood obesity-associated asthma. Scientific Reports. 2013;**3**:2164

[49] Yang Y, Zang HL, Wu J. Role of T regulatory cells in the pathogenesis of asthma. Chest. 2010;**138**:1282-1283

[50] Eller K, Kirsch A, Wolf AM, et al. Potential role of regulatory T cells in reversing obesity-linked insulin resistance and diabetic nephropathy. Diabetes. 2011;**60**:2954-2962

[51] Cipolletta D. Adipose tissue-resident regulatory T cells: Phenotypic specialization, functions and therapeutic potential. Immunology. 2014;**142**:517-525

[52] Han JM, Patterson SJ, Speck M, Ehses JA, Levings MK. Insulin Inhibits IL-10–mediated regulatory T cell function: Implications for obesity. Journal of Immunology. 2013:1302181

[53] Zhang L, Yin Y, Zhang H, Zhong W, Zhang J. Association of asthma diagnosis with leptin and adiponectin: A systematic review and meta-analysis. Journal of Investigative Medicine. 2017;**65**:57-64

[54] O"Donnell CP, Schaub CD, Haines AS, et al. Leptin prevents respiratory depression in obesity. American Journal of Respiratory and Critical Care Medicine. 1999;**159**:1477-1484

[55] Mai X-M, Böttcher MF, Leijon I. Leptin and asthma in overweight children at 12 years of age. Pediatric Allergy and Immunology. 2004;**15**:523-530

[56] Muc M, Todo-Bom A, Mota-Pinto A, Vale-Pereira S, Loureiro C. Leptin and resistin in overweight patients with and without asthma. Allergol Immunopathol (Madr). 2014;**42**:415-421

[57] Ubags ND, Vernooy JH, Burg E, et al. The role of leptin in the development of pulmonary neutrophilia in infection and acute lung injury. Critical Care Medicine. 2014;**42**:e143-e151

[58] Hsu P-S, Wu C-S, Chang J-F, Lin W-N. Leptin promotes $cPLA_2$ gene expression through activation of the MAPK/NF-κB/p300 Cascade. International Journal of Molecular Sciences. 2015;**16**:27640-27658

[59] Lee S-M, Choi H-J, Oh C-H, Oh J-W, Han J-S. Leptin increases TNF-α expression and production through phospholipase D1 in raw 264.7 cells. PLoS One. 2014;**9**:e102373

[60] Giouleka P, Papatheodorou G, Lyberopoulos P, et al. Body mass index is associated with leukotriene inflammation in asthmatics. European Journal of Clinical Investigation. 2011;**41**:30-38

[61] Coffey MJ, Torretti B, Mancuso P. Adipokines and cysteinyl leukotrienes in the pathogenesis of asthma. Journal of Allergy (Cairo). 2014;**42**:415-421

[62] Luo M, Jones SM, Peters-Golden M, Brock TG. Nuclear localization of 5-lipoxygenase as a determinant of leukotriene B_4 synthetic capacity. Proceedings of the National Academy of Sciences of the United States of America. 2003;**100**:12165-12170

[63] Arteaga-Solis E, Zee T, Emala CW, Vinson C, Wess J, Karsenty G. Inhibition of leptin regulation of parasympathetic signaling as a cause of extreme body weight-associated asthma. Cell Metabolism. 2013;**17**:35-48

[64] Suzukawa M, Koketsu R, Baba S, Igarashi S, et al. Leptin enhances ICAM-1 expression, induces migration and cytokine synthesis, and prolongs survival of human airway epithelial cells. American Journal of Physiology. Lung Cellular and Molecular Physiology. 2015;**309**:L801-L811

[65] Radić R, Nikolić V, Karner I, et al. Circadian rhythm of blood Leptin level in obese and non-obese people. Collegium Antropologicum. 2003;**27**:555-561

[66] Assad NA, Sood A. Leptin, adiponectin and pulmonary diseases. Biochimie. 2012;**94**: 2180-2189

[67] Sood A, Qualls C, Schuyler M, et al. Low serum adiponectin predicts future risk for asthma in women. American Journal of Respiratory and Critical Care Medicine. 2012;**186**(1):41-47

[68] Kim KW, Shin HY, Lee KE, Kim ES, Kim KE. Relationship between adipokines and manifestations of childhood asthma. Pediatric Allergy and Immunology. 2008;**19**:535-540

[69] Ohashi K, Parker JL, Ouchi N, et al. Adiponectin promotes macrophage polarization toward an anti-inflammatory phenotype. The Journal of Biological Chemistry. 2010;**285**:6153-6160

[70] Hayashikawa Y, Iwata M, Inomata M, et al. Association of serum adiponectin with asthma and pulmonary function in the Japanese population. Endocrine Journal. 2015;**62**:695-709

[71] Hinks TSC, Brown T, Lau LCK, et al. Multidimensional endotyping in patients with severe asthma reveals inflammatory heterogeneity in matrix metalloproteinases and chitinase 3-like protein 1. The Journal of Allergy and Clinical Immunology. 2016;**138**(1):61-75

[72] Desai D, Newby C, Symon FA, et al. Elevated sputum interleukin-5 and submucosal eosinophilia in obese individuals with severe asthma. American Journal of Respiratory and Critical Care Medicine. 2013;**188**(6):657-663

[73] Lefaudeux D, De Meulder B, Loza MJ, et al. U-BIOPRED clinical adult asthma clusters linked to a subset of sputum-omics. The Journal of Allergy and Clinical Immunology. 2016. DOI: 10.1016/j.jaci.2016.08.048

[74] Li Q, Baines KJ, Gibson PG, Wood LG. Changes in expression of genes regulating airway inflammation following a high-fat mixed meal in asthmatics. Nutrients. 2016;**8**(1):30

[75] Maniscalco M, Paris D, Melck DJ, et al. Coexistence of obesity and asthma determines a distinct respiratory metabolic phenotype. The Journal of Allergy and Clinical Immunology. 2017;**139**(5):1536-1547

[76] van Huisstede A, Rudolphus A, van Schadewijk A, et al. Bronchial and systemic inflammation in morbidly obese subjects with asthma: A biopsy study. American Journal of Respiratory and Critical Care Medicine. 2014;**190**:951-954

[77] Zhang X, Zheng J, Zhang L, et al. Systemic inflammation mediates the detrimental effects of obesity on asthma control. Allergy and Asthma Proceedings. 2018;**39**(1):43-50

[78] Han Y-Y, Forno E, Celedón JC. Adiposity, fractional exhaled nitric oxide, and asthma in U.S. children. American Journal of Respiratory and Critical Care Medicine. 2014;**190**(1): 32-39

[79] Nigro E, Daniele A, Scudiero O, et al. Adiponectin in asthma: Implications for Phenotyping. Current Protein & Peptide Science. 2015;**16**:182-187

[80] Ballantyne D, Scott H, MacDonald-Wicks L, et al. Resistin is a predictor of asthma risk and resistin: Adiponectin ratio is a negative predictor of lung function in asthma. Clinical and Experimental Allergy. 2016;**46**:1056-1065

[81] Bennett WD, Ivins S, Alexis NE, et al. Effect of obesity on acute ozone-induced changes in airway function, reactivity, and inflammation in adult females. PLoS One. 2016;**11**(8):e0160030

[82] Arismendi E, Rivas E, Vidal J, et al. Airway hyperresponsiveness to mannitol in obesity before and after bariatric surgery. Obesity Surgery. 2015;**25**(9):1666-1671

[83] Boulet LP, Boulay ME. Asthma-related comorbidities. Expert Review of Respiratory Medicine. 2011;**5**:377-393

[84] Hampel H, Abraham NS, El-Serag HB. Meta-analysis: Obesity and the risk for gastroesophageal reflux disease and its complications. Annals of Internal Medicine. 2005;**143**(3):199-211

[85] Ekström T, Tibbling L. Influence of theophylline on gastro-oesophageal reflux and asthma. European Journal of Clinical Pharmacology. 1988;**35**:353-365

[86] Bruno A, Pace E, Cibella F, Chanez P. Body mass index and comorbidities in adult severe asthmatics. BioMed Research International. 2014, Article ID 607192:7

[87] Ruigómez A, Rodriguez LA, Wallander MA, et al. Gastroesophageal reflux disease and asthma. Chest. 2005;**128**(1):85-93

[88] Madama D, Silva A, Matos MJ. Overlap syndrome – Asthma and obstructive sleep apnea. Revista Portuguesa de Pneumologia. 2016;**22**(1):6-10

[89] Teodorescu M, Barnet JH, Hagen EW, Palta M, Young TB, Pep- pard PE. Association between asthma and risk of developing obstructive sleep apnea. Journal of the American Medical Association. 2015;**313**:156-164

[90] Ong CW, O'Driscoll DM, Truby H, et al. The reciprocal interaction between obesity and obstructive sleep apnoea. Sleep Medicine Reviews. 2013;**17**:123-131

[91] Devouassoux G, Levi P, Rossini E, et al. Sleep apnea is associated with bronchial inflammation and continuous positive airway pressure–induced airway hyperresponsiveness. The Journal of Allergy and Clinical Immunology. 2007;**119**:597-603

[92] Julien JY, Martin JG, Ernst P, et al. Prevalence of obstructive sleep apnea–hypopnea in severe versus moderate asthma. The Journal of Allergy and Clinical Immunology. 2009;**124**:371-376

[93] Raşcu A, Popa DE, Arghir OC, Otelea MR. Effects of corticosteroid treatment on respiratory muscles function in patients with severe obstructive lung disease. Farmácia. 2016;**64**(6):819-822

[94] Emilsson ÖI, Benediktsdóttir B, Ólafsson Í, et al. Respiratory symptoms, sleep-disordered breathing and biomarkers in nocturnal gastroesophageal reflux. Respiratory Research. 2016;**17**:115

[95] Fenger RV, Gonzalez-Quintela A, Linneberg A, et al. The relationship of serum triglycerides, serum HDL, and obesity to the risk of wheezing in 85,555 adult. Respiratory Medicine. 2013;**107**(6):816-824

[96] Porsbjerg C, Menzies-Gow A. Co-morbidities in severe asthma: Clinical impact and management. Respirology. 2017;**22**:651-661

[97] Akerman MJ, Calacanis CM, Madsen MK. Relationship between asthma severity and obesity. The Journal of Asthma. 2004;**41**:521-526

[98] Ulrik CS. Asthma and obesity: Is weight reduction the key to achieve asthma control? Current Opinion in Pulmonary Medicine. 2016;**22**:69-73

[99] Dixon AE, Pratley RE, Forgione PM, et al. Effects of obesity and bariatric surgery on airway hyperresponsiveness, asthma control, and inflammation. The Journal of Allergy and Clinical Immunology. 2011;**128**:508-515

[100] Livingston E, Chaudhuri R, McMahon AD, et al. Cigarette smoking impairs the therapeutic response to oral corticosteroids in chronic asthma. American Journal of Respiratory and Critical Care Medicine. 2003;**168**:1308-1311

[101] Tai H, Wang M-Y, Zhao Y-P, et al. The effect of alogliptin on pulmonary function in obese patients with type 2 diabetes inadequately controlled by metformin monotherapy. Medicine (Baltimore). 2016;**95**(33):e4541

[102] Mattos ÂZ, Marchese GM, Fonseca BB, et al. Antisecretory treatment for pediatric gastroesophageal reflux disease - A systematic review. Arquivos de Gastroenterologia. 2017;**54**:271-280

[103] Hu Z, Wu J, Wang Z, et al. Outcome of Stretta radiofrequency and fundoplication for GERD-related severe asthmatic symptoms. Frontiers in Medicine. 2015;**9**:437

[104] Sriratanaviriyakul N, Kivler C, Vidovszky TJ, Yoneda KY. Journal of medical case reports: LINX®, a novel treatment for patients with refractory asthma complicated by gastroesophageal reflux disease: A case report. BioMed Central. 2016;**10**

[105] Kew KM, Evans DJ, Allison DE, Boyter AC. Long-acting muscarinic antagonists (LAMA) added to inhaled corticosteroids (ICS) versus addition of long-acting

beta2-agonists (LABA) for adults with asthma. Cochrane Database of Systematic Reviews. 2015;**6**:CD011438

[106] Yuan C, Zhou L, Cheng J, et al. Statins as potential therapeutic drug for asthma? Respiratory Research. 2012;**13**(1):108. DOI: 10.1186/1465-9921-13-108

[107] Peters-Golden M, Swern A, Bird SS, Hustad CM, Grant E, Edelman JM. Influence of body mass index on the response to asthma controller agents. The European Respiratory Journal. 2006;**27**:495-503

[108] Ortega H, Li H, Suruki R, Albers F, et al. Cluster analysis and characterization of response to mepolizumab. A step closer to personalized medicine for patients with severe asthma. Annals of the American Thoracic Society. 2014;**11**(7):1011-1017

[109] Busse WW, Holgate S, Kerwin E, et al. Randomized, double-blind, placebo-controlled study of brodalumab, a human anti–IL-17 receptor monoclonal antibody, in moderate to severe asthma. American Journal of Respiratory and Critical Care Medicine. 2013;**188**:1294-1302

[110] Durham AL, Caramori G, Chung KF, Adcock IM. Targeted anti-inflammatory therapeutics in asthma and chronic obstructive lung disease. Transgenic Research. 2016;**167**:192-203

[111] Taillé C, Poulet C, Marchand-Adam S, et al. Monoclonal anti-TNF-α antibodies for severe steroid-dependent asthma: A case series. Open Respiratory Medicine Journal. 2013;**7**:21-25

13

Use of Omalizumab as Treatment in Patients with Moderate and Severe Non-Atopic Asthma and Associated with Asthma-COPD Overlap Syndrome (ACOS)

Herrera García José Carlos,
Arellano Montellano Ek Ixel,
Jaramillo Arellano Luis Enrique,
Espinosa Arellano Andrea,
Martínez Flores Alejandra Guadalupe and
Caballero López Christopherson Gengyny

Abstract

The asthma syndrome has many manifestations, termed phenotypes that arise by specific cellular and molecular mechanisms termed endotypes. Understanding helps clinicians make rational therapeutic decisions. Omalizumab has been widely used in clinical practice in Europe and America for over a decade as an add-on therapy to treat patients who have severe asthma. These real-world clinical effectiveness studies have confirmed the benefits, cost-effectiveness, and clinical utility. The purpose of this review is to present the effects of anti-IgE treatment in severe non-atopic asthma and in asthma-COPD overlap syndrome (ACOS). This study describes that the use of omalizumab therapy reduces IgE expression and IgE sensitization of target cells within the bronchial mucosa while exerting a favorable effect on lung function in the short term, as assessed by changes in forced expiratory volume in 1 s (FEV1).

Keywords: omalizumab, non-atopic asthma, ACOS, phenotypes, severe asthma

1. Introduction

Severe asthma is a highly heterogeneous and burdensome disease that requires individualized assessment and management. The exact prevalence of severe asthma is unknown, but it has been reported to affect 5–10% of the population with asthma. Although some patients have

Atopic Patient	Non-Atopic Patient
With o without Eosinophilia	With or Without Eosinofilia
Skin prick test positive	Skin prick test negative
IgE > 150 U/L	IgE < 30 U/L
	30-150 U/L
	or > 150 U/L

Figure 1. Definitions.

asthma that remain poorly controlled despite high doses of inhaled corticosteroid (ICS) with or without additional controlled therapies including long-acting muscarinic antagonists and theophylline. Uncontrolled severe asthma significantly affects the activities of daily living, morbidity, mortality, quality of life (QOL), and health care use. Indeed, severe asthma accounts for approximately 50% of all asthma-related health care costs, direct (physician visits, hospitalizations, intensive care, and medications) and indirect (missed school days and work absenteeism). Categorically, uncontrolled and severe asthma remains a health and economic burden in many countries. Nowadays, we have a targeted therapy to control the burden disease with excellent results. In this chapter, we discuss the benefits of the use of omalizumab (OmAb) in patients with non-atopic and asthma COPD overlap syndrome (ACOS) phenotype. [1] (**Figure 1**).

2. Non-atopic asthma and IgE

The concept of asthma in our practice is a complex disease. Atopy is a familiar knowledge but the significance of non-atopic or non-allergic is a new definition to treat the patients with moderate-to-severe asthma. The presence of negative prick test and presence or not of eosinophilia is an opportunity to use biologics to improve symptoms and quality of life [2–3]. The possible association of serum IgE levels with asthma, irrespective of specific allergic sensitization has long been investigated. Burrows et al. revealed that IgE-mediated mechanisms might play a role even in non-atopic asthmatics with no detectable allergen-specific IgE. Some studies have shown that up to 25% of adult asthmatics are non-allergic. We proposed to treat the patients according to different types [4–6] (**Figure 1**).

A minority of asthmatic individuals are not however demonstrably atopic by conventional criteria, which has led to the suggestion that asthma maybe divided clinically into atopic and non-atopic. Recently, there have been major advances in our understanding of the molecular mechanisms of non-atopic. Indeed, the mechanisms of this variant of asthma in which allergens have no obvious role in driving inflammatory process in the airways remain uncertain. This type of research will certainly point towards new types of mechanisms, which will allow a more personalized way to treat asthma [7].

3. Local and peripheral IgE synthesis in severe asthma

Non-atopic asthma patients are typically a late-onset condition, more common in females, and it tends to be more severe than atopic form, requiring higher doses of corticosteroids for

Cell types of epithelial components	Atopic asthma	Non-atopic asthma
Ciliated columnar	Damage ++	Damage +
Desmosomes	Breakdown ++	Breakdown +
Globlet cells	Hyperplasia (+)	Hyperplasia (−)
Basal cells	Damage +	Damage +
Basement membrane	Thickening ++	Thickening +
Eosinophils	Infiltration +++	Inflitration +++
Neutrophils	Inflitration +	Inflitration ++
Mast cells	Inflitration ++	Infiltration +
Lymphocytes	Infiltration +++	Infiltration ++
Macrophages	Infiltration +	Infiltration ++

Table 1. Comparison of bronchial epithelial components in atopic and non-atopic asthma.

adequate control. It often starts following a severe upper or lower respiratory tract infection or during pregnancy, but it also indicates that environmental factors may be more important in the causation of non-atopic asthma. The presence of increased local synthesis of IgE also in non-atopic asthmatics has been demonstrated in more recent studies. Ying et al. showed local expression of epsilon heavy chain of IgE in the bronchial mucosa in atopic and non-atopic asthmatics. Mouthuy et al. confirmed that local IgE production occurs in the bronchial mucosa in atopic asthma and showed for the first time, that this part of IgE is directed towards house dust mite allergens. [8–10].

We described in 2015, the presence of non-atopic phenotype in a population of 10 asthmatics in a cohort with omalizumab treatment in University Hospital of Puebla, Mexico. Since the identification of IgE as a major stimulus in the inflammation cascade, the development of agents to target IgE has thrived. [11] (**Table 1**).

4. Anti-IgE drug omalizumab: mechanism of action

Omalizumab (OmAb) is a recombinant humanized monoclonal antibody that was designed to bind to IgE on the Fc (constant fragment) portion, C epsilon 3 locus, in the same domain where IgE is bound to FcRI. This drug was synthesized with the aim of sequestering free IgE and reducing allergic inflammation. This drug is administered subcutaneously and is absorbed slowly. The peak of serum concentration is reached after 7–8 days and it is eliminated via reticuloendothelial system having a half-life of around 26 days. It has been accepted for a long time that OmAb acts on the free IgE and abolish the binding of IgE to FcRI or FcRII, CD23 cells, B-cells, dendritic cells (DC), eosinophils (Eo), and monocytes. In several real-life studies, the use of OmAb has been associated with an absence of exacerbations and improvement in the quality of life, which is reflected in reduced hospital admissions and emergency visits but not in pulmonary function. The standard duration of treatment with OmAb has not been established to date. A follow-up study showed that after 6 years of OmAb treatment, most patients have mild and stable asthma in the ensuing 3 years after treatment discontinuation, it has been suggested that the persistence of the effects of OmAb may be due to its ability to curtail airway remodeling in patients with asthma. In fact, it has been found that OmAb significantly decreased the airway wall area. After 1 year of omalizumab treatment, a significant mean reduction in eosinophilic infiltration was recorded as well as a reduction in the reticular base membrane in bronchial biopsies from patients with severe persistent allergic asthma was observed. These findings indicate that OmAb may modify the course of the disease due to their possible influence curtailing airway remodeling [12].

5. Anti-Immunoglobulin E in non-atopic asthma with omalizumab

In an attempt to elucidate the drug's mechanism of action, OmAb regulated FcRI expression negatively on basophils and plasmacytoid dendritic cells and increased forced expiratory volume in the first minute (FEV1) compared with baseline after 16 weeks in patients with severe non-atopic asthma demonstrated the possible role of IgE in non-atopic asthmatics [12–14]. The concept of Omalizumab treatment in non-atopic asthma is a new provocative idea and initially, some reports cases and data from severe asthma registries gave food for thought and discussion [15–16].

We concluded the functional role of local polyclonal IgE in airway mucosal tissue also in view of the finding of eosinophilic inflammation in nasal polyps with increased local tissue IgE levels independently of the allergic status of the patients. We presented the same case to Mexican female patient in University hospital of Puebla and showed the benefits of omalizumab in symptoms, QOL, and acute exacerbations, not in pulmonary function [13, 17].

6. Effects of omalizumab in non-atopic asthma patients

Eosinophilic asthma has been considered a phenotype of severe asthma. Allergic asthma can present with normal or increased numbers of eosinophils. The guidelines generally do not distinguish between the pathways responsible for the eosinophilia (atopic or non-atopic). Omalizumab can decrease the number of eosinophils in sputum on the bronchial mucosa and to a lesser extent in peripheral blood, in some cases, omalizumab fails to improve allergic asthma, this in probably due to the fact that the predominant physiopathological dysregulation comer initially from adaptive immunity, probably as a consequence of the highly intense activity of the allergic cascade. [18–19].

As a result of all these different modes of action, omalizumab has also been shown to interfere in certain stages of the remodeling process. [20–23]. Kutlu et al. described a case with 34 years old male patient the use of omalizumab with negative skin prick test and IgE in 203 U/L, they use omalizumab a dose of 225 mg every 2 weeks and after 6 months the patient was scored as 7 to 25 points at the asthma control test before the treatment of anti-IgE. We described and showed the improvement or non-atopic patients with omalizumab and started with 150 mg of omalizumab in our asthma Clinic in Puebla and increased the doses with excellent results [20–24].

7. Asthma-COPD overlap syndrome

Asthma and chronic obstructive pulmonary disease (COPD) are two common respiratory disorders which are associated with chronic inflammation or the airways. In text books, the two are described as distinct disorders, however, there is increasing awareness that in clinical practice many patients may have features of both. ACOS is a subset of patients with persistent airflow limitation who have clinical features of both asthma and COPD. (25).

Patients with ACOS have largely excluded from studies and hence information on their epidemiology, pathogenesis and treatment is sparse, we described in a COPD cohort from pneumology department in our asthma COPD clinic prevalence was 10 and 25% in asthma cohort. Another study described in COPD cohort has 15% of them fulfilling criteria for ACOS. Another study done in asthmatics who were smokers, found that 27% of them had ACOS. However, another study done showed that only 7% of asthma/COPD patients had ACOS. This wide variation can be partly attributed to the difference in the criteria used to diagnose ACOS in the above studies. The lack of consensus on a definition for ACOS has led to the wide range in prevalence varying between 11 and 56% among COPD, 13 and 61% among asthma, and 2% among the general population [25–30] (**Tables 2** and **3**).

Major criteria	Minor criteria
1. Persistent airflow limitation (post bronchodilator FEV1/ FVC ratio < 0.70 of lower limit of normal) in individuals aged 40 years or older.	1. Documented history of atopy or allergic rhinitis.
2. At least 10 pack years of tobacco smoking or equivalent exposure to indoor of outdoor pollutants (biomass).	2. Bronchodilator response (BDR) using 400 mcg of albuterol/salbutamol >200 ml and 12% from baseline values on 2 or more visits.
3. Documented history of asthma before the age of 40 years or BDR >400 ml in forced expiratory volume in 1 s (FEV1).	3. Peripheral blood eosinophil count >300 cells/μL.
FVC = Forced vital capacity	

The criteria for diagnosis of ACOS consist of 3 major and 3 minor criteria. To diagnose ACOS, it is necessary to have 3 major criteria and at least 1 minor criteria.

Table 2. Expert consensus major and minor criteria for ACOS.

Major criteria	Minor criteria
1. Very positive bronchodilator test (increase in FEV1 > 15% and >400 ml	1. High Level of total IgE
2. Sputum eosinophils	2. Personal history of atopy
3. History of asthma	3. Positive bronchodilator test on at least 2 occasions (increase of FEV1 > 12% and 200 ml).

For diagnosis at least 2 major criteria of 1 major criteria with 2 minor criteria.

Table 3. SEPAR criteria for mixed COPD/asthma phenotype in COPD.

8. Recently use of biologicals for ACOS

In the past decade, interest in the clinical characteristics, importance and consequences for patients with overlapping features of asthma and COPD has been renewed. In their purest forms, asthma and COPD are distinct and readily recognizable clinical entities. Furthermore, guidelines for treatment of asthma and COPD are well established and evidence-based.

The unknowns continue to mount for patients in this overlap syndrome group who are unresponsive to existing treatments but continue to be symptomatic and at increased risk for exacerbations. The absence of treatment guidelines becomes particularly problematic when the use of biological is being considered. Experience with biological is most extensive with asthma, but studies of asthma treatments often exclude subjects with a history of smoking. Furthermore, in studies in COPD, a history of asthma is usually and exclusion criterion. Therefore, well recognized evidence-based guidance is largely absent as to what might be the best therapeutic approach, what patient characteristics are most predictive in selecting a specific next treatment of what outcomes are most likely to reflect treatment responsiveness. As many patients with asthma-COPD overlap syndrome might not achieve disease control with existing treatments, the consideration for and selection of a biological agent is an important unmet clinical need, both for the clinician and the affected patient [31].

Chest, Steven Maltby and colleagues at the University of Newcastle in Australia began to address this largely open question. What are the effects of omalizumab in this patient cohort? The Australian Xolair Registry was used to evaluate the real world use of omalizumab for severe uncontrolled allergic asthma. A total of 177 participants were evaluated and 17 of these had a doctor diagnosis of COPD. Omalizumab was found to be equivalently effective in patients with severe allergic asthma and a physician diagnosis of COPD, as well as severe asthma without COPD. In severe asthma and COPD, the asthma control questionnaire (ACQ) improved from 3.68 to 1.69 with the addition of omalizumab [31].

Initial studies have shown that omalizumab may be useful in patients with ACOS. It has been shown to improve symptoms, reduce exacerbations and hospitalization, and improve lung function parameters and reduced steroid requirement in these patients. However, larger randomized trial is required to further validate this observation. We presented the effects of omalizumab in ACOS patients with an excellent result in a group of 5 patients of the asthma COPD cohort clinic in University hospital of Puebla and showed improved lung function and symptoms [31–33].

Nayci et al. published the effectiveness of omalizumab treatment in asthma-COPD overlap syndrome in 2016 and described a clinical reduction in exacerbations and steroid requirement and improved symptoms and pulmonary function parameters in 6 patients. Dammert et al. published the use of Omalizumab in patients with COPD and atopic phenotypes in 7 cohort patients with positive allergy test and showed that omalizumab reduced the number of exacerbations, hospitalizations, and improved symptoms [34–35].

9. Conclusion

To conclude, there is now evidence suggesting that omalizumab improves patients with severe non-atopic asthma and ACOS. Therefore, it is important to review each patient meticulously and regularly and provide personalized and targeted treatment. In the case of using omalizumab to treat non atopic severe asthma, the evidence is conclusive in these phenotypes. In the era of personalized and targeted medicine, it is important to fully characterize our patients and prescribe treatment that aims at treating the particular patient to consider the cost-effectiveness. In this chapter, we described that omalizumab is efficient and safe to treat and improves and increases the quality of life.

Acknowledgements

First, I want to thank my parents for supporting me in my career, and also thank my wife Ek who has been my companion and confidant in this way of research, my sons Karla and Joss for being my motors in life and finally God for making this dream of life possible. Thank you. I would also like to thank the Universidad Hospital of Puebla and Novartis for their support in the publication.

Author details

Herrera García José Carlos[1*], Arellano Montellano Ek Ixel[1], Jaramillo Arellano Luis Enrique[3],
Espinosa Arellano Andrea[3], Martínez Flores Alejandra Guadalupe[1] and
Caballero López Christopherson Gengyny[2]

*Address all correspondence to: jchg10@yahoo.com.mx

1 Asthma-COPD Clinic-University Hospital of Puebla, Mexico

2 University Hospital of Puebla, Mexico

3 Benemerita Autonomous University of Puebla, Mexico

References

[1] Borriello EM, Vatrella A. Does non-allergic asthma still exist? Shortness of Breath. 2013; **2**(2):55-60

[2] Ishizaka K, Ishizaka T, Hornbrook MM. Physicochemical properties of human reaginic antibody. IV. Presence of a unique immunoglobulin as a carrier of reaginic activity. Journal of Immunology. Jul 1966;**97**(1):75-85

[3] Brown WG, Halonen MJ, Kaltenborn WT, Barbee RA. The relationship of respiratory allergic, skin test reactivity and serum IgE in a community population sample. Journal ofAllergy and Clinical Immunology. May 1979;**63**(5):328-335

[4] Burrows B, Martinez FD, Halonen M, Barbee RA, Cline MG. Association of asthma with serum IgE levels and skin test reactivity to allergens. The New England Journal of Medicine. Feb 1989;**320**(5):271-277

[5] Sunyer J, Antó JM, Castellsague J, Soriano JB, Roca J. Total serum IgE is associated with asthma independently of specific IgE levels. The Spanish Group of the European Study of Asthma. The European Respiratory Journal. Sep 1996;**9**(9):1880-1884

[6] Beeh KM, Ksoll M, Buhl R. Elevation of total serum immunoglobulin E is associated in non-allergic individuals. The European Respiratory Journal. Oct 2000;**16**(4):609-614

[7] Humbert M, Menz G, Ying S, et al. The Immunopathology of extrinsic (atopic) and intrinsic (non-atopic) asthma: More similarities than differences. Immunology Today. 1999;**20**:528-533

[8] Humbert M, Grant JA, Taborda-Barata L, Durham SR, Pfister R, Menz G, Barkans J, Ying S, Kay AB. High affinity IgE receptor bearing cells in bronchial biopsies from atopic and non-atopic asthma. American Journal of Respiratory and Critical Care Medicine. Jun 1996;**153**(6):1931-1937

[9] Ying S, Humbert M, Meng Q, Pfister R, Menz G, Gould HJ, Kay AB, Durham SR. Local expression of epsilon germline gene transcripts and RNA for the epsilon heavy chain of IgE in the bronchial mucosa in atopic and non-atopic asthma. The Journal of Allergy and Clinical Immunology. Jan 2007;**119**(1):213-218

[10] Mouthuy J, Detry B, Sohy C, Pirson F, Pilette C. Presence in sputum of functional dust mite specific IgE antibodies in intrinsic asthma. American Journal of Respiratory and Critical Care Medicine. 2011 Jul 15;**184**(2):206-214

[11] Herrera-García JC, Sánchez-Casas GA, Arellano-Jaramillo LE, Lechuga-Hernández S, et al. Omalizumab in the treatment of moderate to severe persistent asthma in the context of allergic and non-allergic asthma. Medicina Interna de México. 2015;**31**: 693-700

[12] Gaga M, Zervas E, Humbert M. Targeting immunoglobulin E in non-atopic asthma: crossing the red line? The European Respiratory Journal. 2016;**48**:1538-1540. DOI: 10.1183/13993003.01797-2016

[13] Herrera J et al. Successful use of omalizumab as a patient treatment with chronic rino-sinusitis, nasal polyps and severe asthma. National Congress of Pneumology in Puebla, Mexico. April 17th to 21st 2017

[14] Navines-Ferrer A, Serrano-Candelas E, Molina Molina GJ, Martin M. IgE-related chronic diseases and anti-IgE based treatments. Journal of Immunology Research. Hindawi Publising Corporation. 2016;**2016**:1-12. http://dx-doi.org/10-1155/2016/8163803

[15] Pillai P, Chan Y-C, Wu S-Y, et al. Omalizumab reduces bronchial mucosal IgE and improves lung function in non-atopic asthma. The European Respiratory Journal. 2016; **48**:1593-1601

[16] Garcia G, Magnan A, Chiron R, et al. A proof of concept, randomized, controlled trial of omalizumab in patients with severe, difficult to control, nonatopic asthma. Chest. 2013;**144**:411-419

[17] Menzella F, Piro R, Facciolongo N, et al. Long term benefits of omalizumab in patient with severe non-allergic asthma. Allergy, Asthma and Clinical Immunology. 2011;**7**:9

[18] Lynch JP, Mazzone SB, Rogers MJ, Arikkatt JJ, Loh Z, Pritchard AL, Upham JW, Phipps S. The plasmacytoid dendritic cell: at the cross–roads in asthma. The European Respiratory Journal. 2014;**43**:264-275

[19] Domingo C. Overlapping effects of new monoclonal antibodies for severe asthma. Drugs. Springer International Publishing. 2017;**77**:1769. https://doi.org/10.1007/s40265-017-0810-5. Version Online ISSN: 1179-1950

[20] Van den Berge M, Pauw RG, de Monchy JG, van Minnen CA, Postma DS, Kerstjens HA. Beneficial effects of treatment with anti-IgE antibodies (omalizumab) in a patient with severe asthma and negative skin prick test results. Chest. 2011;**139**:190-193

[21] Domingo C, Pomares X, Angril N, Rudi N, Amengual MJ, Mirapeix RM. Effectiveness of omalizumab in non-allergic severe asthma. Journal of Biological Regulators and Homeostatic Agents. 2013;**27**:45-53

[22] De Llano LP, Vennera Mdel C, Alvarez FJ, Medina JF, Borderias L, Pellicer C, Gonzalez H, Guillón JA, Martinez Moragón E, Sabadell C, Zamarro S, Picado C. Effects of omalizumab in non-atopic asthma: Results from a Spanish multicenter registry. The Journal of Asthma. 2013;**50**:296-301

[23] Herrera J, Arellano EK, Jaramillo E, Espinosa A, Martinez AG, Caballero CG. Succesfful use of omalizumab in patients with moderate to severe non atopic asthma. National Congress of Pneumology in Puebla, Mexico. April 17th to 21st 2017

[24] Kutlu A, Demirer E, Ozturk S, Gunes A, Kartal O, Sezer O, Kartaloglu Z. Can anti-IgE treatment be used in non-atopic asthma patients: throughts of a case about the role of IgE in asthma. Gülhane Tıp Dergisi. 2014;**56**:46-44. DOI: 10.5455/gullhane.11713

[25] Postma DS, Rabe KF. The asthma-COPD overlap syndrome. The New England Journal of Medicine. 2015;**373**:1241-1249

[26] Sin DD et al. What is asthma-COPD overlap syndrome? Towards a consensus definition from a round table discussion. The European Respiratory Journal. 2016. DOI: 10.1183/13993003.00436-2016

[27] Cosio et al. Definiting the asthma-COPD overlap syndrome in COPD cohort. Chest. Jan 2016;**149**(1):45-52

[28] Kiljander T, Helin T, Venho K, Jaakkola A, Lehtimäki L. Prevalence of asthma–COPD overlap syndrome among primary care asthmatics with a smoking history: A cross-sectional study. NPJ Primary Care Respiratory Medicine. 2015;**25**:15047. DOI: 10.1038/npjpcrm.2015.47

[29] Rodrigues D, Galego MA, Teixeira M, Vaz AP, Ferreira J. Characterization of ACOS patients in pulmonary outpatient consultation-applying the questionnaire by GINA/GOLD consensus. The European Respiratory Journal. 2016. DOI: 10.1183/13993003.congress-2016.PA869

[30] Herrera J, et al Prevalence of asthma-COPD patients in pulmonary department and asthma/COPD clinic consultation: A cohort study: IN PRESS

[31] Yalcin AD, Celik B, Yalcin AN. Omalizumab anti-IgE therapy in the asthma-COPD overlap syndrome (ACOS) and its effects on circulating cytokine levels. Immunopharmacology and Immunotoxicology. Jun 2016;**38**(3). DOI: 10.3109/08923973.2016.1173057

[32] Herrera J, Arellano EK, Jaramillo L, Espinosa A, Martinez A, Caballero C. Use of omalizumab in 5 patients with ACOS in terciary hospital of Puebla: A cohort study. In: National Pneumology Congress: 17-21 April 2017. IN PRESS

[33] Busse WW et al. Clinical preview, biologicals for asthma in patients with asthma-COPD overlap syndrome. The Lancet. March 2017;**5**:176-177

[34] Nayci SA, Ozgur E, Tastekin E, Ozge C. Effectiveness of omalizumab treatment in Asthma-COPD Overlap syndrome In: Chest Annual Meeting 2016. 22-26 Los Angeles, Cal. DOI: http//dx-doi.org/10-1016/j.chest.2016.08.967

[35] Dammert P, Jawahar D. Omalizumab in patients with COPD and atopic phenotype: A case series. American Journal of Respiratory and Critical Care Medicine. 2016;**193**:A6246

14

Cough Variant Asthma as a Phenotype of Classic Asthma

Sanela Domuz Vujnović, Adrijana Domuz and
Slobodanka Petrović

Abstract

Cough variant asthma (CVA) was first described by Glauser. CVA was described as the isolated chronic cough as the only presenting symptom responsive to bronchodilator therapy. The authors now suggest that CVA is present with airway hyperresponsiveness, eosinophilic inflammation of central and peripheral airways and bronchodilator respon sive coughing without typical manifestation of asthma such as wheezing or dyspnea. Pathologically, CVA shares common features such as eosinophilic inflammation and remodeling changes with classic asthma. Because of that, CVA is clinically considered as a variant type of asthma, a phase at the beginning of asthma pathogenesis or as a pre cursor of classic asthma. Nearly 30% of patients with CVA eventually develop intermit tent wheezing, an average of 3–5 years. It is clinically very important to recognize CVA because long-term inhaled corticosteroids can significantly decrease the development of classic asthma in these patients.

Keywords: asthma, cough variant asthma, airway hyperresponsiveness, chronic cough, airway remodeling, airway inflammation

1. Introduction

Asthma could be defined more as a syndrome characterized by several different phenotypes [1–3]. Therefore, one of the possible definitions describing the characteristics of the disease and unifying more different definitions could define asthma as chronic inflammatory disease characterized by acute variable onset of symptoms (coughing, air deficiency, chest tightening) with bronchoconstriction (clinical definition) reversible and passes spontaneously or under the impact of therapy (pharmacological definition), followed by bronchial hyperactivity on different stimulants (functional definition) and the inflammation of different stage, duration and difficulty (biological definition) [1]. Cough variant asthma (CVA) is defined as a phenotype of asthma, which characterized by cough as the sole symptom and airway hyperreactivity (AHR) [4]. Corrao and colleagues first defined "cough variant asthma" as AHR, chronic cough and absence of wheezing [5].

The authors agree that CVA and classic asthma have the same pathophysiological and immunological mechanisms, so CVA is considered a precursor of classic asthma [6–8].

Case 1 [9]: A 5-year-old boy presented to the clinic because of prolonged dry coughing with no history of wheezing. Because boy could not do spirometry, a forced oscillation technique was made. The total respiratory resistance was decreased by −20.4% after beta-2-agonist inhalation. At the first visit, 2-week therapy of inhaled beta-2-agonist was started. This treatment was clearly effective against his cough. The CVA was diagnosed, and his treatment with leukotriene receptor antagonist (Montelukast) and LABA (tulobuterol patch) was started for next 8 weeks. Eight months later, boy has the same symptoms. The same treatment was restarting. Three years later, boy has another episode of a dry cough with no complaints of wheezing. A physician confirmed a wheeze during expiration by auscultation. The treatment with inhaled steroid (Fluticasone), LABA (Salmeterol) and leukotriene receptor antagonist (Montelukast) was started. Over time, after boy developed recurrent wheezing, the diagnosis of asthma was set.

Case 2 [10]: "A 64-year-old female presented to the clinic as a self-referral complaining of a persistent cough." She said that the symptoms last for almost 17 years. The patient had diagnosed seasonal rhinosinusitis with positive skin prick test. Previous evaluations were all unremarkable. She underwent a methacholine challenge test. Spirometry showed increase in FEV1 with a 13% change from baseline. The patient was diagnosed with CVA and therapy with a combination of medium dose inhaled steroid and long-acting beta-2-agonist (Mometasone/Formoterol) was started.

Case 3 [11]: "A 32-year-old women presented with an intermittent nonproductive hacking cough that had lasted several days." Her medical history was unremarkable, and previous evaluations were normal. Results of a methacholine challenge test showed severe airway hyperreactivity. The patient was diagnosed with CVA, and bronchodilator with ICS treatment was started.

The prevalence of CVA is unknown, and from these cases it can be noticed that patients with chronic cough, as the only symptom, remain unrecognized as asthma for a long-time period.

The isolated cough is less common than other clinical manifestations of classic asthma [11]. Diagnosis of CVA may prove to be a challenge for the physicians. Therefore, evaluation results of patients with CVA are usually normal (spirometry, skin prick test, chest radiography, blood test) [12]. Previous clinical history is also normal in these patients [2, 11, 13].

Clinical feature of CVA is a good response to bronchodilator and ICS therapy [12, 13]. Studies have shown that the ICS therapy in CVA patients prevents the development of classic asthma [3, 7, 12]. Namely, it has been noticed that an average of 30% of patients with CVA without treatment develop classic asthma with wheezing [3]. A smaller number, about 10% of patients with CVA and with adequate therapy (bronchodilator, ICS or Montelukast) develop classic asthma. A good response of chronic cough to the therapy with ICS cannot be used to distinguish other cough present diseases (atopic cough, non-asthmatic eosinophilic bronchitis) from CVA [2, 8].

It should be emphasized that in patients with chronic cough, a diagnostic evaluation for asthma should be performed.

2. Pathological mechanism underlying CVA

The main underlying pathophysiological mechanism of CVA is airway hyperresponsiveness (AHR) [3]. Airway hyperresponsiveness in CVA patients is milder than in patients with classic asthma. AHR is defined by two basic parameters: bronchial sensitivity and bronchial reactivity.

Airway remodeling is milder in CVA than in classic asthma [14, 15]. The more important is their airway sensitivity (threshold dose of methacholine to increase respiratory resistance) and airway reactivity (slope of respiratory resistance response curves), which are tested by challenge tests [15]. The difference in the challenge test between CVA and classic asthma patients was only in airway reactivity. Since bronchial reactivity is the one that is crucial in patients with CVA, there is a normal baseline result in these patients, but only challenge tests are positive [15, 16]. Airway reactivity is lower in CVA patients mostly because bronchoconstriction is lower and limited in CVA. Niimi et al. suggested that airway remodeling does not protect against bronchial sensitivity but against bronchial reactivity [15]. Bronchial hyperreactivity plays a significant role in the pathophysiology of CVA development. Cough reflex sensitivity does not change in patients with CVA, and it is not essential in pathophysiology in CVA [7, 8].

An important role in the pathophysiology of CVA has eosinophilic inflammation [3]. The results of studies have shown that BAL and sputum in patients with CVA contain an increased percentage of eosinophils [2]. Also, the studies showed that there was no significant difference between CVA and classic asthma in the sputum levels of eosinophilic cationic protein, interleukin 8 (IL-8) and levels of exhaled nitric oxide (FeNO) [2, 7, 12, 17, 18]. Studies have suggested that the basic pathophysiological characteristics of CVA are eosinophilic inflammation and AHR [3].

Bronchoconstriction is milder in CVA than in classic asthma patients, and this can be a possible reason why these patients do not have wheezing as a symptom [16]. The main puzzle in the clinical feature of CVA is the absence of wheezing. One of the possible mechanisms may be slower and limited bronchoconstriction. The possible cause of this slower bronchoconstriction may be airway remodeling [12] and variations in cytokine production [16].

The bronchodilatory test in patients with CVA is often negative because baseline FEV1 values are normal in CVA patients [12]. Corrao and colleagues defined "cough variant asthma" as AHR, chronic cough and absence of wheezing [5]. The peak expiratory flow (PEF) assessment does not show any variability in CVA patients [2]. The spirometric measurements are normal in patients with CVA [2].

Structural changes such as subepithelial thickening, goblet cell hyperplasia and vascular proliferation in the bronchial tree were noticed in patients with CVA [12]. These changes are less expressed than in patients with classic asthma and most commonly associated with airway inflammation. An important role in the development of cough in CVA patients has inflammatory mediators such as histamine, prostaglandins D2 and E2, leukotrienes C4, D4 and E4 [12, 19]. The study by Liu et al. showed similarities between AHR and the level of inflammatory biomarkers (IL-5, IL-10 and eosinophils in induced sputum) [3].

Because of this, researchers agree that early anti-inflammatory treatment in patients with CVA can prevent the development of classical asthma in these patients [7, 15].

The pathophysiological aspects of CVA are similar to classical asthma [7, 16]. The study of Fujimura et al. also showed that the use of ICS prevents the development of classical asthma in patients with CVA [7].

It is necessary to emphasize that further investigations in this matter are necessary.

3. Biomarkers and diagnostic criteria

Patients with CVA frequently report that cough is provoked by trivial stimuli (cold air, talking, etc.) and do not respond to the antitussive preparations [3].

Mochizuki and associates in their study showed that children with CVA have slower bronchoconstriction against non-specific airway stimuli, but have significant bronchial sensitivity as well as children with classical asthma [16]. Children with CVA show latent bronchoconstriction without wheezing [16].

Bronchodilatatory test, spirometry and chest radiography are usually normal in patients with CVA. The bronchodilatory test in patients with CVA is often negative because baseline FEV1 values are normal in CVA patients [12]. Methacholine testing has a positive predictive value up to 90, a negative predictive value of 100 for CVA [11, 20].

The more important is their airway sensitivity (threshold dose of methacholine to increase respiratory resistance) and airway reactivity (slope of respiratory resistance response curves), which are tested by challenge tests [15]. The difference in the challenge test between CVA and classic asthma patients was only in airway reactivity. Airway reactivity is lower in CVA patients mostly because bronchoconstriction is lower and limited in CVA [12].

Positive challenge test and good response on bronchodilator or ICS therapy can be criteria for diagnosis of CVA [11]. Improvement of chronic cough with bronchodilators is the essential diagnostic feature of CVA [12, 13, 21].

The study by Liu and et al. showed similarities between AHR and the level of inflammatory biomarkers (IL-5, IL-10 and eosinophils in induced sputum) [3]. The improvement of these criteria was lower in the classic asthma group with the ICS therapy. The IL-5 level in the CVA group decreased after 3 months of treatment, while in the classic asthma group decreased after 6 months of treatment. The percentage of eosinophils in the sputum decreased after 6 months of ICS treatment in the CVA group and after 12 months in the classic asthma group.

Biomarkers that can be used in diagnosis of CVA do not differ from biomarkers in classic asthma. Studies have shown that there are elevated sputum markers (eosinophils, IL-5, IL-10, prostaglandins D2 and E2, leukotrienes C4, D4 and E4) in patients with CVA [12]. Patients with CVA have structural changes in the bronchial epithelium such as subepithelial thickening, goblet cell hyperplasia and vascular proliferation [12]. These changes are less expressed than in patients with classic asthma.

Fractional exhaled nitric oxide (FeNO) is a biomarker that is related to allergic cough [1]. FeNo levels were significantly higher in patients with CVA or classic asthma than in healthy controls in the study by Shimoda et al. [22]. Patients with CVA have significantly lower FeNO than patients with classic asthma. In this study, FeNO values correlated with the severity of asthma symptoms [22]. Asano et al. had the same results in their study [23].

Another significant marker that is listed in the literature as a useful marker of inflammation in classic asthma is serum high sensitivity C-reactive protein (hs-CRP). Serum hs-CRP levels were significantly higher in patients with CVA and classic asthma. However, no significant difference was detected between CVA and classic asthma patients. Studies have shown that the levels of FeNO rise in patients with CVA and classic asthma. Serum hs-CRP is considered inappropriate as a marker of airway inflammation. Namely, this marker is higher in men than in women, also its values are elevated in other various systemic inflammations, arterial hypertension, diabetes and cardiovascular disease. The values of hsCRP are also elevated in smokers [22].

The authors of CVA studies agree that the criteria proposed by the Japanese Cough Research Society are adequate for diagnosing CVA [6, 8, 13]. The above criteria are as follows [13]:

- isolated chronic non-productive cough lasting more than 8 weeks;
- absence of a history of wheeze or dyspnea, and no adventitious lung sounds on physical examination;
- absence of postnasal drip to account for the cough;
- FEV1, FVC, and FEV1/FVC ratio within normal limits;
- presence of bronchial hyperresponsiveness (PC20 < 10 mg/mL);
- cough reflex sensitivity within normal limits (C5 > 3.9 mmol/L);
- no abnormal findings indicative of cough etiology on chest radiograph and
- relief of cough with bronchodilator therapy.

If all the criteria are fulfilled, a diagnosis of CVA can be made. However, if some of the criteria are not presented, the diagnosis of CVA can be set if the following criteria are fulfilled [13]:

- cough without wheezing lasting 8 weeks or more and no wheezing on auscultation
- no upper respiratory tract infection and
- relief of cough with bronchodilator therapy.

The most important criterion is the response to bronchodilator therapy that can be excellent when cough was totally resolved, good when sleep and daytime quality of life were improved, fairly good when severity and frequency of cough were somewhat decreased and poor when cough was unchanged [6].

4. Therapy

Therapeutic approach for CVA is similar to the treatment for classic asthma [10, 12]. Therapy with short-acting bronchodilators can be useful in patients with intermittent cough. Most of researchers agree that eosinophilic inflammation and remodeling require ICS therapy especially in patients with persistent cough [12].

The choice of ICS, its dose and duration of therapy should be as in patients with classic asthma. The results of the studies show that early application of ICS therapy reduces the risk of progression of CVA to classical asthma [8, 12, 21]. Namely, an average of 30% of patients with CVA without treatment develop classic asthma with wheezing in the future [3, 7]. A smaller number, about 10% of patients with CVA and adequate therapy (bronchodilator, ICS or Montelukast) develop classic asthma [12].

The study by Liu and et al. showed similarities between AHR and the level of inflammatory biomarkers (IL-5, IL-10 and eosinophils in induced sputum). The IL-5 level in the CVA group decreased after 3 months of ICS treatment, while in the classic asthma group decreased after 6 months of treatment. The percentage of eosinophils in the sputum decreased after 6 months of ICS treatment in the CVA group and after 12 months in the classic asthma group [3].

A fact that significantly influences the therapeutic response in children is described by Hutton et al. The fact is that "the parents who wanted medicine at the initial visit reported more improvement at follow-up regardless of whether the child received a drug, placebo or no treatment" [24, 25].

5. Differentiation of the reactive airway diseases

Whether CVA represents a self-standing airway disease is still the object of debate. CVA is pathophysiologically similar to asthma, but with mild bronchial hyperreaction and eosinophilic inflammation [6, 7]. CVA has been considered a precursor of classic asthma [6, 7].

Reaction to bronchodilator therapy could be a pathognomic feature in the differential diagnosis of CVA [7]. Namely, in conditions such as postnasal drip induced cough, gastroesophageal reflux associated cough and atopic cough bronchodilators have no antitussive effect [7, 26].

The presence of eosinophilia in the sputum, bronchial hyperactivity and a positive bronchodilator test is a sign of a stronger immune response of the respiratory tract. In essence, the differences between CVA and classical asthma are in the immune system's response to different stimuli [27].

6. Evaluation of chronic cough in children

A cough is a natural and universal occurrence, and it is a part of the body's defense mechanism of the respiratory system. Chronic cough is defined as lasting more than 4 weeks in children and more than 8 weeks for adults [26, 28–30]. Diagnosis and management of patients with chronic cough are challenging for clinicians. Chronic cough can be a primary symptom of a variety of underlying conditions [25, 31]. The most common conditions that cause chronic

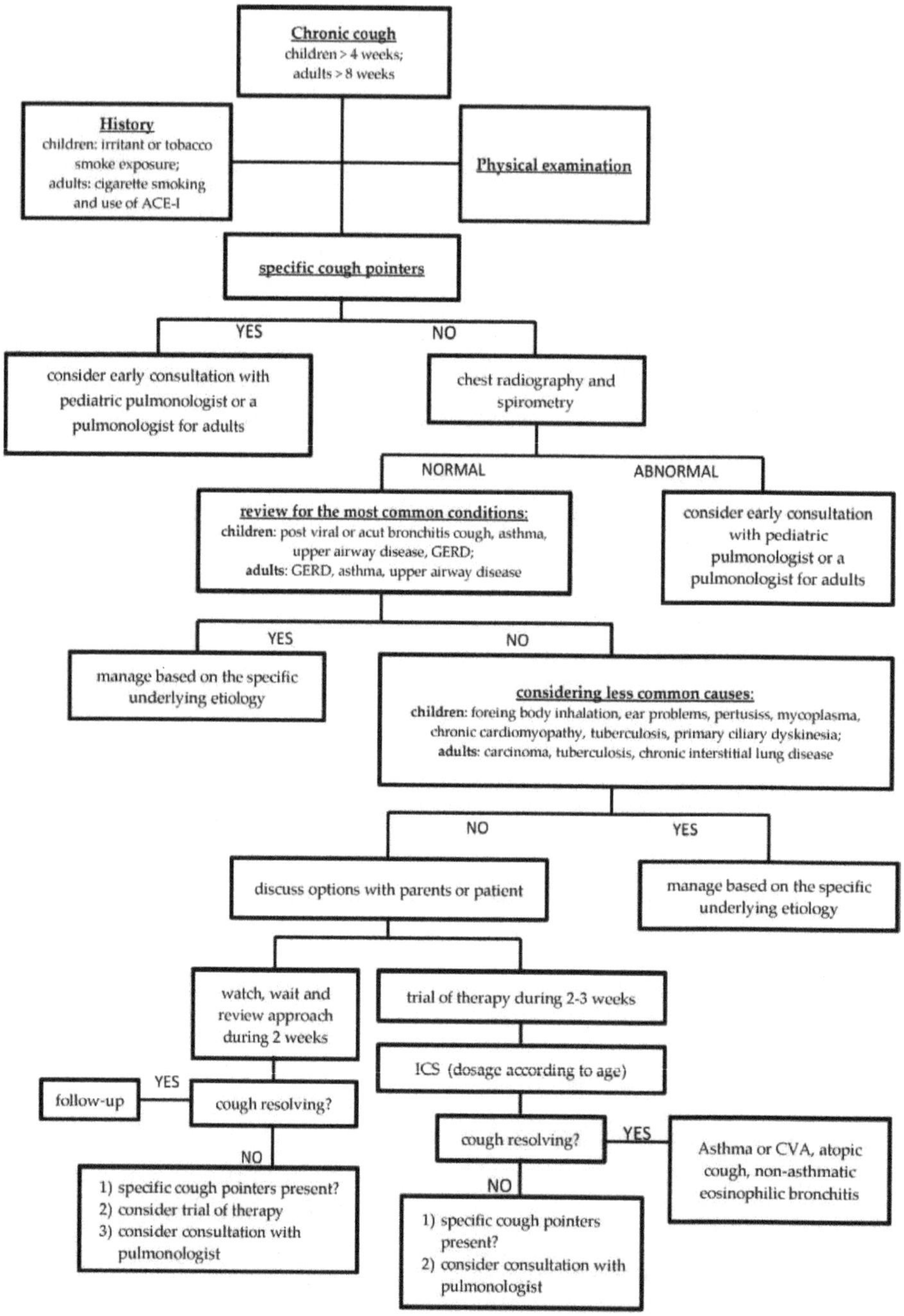

Figure 1. Algorithm for evaluation of chronic cough in children and adults for primary level doctors (general practitioner, pediatrician, family doctor, etc.).

cough in children under 14 are CVA, atopic cough, gastroesophageal reflux disease (GERD) and upper airway cough syndrome (formerly postnasal drip cough) [28–30]. CVA should be considered when chronic cough is exacerbated by cold or exercise [30]. Besides asthma and CVA in adult patients with chronic cough in the differential diagnosis, smoking and ACE-I induced a cough should always be considered [30]. Less common conditions include heart failure, interstitial lung disease, tuberculosis and primary lung cancer [26, 29, 31].

A few algorithms of the evaluation of chronic cough in adults and children are available in the literature [25, 30–32]. The use of these protocols or algorithms can improve clinical outcomes [28]. Most appropriated algorithm for adults can be found in a review article by Terasaki et al. [31]. In adults, the clinicians need to be attentive to two high-yield elements of the history patients: the use of an angiotensin-converting enzyme inhibitor (ACE-I) and cigarette smoking. Of equal importance is to inquire about exposure to second-hand smoke in children [25, 26, 31]. Most appropriated algorithm for children can be found in a review article by Chang et al. [25]. We have designed one of the algorithms that can be used as a guide for the primary level physicians (**Figure 1**).

Initial diagnostic evaluation should include the chest radiograph and pulmonary function testing in patients with chronic cough [25, 29–31]. It is not recommended to routinely performing additional tests (skin prick test, bronchoscopy, chest CT) for all children with chronic cough. Additional tests should be individualized and undertaken in accordance with the clinical symptoms and signs [29]. Chronic cough suggestive of serious underlying lung disease includes neonatal onset of cough [30].

It is recommended that in case of inadequate response to inhalation therapy, it should try with the inhalation therapy through an aerochamber which can help to maximize drug delivery to the lungs [31].

In a clinical evaluation of patients with chronic cough, it can be tried with the diagnosis *ex juvantibus*. There are no agreement about recommendations how long to use a particular therapy and wait for a therapeutic response to confirm the diagnosis *ex juvantibus* [25, 29, 31].

7. Conclusion

The CVA has the same pathophysiological features as classical asthma but in a mild form. The main pathophysiology of CVA is bronchial hyperreactivity.

Since a large percentage of patients with CVA develop classical asthma and wheezing over time, ICS treatment in these patients is very important because of the prevention of classical asthma development. One very important diagnostic criterion in CVA patients is an improvement of the symptoms after bronchodilator therapy. The positive therapeutic effect of ICS on cough in children with CVA should not be considered as a diagnostic criterion because the positive therapeutic effect also has patients with atopic cough [8].

"In children with chronic cough parental expectations should be determined, and the specific concerns of the parents should be sought and addressed" [25].

Author details

Sanela Domuz Vujnović[1]*, Adrijana Domuz[2] and Slobodanka Petrović[3]

*Address all correspondence to: drdomuz@gmail.com

1 School of Applied Medical Sciences, Prijedor, Republic of Srpska, Bosnia and Herzegovina

2 Primary Health Center, Ribnik, Republic of Srpska, Bosnia and Herzegovina

3 Institute for Child and Youth Health Care of Vojvodina, Novi Sad, Republic of Srbija

References

[1] Domuz S. Prevalence of asthma symptoms in children aged 6 to 15 years in the territory of Republic of Srpska [dissertation]. Novi Sad: Medical Faculty; 2016. 156 p

[2] Morjaria BJ, Kastelik AJ. Unusual asthma syndromes and their management. Therapeutic Advances in Chronic Disease. 2011;**2**(4):249-264. DOI: 10.1177/2040622311407542

[3] Liu M, Liu K, Zhu N, Xia J, Chen X. Inflammatory mediators in induced sputum and airway hyperresponsiveness in cough variant asthma during long-term inhaled corticosteroid treatment. Mediators of Inflammation. 2012;**2012**:403868. DOI: 10.1155/2012/403868

[4] Ioan I, Poussel M, Coutier L, Plevkova J, Poliacek I, Bolser CD, et al. What is chronic cough in children? Frontiers in Physiology. 2014;**5**:322. DOI: 10.3389/FPHYS.2014.00322

[5] Corrao WM, Braman SS, Irwin RS. Chronic cough as the sole presenting manifestation of bronchial asthma. The New England Journal of Medicine. 1979;**300**:633-637

[6] Magni C, Chellini E, Zanasi A. Cough variant asthma and atopic cough. Multidisciplinary Respirator Medicine. 2010;**5**(2):99-103. DOI: 10.1186/2049-6958-5-2-99

[7] Fujimura M, Hara J, Myou S. Change in bronchial responsiveness and cough reflex sensitivity in patients with cough variant asthma: Effect of inhaled corticosteroids. Cough. 2005;**1**:5. DOI: 10.1186/1745-9974-1-5

[8] Fujimura M, Ogawa H, Nishizawa Y, Nishi K. Comparison of atopic cough with cough variant asthma: Is atopic cough a precursor of asthma? Thorax. 2003;**58**:14-18. DOI: 10.1136/thorax.58.1.14

[9] Imai E, Enseki M, Nukaga M, Tabata H, Hirai K, Kato M, et al. A lung sound analysis in a child thought to have cough variant asthma: A case report. Allergology International. 2017;**67**(1):150-152. DOI: 10.1016/j.alit.2017.06.004

[10] Sridaran S, Gonzalez-Estrada A, Aronica AM. A case of cough variant asthma undiagnosed for 16 years. Operation and Maintenance Center – Radio. 2014;**2014**(2):29-30. DOI: 10.1093/omcr/omu012

[11] D'Urzo A, Jugovic P. Case Report: Cough variant asthma. Canadian Family Physician. 2002;**48**:1323-1325

[12] Niimi A. Cough and asthma. Curent Respiratory Medicine Reviews. 2011;**7**(1):47-54. DOI: 10.2174/157339811794109327

[13] Ichinose M, Sugiura H, Nagase H, Yamaguchi M, Inoue H, Sagara H, et al. Japanese guidelines for adult asthma 2017. Allergology International. 2017;**66**(2):163-189. DOI: 10.1016/j.alit.2016.12.005

[14] Arakawa H, Hamasaki Y, Kohno Y, Ebisawa M, Kondo N, Nishima S, et al. Japanese guidelines for childhood asthma 2017. Allergology International. 2017;**66**(2):190-204. DOI: 10.1016/j.alit.2016.11.003

[15] Niimi A, Matsumoto H, Takemura M, Ueda T, Chin K, Mishima M. Relationship of airway wall thickness to airway sensitivity and airway reactivity in asthma. American Journal of Respiratory and Critical Care Medicine. 2003;**168**(8):983-988. DOI: 10.1164/rccm.200211-1268OC

[16] Mochizuki H, Arakawa H, Tokuyama K, Morikawa A. Bronchial sensitivity and bronchial reactivity in children with cough variant asthma. Chest. 2005;**128**(4):2427-2434. DOI: 10.1378/chest.128.4.2427

[17] De Diego A, Martinez E, Perpina M, Nieto L, Compte L, Macian V, et al. Airway inflammation and cough sensitivity in cough-variant asthma. Allergy. 2005;**60**(11):1407-1411. DOI: 10.1111/j.1398-9995.2005.00609.x

[18] Kanazawa H, Eguchi Y, Nomura N, Yoshikawa J. Analysis of vascular endothelial growth factor levels in induced sputum samples from patients with cough variant asthma. Annals of Allergy, Asthma & Immunology. 2005;**95**(3):266-271. DOI: 10.1016/S1081-1206(10)61224-0

[19] Birring SS, Parker D, Brightling CE, Bradding P, Wardlaw AJ, Pavord ID. Induced sputum inflammatory mediator concentrations in chronic cough. American Journal of Respiratory and Critical Care Medicine. 2004;**169**(1):15-19. DOI: 10.1164/rccm.200308-1092OC

[20] McGarvey LP, Heaney LG, Lawson JT, Johnston BT, Scally CM, Ennis M, et al. Evaluation and outcome of patients with chronic non-productive cough using a comprehensive diagnostic protocol. Thorax. 1998;**53**(9):738-743

[21] Matsumoto H, Niimi A, Takemura M, Ueda T, Tabuena R, Yamaguchi M, et al. Prognosis of cough variant asthma: A retrospective analysis. The Journal of Asthma. 2006;**43**(2):131-135. DOI: 10.1080/02770900500498477

[22] Shimoda T, Obase Y, Kishikawa R, Iwanaga T, Miyatake A, Kasayama S. The fractional exhaled nitric oxide and serum high sensitivity C-reactive protein levels in cough variant asthma and typical bronchial asthma. Allergology International. 2013;**62**(2):251-257. DOI: 10.2332/allergolint.12-OA-0515

[23] Asano T, Takemura M, Fukumitsu K, Takeda N, Ichikawa H, Hijikata H, et al. Diagnostic utility of fractional exhaled nitric oxide in prolonged and chronic cough according to atopic status. Allergology International. 2017;**66**(2):344-350. DOI: 10.1016/j.alit.2016.08.015

[24] Hutton N, Wilson MH, Mellits ED, Baumgardner R, Wissow LS, Bonuccelli C, et al. Effectiveness of an antihistamine-decongestant combination for young children with the common cold: A randomized, controlled clinical trial. The Journal of Pediatrics. 1991; **118**(1):125-130

[25] Chang AB, Glomb WB. Guidelines for evaluating chronic cough in pediatrics: ACCP evidence-based clinical practice guidelines. Chest. 2006;**129**(1 Suppl):260S-283S. DOI: 10.1378/chest.129.1_suppl.260S

[26] Bergamini M, Kantar A, Cutrera R, Interest Group IPC. Analysis of the literature on chronic cough in children. Open Respiratory Medicine Journal. 2017;**11**:1-9. DOI: 10.2174/1874306401711010001

[27] Adnyana IGANS, Suwendra P, Santoso H. Prevalence and associated factors of airway hyperresponsiveness in children with recurrent chronic cough. Paediatrica Indonesiana. 2004;**44**(9-10):181-187. DOI: 10.14238/pi44.5.2004.181-7

[28] Kantar A. Phenotypic presentation of chronic cough in children. Journal of Thoracic Disease. 2017;**9**(4):907-913. DOI: 10.21037/jtd.2017.03.53

[29] Chang AB, Oppenheimer JJ, Weinberger MM, Rubin BK, Weir K, Grant CC, et al. Use of management pathways or algorithms in children with chronic cough: CHEST guideline and expert panel report. Chest. 2017;**151**(4):875-883. DOI: 10.1016/j.chest.2016.12.025

[30] Benich JJ, Carek PJ. Evaluation of the patient with chronic cough. American Family Physician. 2011;**84**(8):887-892

[31] Terasaki G, Paauw DS. Evaluation and treatment of chronic cough. Medical Clinics of North America. 2014;**98**(3):391-403. DOI: 10.1016/j.mcna.2014.01.002

[32] Gedik AH, Cakir E, Torun E, Demir AD, Kucukkoc M, Erenberk U, et al. Evaluation of 563 children with chronic cough accompanied by a new clinical algorithm. Italian Journal of Pediatrics. 2015;**41**:73. DOI: 10.1186/s13052-015-0180-0

Permissions

All chapters in this book were first published in ADMABPE, by InTech Open; hereby published with permission under the Creative Commons Attribution License or equivalent. Every chapter published in this book has been scrutinized by our experts. Their significance has been extensively debated. The topics covered herein carry significant findings which will fuel the growth of the discipline. They may even be implemented as practical applications or may be referred to as a beginning point for another development.

The contributors of this book come from diverse backgrounds, making this book a truly international effort. This book will bring forth new frontiers with its revolutionizing research information and detailed analysis of the nascent developments around the world.

We would like to thank all the contributing authors for lending their expertise to make the book truly unique. They have played a crucial role in the development of this book. Without their invaluable contributions this book wouldn't have been possible. They have made vital efforts to compile up to date information on the varied aspects of this subject to make this book a valuable addition to the collection of many professionals and students.

This book was conceptualized with the vision of imparting up-to-date information and advanced data in this field. To ensure the same, a matchless editorial board was set up. Every individual on the board went through rigorous rounds of assessment to prove their worth. After which they invested a large part of their time researching and compiling the most relevant data for our readers.

The editorial board has been involved in producing this book since its inception. They have spent rigorous hours researching and exploring the diverse topics which have resulted in the successful publishing of this book. They have passed on their knowledge of decades through this book. To expedite this challenging task, the publisher supported the team at every step. A small team of assistant editors was also appointed to further simplify the editing procedure and attain best results for the readers.

Apart from the editorial board, the designing team has also invested a significant amount of their time in understanding the subject and creating the most relevant covers. They scrutinized every image to scout for the most suitable representation of the subject and create an appropriate cover for the book.

The publishing team has been an ardent support to the editorial, designing and production team. Their endless efforts to recruit the best for this project, has resulted in the accomplishment of this book. They are a veteran in the field of academics and their pool of knowledge is as vast as their experience in printing. Their expertise and guidance has proved useful at every step. Their uncompromising quality standards have made this book an exceptional effort. Their encouragement from time to time has been an inspiration for everyone.

The publisher and the editorial board hope that this book will prove to be a valuable piece of knowledge for researchers, students, practitioners and scholars across the globe.

List of Contributors

F. Muñoz-López
Former Head of the Department of Pediatric Immunoallergology,Clínic Hospital - Sant Joan de Déu Hospital, Faculty of Medicine University of Barcelona, Spain

Yousser Mohammad
Department of Pulmonary and Family Medicine, Syrian Private University, Damascus, Syria
Department of Pulmonary, Damascus University, Damascus, Syria
Center for Research and Training for CRD, Tishreen University, Latakia, Syria

Basim Dubaybo
Department of Internal Medicine, Wayne State University School of Medicine, Detroit, Michigan, USA

Mirjana Turkalj and Damir Erceg
Srebrnjak Children's Hospital, Zagreb, Croatia
Medical School University of Osijek, Osijek, Croatia
Catholic University of Croatia, Zagreb, Croatia

Iva Dumbović Dubravčić
Institute for Anthropological Research, Zagreb, Croatia

Sanela Domuz Vujnovic
School of Applied Medical Sciences, Prijedor, Republic of Srpska, Bosnia and Herzegovina

Adrijana Domuz
Primary Health Center, Republic of Srpska, Bosnia and Herzegovina

Francisco Muñoz-López
Department of Pediatric Immunoallergology, Faculty of Medicine, University of Barcelona, Clínic Hospital-Sant Joan de Déu Hospital, Spain

Frantisek Lopot, David Skalicky and Karel Jelen
Department of Anatomy and Biomechanics, Faculty of Sports and Physical Education, Charles University, Praha, Czech Republic
Department of Biomathematics, Institute of Physiology, Czech Academy of Sciences, Praha, Czech Republic

Vaclav Koucky
Second Faculty of Medicine, Charles University, Praha, Czech Republic
Department of Biomathematics, Institute of Physiology, Czech Academy of Sciences, Praha, Czech Republic

Daniel Hadraba
Department of Anatomy and Biomechanics, Faculty of Sports and Physical Education, Charles University, Praha, Czech Republic
Department of Paediatrics, University Hospital Motol, Praha, Czech Republic
Department of Biomathematics, Institute of Physiology, Czech Academy of Sciences, Praha, Czech Republic

Drew A. Harris, Caitlin Welch, Morgan Soper and Yun Michael Shim
Department of Medicine, Division of Pulmonary and Critical Care, Complex Airways Diseases Program, University of Virginia, Charlottesville, Virginia, USA

Jan Beute and Alex KleinJan
Department of Pulmonary Medicine, Erasmus MC Rotterdam, Rotterdam, The Netherlands

Vincent Manganiello
Cardiovascular Pulmonary Branch, NHLBI, National Institutes of Health, Bethesda, Maryland

Yong Chul Lee and So Ri Kim
Division of Respiratory Medicine and Allergy, Department of Internal Medicine, Chonbuk National University Medical School, Jeonju, South Korea

Marcia Regina Piuvezam and Claudio Roberto Bezerra-Santos
Department of Physiology and Pathology, Federal University of Paraíba, João Pessoa Paraiba, Brazil

Laércia Karla Diega Paiva Ferreira and Talissa Mozzini Monteiro
Federal University of Paraíba, João Pessoa, Paraiba, Brazil

Giciane Carvalho Vieira
Department of Morphology, Center of Health Science, Federal University of Paraíba, João Pessoa, Paraiba, Brazil

Dolly V. Rojas, Diana L. Silva and Carlos D. Serrano
Allergy Unit, Fundación Valle del Lili, Faculty of Health Sciences, ICESI University, Cali, Colombia

Marina Ruxandra Otelea
University of Medicine and Pharmacy "Carol Davila", Bucharest, Romania

Agripina Rascu
University of Medicine and Pharmacy "Carol Davila", Bucharest, Romania
Colentina Clinical Hospital, Occupational Medicine Department, Bucharest, Romania

Herrera García José Carlos, Arellano Montellano Ek Ixel and Martínez Flores Alejandra Guadalupe
Asthma-COPD Clinic-University Hospital of Puebla, Mexico

Jaramillo Arellano Luis Enrique and Espinosa Arellano Andrea
Benemerita Autonomous University of Puebla, Mexico

Caballero López Christopherson Gengyny
University Hospital of Puebla, Mexico

Sanela Domuz Vujnović
School of Applied Medical Sciences, Prijedor, Republic of Srpska, Bosnia and Herzegovina

Adrijana Domuz
Primary Health Center, Ribnik, Republic of Srpska, Bosnia and Herzegovina

Slobodanka Petrović
Institute for Child and Youth Health Care of Vojvodina, Novi Sad, Republic of Srbija

Index

www.ingramcontent.com/pod-product-compliance
Lightning Source LLC
LaVergne TN
LVHW061511220926
848485LV00017B/797
9781639890637